Advanced Photonics Methods for Biomedical Applications

Advanced photonics methods for biomedical applications give researchers in universities and industries, and clinicians an overview of the novel tools for cancer diagnostics and treatment. This book provides researchers and professionals in the area of biomedical photonics with a toolbox of novel methodologies for biomedical applications, including health diagnostics, cancer detection, and treatment. It covers the theory, modeling, and design of each method, alongside their applications, fabrication, characterization, and measurements in clinical practice. A wide scope of concepts concerning innovative science and technologies of medicine will be covered, providing the readers with the latest research, developments, and technologies. It will also be a valuable resource for students and early-career researchers, alongside those involved in the design of the novel photonics-based techniques for health diagnostics and cancer detection and treatment.

Key features

- Discusses novel methods of cancer diagnostics and cancer treatment.

- Details non- and minimally invasive photonics techniques.

- Explores the applications of machine learning and artificial intelligence to these novel techniques.

Edik Rafailov received a PhD degree from the Ioffe Institute in 1992. In 1997 he moved to St Andrews University (UK) and in 2005 he established a new group at Dundee University. In 2014 he and his Optoelectronics and Biomedical Photonics Group moved to Aston University (UK). He has authored and co-authored over 450 articles in refereed journals and conference proceedings, including two books, ten invited chapters, and numerous invited talks. He coordinated the €14.7M FP7 FAST-DOT project development of new ultrafast lasers for biophotonics applications and the €12.5M NEWLED project, which aims to develop a new generation of white LEDs. He coordinates the H2020 FET Mesa-Brain (which aims to develop 3D nano-printing technology for functional three-dimensional human stem cell-derived neural networks), NEUROPA (which aims to develop novel non-invasive theragnostic approaches), the H2020 PLATFORMA project, and the EPSRC (EP/R024898/1) proposal. He also leads a few other projects funded by the EU and EPSRC (UK). His current research interests include high-power CW and ultrashort-pulse lasers; generation of UV/visible/IR/MIR and THz radiation nano-structures; nonlinear and integrated optics; and biomedical photonics.

Tatjana Gric's research career has been focused on the investigation of waveguide devices (waveguide modulators, filters, etc.), namely on proposing their electrodynamical analysis. Applied research includes the design of microwave frequency selective structures, waveguide modulators, and filters. Fundamental research is primarily concerned with developing rigorous computational methods for the electrodynamical analysis of the waveguide structures. Another major goal of her studies is plasmonics as the examination of the interaction between electromagnetic field and free electrons in a metal. The optically active nanostructures have been simulated, and their fundamental photonic properties have been explored. Moreover, the broad scope of research carried out by Dr. Gric has included investigations into the new fascinating properties of novel materials. Dr. Gric is involved in development of unusual materials and structures that can manipulate the flow of light in ways that are useful in optical sensing, photovoltaics, solid-state lighting, fiber optics, and other applications. Dr. Gric has published extensively in her field of investigation with more than 50 peer-reviewed papers in top journals in physics, electrodynamics, and optics and has written one book and two book chapters. It is worth noting that her recent publication rate as the first author is increasing.

Advanced Photonics Methods for Biomedical Applications

Edited by
Edik Rafailov and Tatjana Gric

CRC Press
Taylor & Francis Group
Boca Raton London New York

CRC Press is an imprint of the
Taylor & Francis Group, an **informa** business

Designed cover image: Shutterstock_775583890 and Shutterstock_1666018906

First edition published 2024
by CRC Press
6000 Broken Sound Parkway NW, Suite 300, Boca Raton, FL 33487-2742

and by CRC Press
4 Park Square, Milton Park, Abingdon, Oxon, OX14 4RN

CRC Press is an imprint of Taylor & Francis Group, LLC

Library of Congress Cataloging-in-Publication Data
Names: Rafailov, Edik U., editor. | Gric, Tatjana, editor.
Title: Advanced photonics methods for biomedical applications / edited by Edik Rafailov and Tatjana Gric.
Description: First edition. | Boca Raton : CRC Press, 2023. |
Includes bibliographical references and index.
Identifiers: LCCN 2022055688 | ISBN 9781032128429 (hardback) |
ISBN 9781032133812 (paperback) | ISBN 9781003228950 (ebook)
Subjects: MESH: Spectrum Analysis—methods | Fluorometry—methods |
Neoplasms—diagnostic imaging | Terahertz Radiation
Classification: LCC R857.M3 | NLM QY 90 | DDC 610.28/4—dc23/eng/20230429
LC record available at https://lccn.loc.gov/2022055688

ISBN: 9781032128429 (hbk)
ISBN: 9781032133812 (pbk)
ISBN: 9781003228950 (ebk)

DOI: 10.1201/9781003228950

Typeset in Minion
by codeMantra

Contents

Contributors

A. Bykov
Opto-Electronics and
  Measurement Techniques
University of Oulu
Oulu, Finland

Viktor Dremin
College of Engineering and
  Physical Sciences
Aston University
Birmingham, UK
And
Research & Development Center of
  Biomedical Photonics
Orel State University
Orel, Russia

Andrey Dunaev
Research and Development Center
  of Biomedical Photonics
Orel State University
Orel, Russia

Andrei Gorodetsky
School of Physics and Astronomy
University of Birmingham
Birmingham, UK

Tatjana Gric
College of Engineering and
  Physical Sciences
Aston University
Birmingham, UK

I. Meglinski
College of Engineering and
  Physical Sciences
Aston University
Birmingham, UK

M. Peyvasteh
Opto-Electronics and
  Measurement Techniques
University of Oulu
Oulu, Finland

Elena Potapova
Research and Development Center
  of Biomedical Photonics
Orel State University
Orel, Russia

Edik Rafailov
Institute of Photonics Technologies
Aston University
Birmingham, UK

Sergei Sokolovski
College of Engineering and
    Physical Sciences
Aston University
Birmingham, UK

Amit Yadav
Institute of Photonics Technologies
    Aston University
Birmingham, UK

Elena Zharkikh
Research and Development Center
    of Biomedical Photonics
Orel State University
Orel, Russia

Evgenii Zherebtsov
Optoelectronics and Measurement
    Techniques
University of Oulu
Oulu, Finland
And
Research and Development Center
    of Biomedical Photonics
Orel State University
Orel, Russia

CHAPTER 1

In Vivo Fluorescence Measurements of Biological Tissue Viability

Viktor Dremin, Sergei Sokolovski, and Edik Rafailov
Aston University

Elena Zharkikh, Elena Potapova, and Andrey Dunaev
Orel State University

Evgenii Zherebtsov
University of Oulu

CONTENTS

DOI: 10.1201/9781003228950-1

1.1 INTRODUCTION

Noninvasive optical methods are increasingly used in biomedical diagnostics. Fluorescence spectroscopy, in particular, has found its application in chemistry, biology, and various fields of medicine. This method is highly sensitive and allows one to evaluate such complex biochemical processes as tissue metabolism (Mycek and Pogue, 2003; Lakowicz, 2006). The most perspective area of application of fluorescence spectroscopy is optical diagnostics in such fields as oncology, cosmetology, surgery and transplantation. Fluorescence spectroscopy is a reliable method for distinguishing benign and malignant tumors of various origins, offering several benefits over traditional diagnostic methods (Potapova et al., 2020; Zherebtsov et al., 2022; Zherebtsov et al., 2020).

Despite the undoubted advantages of the method, there are unresolved problems that limit its use at present. The main difficulty in interpreting the fluorescence spectrum of biological tissues is identifying the contribution of individual fluorophores to the resulting spectrum since many tissue fluorophores have overlapping absorption and emission spectra. The reliability and reproducibility of fluorescence spectroscopy results depend on many factors, including temperature, topological heterogeneity, and various optical and physicochemical properties of samples. Various parameters of measuring systems, such as the sensitivity of a photodetectors and the features of an optical fiber, also contribute to the accuracy of the measurement results. Thus, to achieve clinically significant and reliable results, issues of accuracy, convergence and dispersion measurement also need to be addressed.

1.2 INDIVIDUAL VARIABILITY OF MEASURED PARAMETERS

The aim of this part of the study was to evaluate the individual long-term variability of parameters in fluorescence spectroscopy, as well as to analyze its possible causes (Dunaev et al., 2015).

Experimental studies were conducted with the participation of three conditionally healthy volunteers: male 35 years (for 9 months) – volunteer number 1, male 22 years (5 months) – volunteer number 2, and woman 24 years (3 months) – volunteer number 3. Measurements were carried out at two points of the biotissue: on the pads skin (volar surface) of the middle finger of the right hand, that is, in the area saturated with arterio-venous anastomoses (AVA), and on the right forearm, in the zone almost devoid of AVAs.

All measurements were made on working days, mostly in the morning, when the volunteer was at rest. A total of 200 spectral records were recorded from the fingertip when fluorescence was excited by 365 nm light, 20 at 532 nm and 50 at 637 nm. In addition, 150 fluorescence spectral records were taken when excited by 365 nm light from the forearm. For experimental studies, a multifunctional laser noninvasive diagnostic system (LAKK-M, LAZMA Ltd., Russia) was used, which implements a fluorescence spectroscopy channel with four excitation sources. Fluorescence was excited by sources with wavelengths of 365, 420, 532 and 637 nm. These wavelengths trigger the fluorescence of elastin, collagen, pyridoxine, keratin, NADH, flavins, lipofuscin, carotene and porphyrins.

The intensity of amplitude at the maximum of the fluorescence spectrum $I_f(\lambda)$ for different wavelengths of registration and the intensity of the backscattered radiation $I_{bs}(\lambda)$ were analyzed. On the basis of the recorded data, the redox ratio (RR) was calculated and analyzed. The redox ratio was calculated using the following formula:

$$RR = I_{NADH}/I_{FAD}. \tag{1.1}$$

All analyzed parameters were averaged over the whole study period, and the arithmetic mean M_n, the standard deviation σ from the M_n and the coefficient of variation or the relative scatter of the measurement results δ as a percentage to the mean were calculated. Additionally, for the measured values and calculated parameters, probability density distribution functions were constructed. Figure 1.1 shows histograms of fluorescence intensity distributions for the finger (Figure 1.1a) and forearm (Figure. 1.1b) surfaces of three volunteers.

The results of the calculation of the coefficients of variation (variation of the measurement results) for the fluorescence intensities $I_f(\lambda)$ for the case under consideration are summarized in Table 1.1.

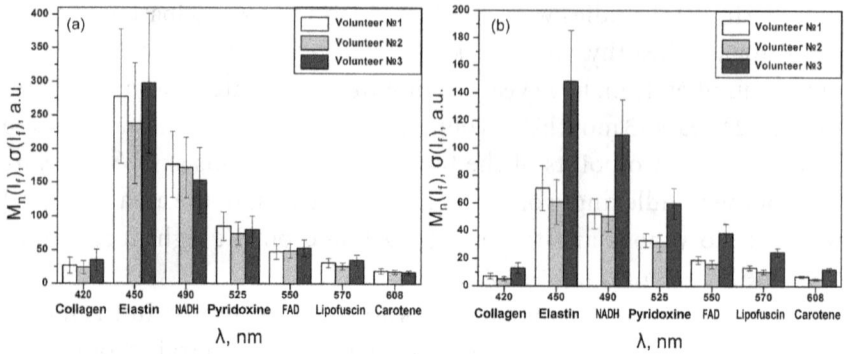

FIGURE 1.1 Histograms of the fluorescence intensity distribution for the surface of the finger (a) and forearm (b). (Reprinted with permission from Dunaev et al. (2015) © Elsevier.)

TABLE 1.1 Coefficients of Variation ($\delta(I_f)$, %) for Fluorescence Intensity $I_f(\lambda)$

| | | Volunteer No. | | | | | |
| | | 1 | 2 | 3 | 1 | 2 | 3 |
Type of Fluorophore	Emission Wavelength (nm)	Finger			Forearm		
Collagen	420	43.42	40.51	44.93	28.07	31.25	29.94
Elastin	450	35.95	37.79	34.88	22.90	26.66	24.79
NADH	490	27.91	26.39	32.29	20.62	21.43	23.10
Pyridoxine	525	24.84	23.11	25.14	15.14	19.32	18.67
FAD	550	24.09	21.54	23.70	15.44	18.34	16.88
Lipofuscin	570	22.30	19.34	22.61	12.92	16.68	11.99
Carotene	608	21.15	18.99	17.75	10.24	14.39	9.037

The results of the calculation of the RR for the finger surface are as follows: $RR_1 = 3.1 \pm 0.75$ AU for volunteer No. 1, $RR_2 = 2.9 \pm 0.71$ AU for volunteer No. 2, and $RR_3 = 3.3 \pm 0.74$ AU for volunteer No. 3. The dispersion of the obtained values for the three volunteers did not exceed 25%. A comparative analysis of the results obtained shows that the relative error (dispersion) of the measurements for three volunteers is at the same level and, depending on the biomarker, the fluorescence intensity varies mainly in the range from 20% to 40%.

The relative dispersion of the measurement results for the forearm was 1.5–2 times less than for the volar surface of the finger, which confirms the effect of tissue blood supply on the individual variability of the measured biotissue parameters. Obviously, skin blood filling is one of the main factors that influences the FS measurement results.

TABLE 1.2   Statistical Evaluation of the Measurement Results for Green and Red
Fluorescence Excitation Wavelengths

The Laser Wavelength (nm)	Emission Wavelength (nm)	The Recorded Fluorescence Intensity $I_f(\lambda)$ (AU)		
		M_n	σ	$\delta, \%$
532	570	35.21	13.45	38.20
	608	55.76	16.18	29.02
	640	38.85	9.12	23.48
	680	18.66	4.73	25.35
637	670	0.84	1.14	134.92
	710	25.41	15.34	60.37

For volunteer No. 1, similar variability studies were conducted at the green (532 nm) and red (637 nm) fluorescence excitation wavelengths. The results of the statistical processing of the data obtained are presented in Table 1.2.

The data obtained show that the relative dispersion is minimal at certain wavelengths. The enormous variability of parameters at a wavelength of 670 nm for carotene analysis upon excitation with red light makes its application problematic.

The analysis of the distribution of the measurement results for the three volunteers showed that the distribution function of the fluorescence intensity deviations for the ultraviolet (UV) excitation line is normal in general. This distribution did not correspond to the wavelength of 704 nm, in which the greatest dispersion of results was observed.

Figure 1.2 shows an example of the obtained density distribution of fluorescence intensity values for NADH at 494 nm for volunteer No. 1. The distribution for NADH is a truncated normal distribution due to the limited range of possible values. The correctness check of the distribution selection was carried out according to the Kolmogorov criterion and the Pearson criterion. Both criteria with a confidence level of 0.95 confirmed the correctness of the distribution selection. In general, it can be concluded that the distribution of the fluorescence parameters can also depend on such parameters as individual characteristics of the biological tissues studied, the type of specific fluorophore, etc. This is also possibly due to the uneven sensitivity of the photodetector-measuring channel in the range of recording endogenous fluorescence spectra.

As is known, the greater the value of the variation coefficient, the relatively greater the scatter and the less evenness of the studied values. It is considered that if the coefficient of variation is less than 33%, then the population is homogeneous. Analyzing the data obtained from the individual

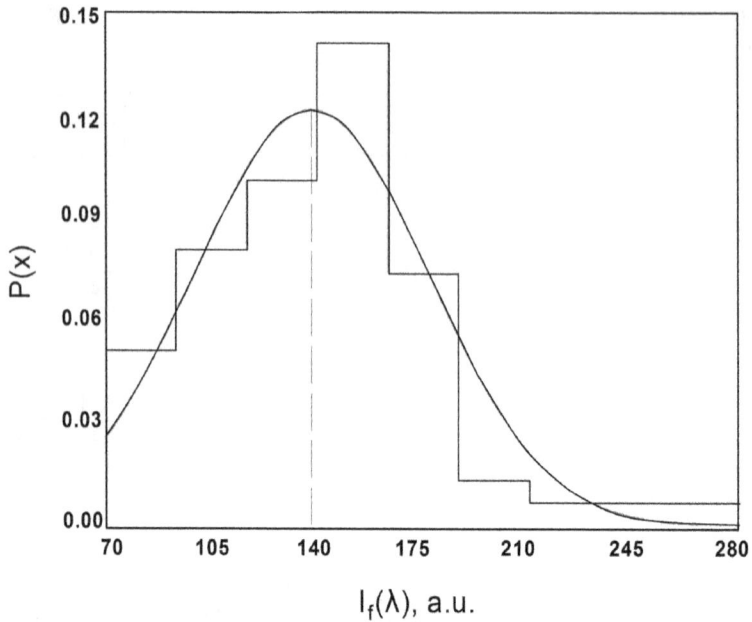

FIGURE 1.2 Probability density distributions of fluorescence intensity values for NADH. (Reprinted with permission from Dunaev et al. (2015) © Elsevier.)

long-term variability of the measured and calculated FS parameters, it can be concluded that most of the biomarkers studied have a variation that is acceptable for diagnostic purposes.

Several factors were also found to influence the final result. Inside a biological tissue, the incoming radiation undergoes multiple scattering (rereflections) at the boundaries of the anatomical and cellular structure heterogeneities and is partially absorbed by the components of the biological tissue substances: water, melanin, hemoglobin, etc. As a result, it becomes necessary to take into account this effect on the recorded fluorescence spectra. A number of experimental studies were conducted aimed at studying the effect of the main absorbing chromophores of the skin on the recorded fluorescence signals and presented in the following sections.

1.2.1 The Study of the Effect of Melanin on Recorded Signals

This section is devoted to the study of the influence on the recorded fluorescence signal of a biological tissue chromophore, melanin, which is one of the most common natural pigments and largely responsible for the optical properties of the skin (Dunaev et al., 2015; Dremin and Dunaev, 2016).

The skin pigment melanin is an important absorbing chromophore. The melanocytes located in the basal layer of the cell produce melanin and transfer it to neighboring cells of the epidermis keratinocytes to protect their nucleus from UV radiation. Regardless of ethnicity, the amount of melanocytes on the skin of each person is the same, but the amount of melanin these cells produce is different.

The amount of melanin produced determines the color of the skin and its sensitivity to light. In people with different ethnic skin types, the melanin concentration varies approximately in the range of 1.3% to 43%. In low-pigmented skin, the melanin content is 1.3%–1.6%, in middle-pigmented it is 11%–16%, and in blacks, it is 18%–43% (Jacques, 2013).

Evaluation modeling of the contribution of scattering and absorption to the total attenuation of probe radiation was carried out on the basis of the published optical properties of human biological tissues by adding different melanin contents.

Skin was considered as a multilayer structure; the absorption coefficients of the layers taking into account the concentration of blood C_{blood}, water C_{H_2O} and melanin C_{mel} and were defined as follows (Petrov et al., 2012; Zherebtsov et al., 2019):

$$\mu_a^{Stratum\ corneum}(\lambda) = C_{H_2O}\mu_a^{H_2O}(\lambda) + (1 - C_{H_2O})\mu_a^{baseline}(\lambda), \qquad (1.2)$$

$$\mu_a^{Epidermis}(\lambda) = (1 - C_{H_2O})\left(C_{mel}\mu_a^{mel}(\lambda) + (1 - C_{mel})\mu_a^{baseline}(\lambda)\right)$$
$$+ C_{H_2O}\mu_a^{H_2O}(\lambda), \qquad (1.3)$$

$$\mu_a^{Dermis}(\lambda) = (1 - C_{H_2O})\left(C_{blood}\mu_a^{blood}(\lambda) + (1 - C_{blood})\mu_a^{baseline}(\lambda)\right)$$
$$+ C_{H_2O}\mu_a^{H_2O}(\lambda), \qquad (1.4)$$

where $\mu_a^{H_2O}(\lambda)$ is the water absorption coefficient, $\mu_a^{mel}(\lambda)$ is the melanin absorption coefficient, $\mu_a^{blood}(\lambda)$ is the blood absorption coefficient and $\mu_a^{baseline}(\lambda)$ is the absorption coefficient of other anhydrous tissues.

The scattering coefficients of the layers were calculated taking into account the combination of Mie and Rayleigh scattering proposed in

$$\mu_s^{Rayleigh}(\lambda) = 2 \cdot 10^{12} \lambda^{-4}, \qquad (1.5)$$

$$\mu_s^{Mie}(\lambda) = 2 \cdot 10^5 \lambda^{-1,5}, \qquad (1.6)$$

$$\mu_s = \mu_s^{Rayleigh} + \mu_s^{Mie}. \qquad (1.7)$$

The overall attenuation coefficient is calculated as follows:

$$\mu_t = \mu_a^{Stratum\ corneum} + \mu_a^{Epidermis} + \mu_a^{Dermis} + \mu_s. \qquad (1.8)$$

As a result, graphical dependences explaining the contribution of scattering and absorption to the total attenuation of radiation in the skin for different levels of melanin are presented in Figure 1.3.

From the graphical dependences obtained, it can be seen that when approaching the near-infrared range, the main contribution to the damping of the probe radiation when the melanin content is of the order 10% is made more by the scattering effect. With a further increase in skin pigmentation, absorption becomes dominant.

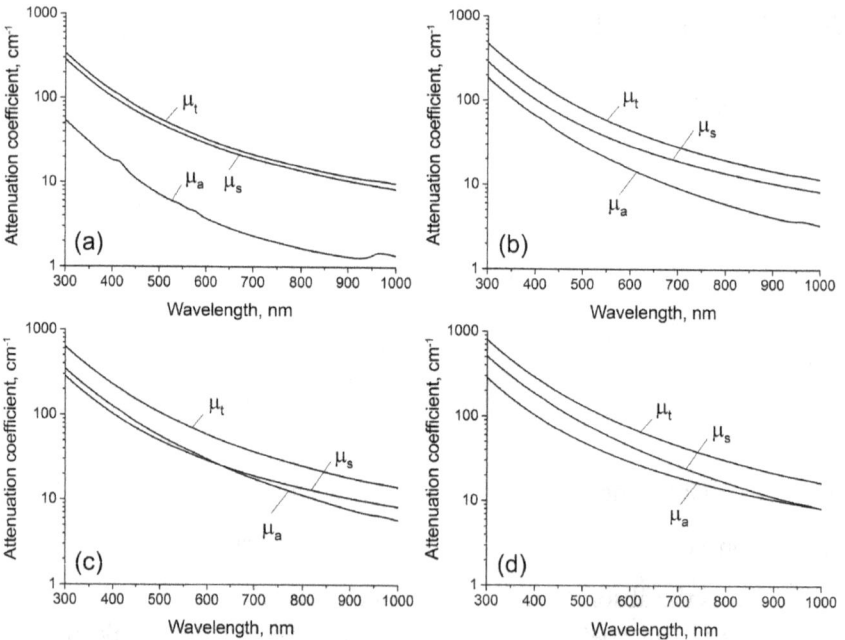

FIGURE 1.3 Graphic dependencies of the contribution of scattering and absorption to the total attenuation of the probe radiation for $C_{mel} = 1\%$ (a), $C_{mel} = 5\%$ (b), $C_{mel} = 10\%$ (c), and $C_{mel} = 15\%$ (d).

To confirm the obtained theoretical dependencies, experimental studies were conducted. For experimental studies, the LAKK-M device was also used. Experimental test studies were conducted with the participation of eight conditionally healthy volunteers. The effect of melanin was studied on various ethnic skin types, including European ($m = 3$), Indian ($m = 1$), Middle Eastern ($m = 1$) and African ($m = 3$). Measurements were carried out at two points of biotissue: on the skin pads of the right hand middle finger – a weakly pigmented area for all volunteers and on the outside of the forearm with marked differences in melanin content for each skin type. The analyzed parameters were the fluorescence intensity of NADH (I_{NADH}) and FAD (I_{FAD}) when excited by UV light (365 nm), as well as the tissue oxygen metabolism indicator (RR), calculated in Eq. (1.1).

The presented parameters were averaged with the calculation of the arithmetic mean M_n and the standard deviation σ. From Figure 1.4 and Table 1.3, it can be seen that the intensity decreases for the forearm area

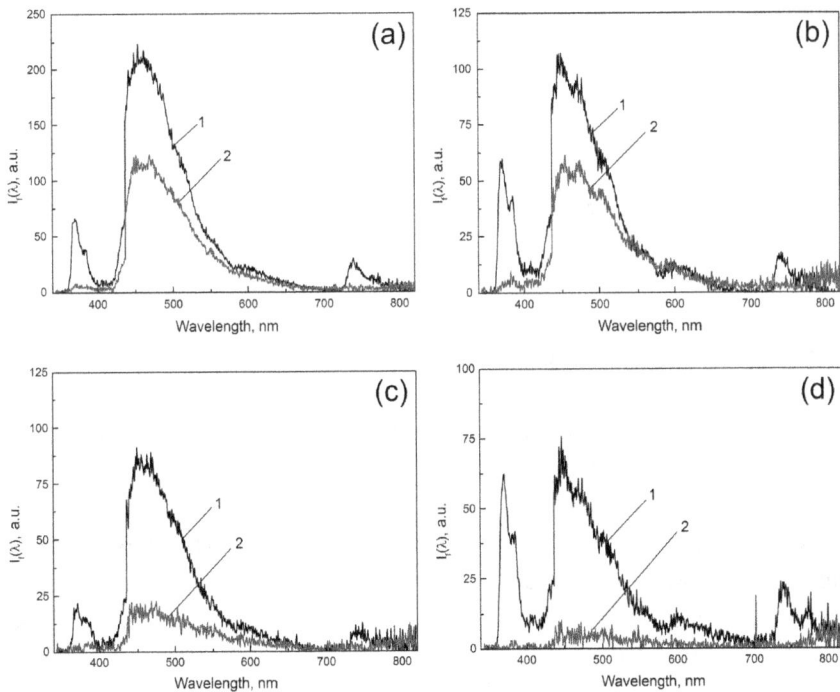

FIGURE 1.4   Examples of fluorescence spectra of skin of various ethnic types on the surface of the finger (1) and forearm (2): (a) European, (b) Indian, (c) Arabic, (d) African. (Reprinted with permission from Dremin and Dunaev (2016) © Optica.)

TABLE 1.3 The Results of Experimental Studies

	$M_n \pm \sigma$ (AU)					
	Finger			Forearm		
Ethnic Skin Type	**NADH**	**FAD**	**RR**	**NADH**	**FAD**	**RR**
Caucasian, $n = 50$	220.2 ± 48.9	49.2 ± 11.8	4.4 ± 0.5	120.1 ± 11.8	21.3 ± 3.3	5.6 ± 0.6
Indian, $n = 27$	110.1 ± 22.3	25.2 ± 6.6	4.9 ± 0.7	60.9 ± 14.2	15.4 ± 5.1	4.0 ± 0.5
Middle Eastern, $n = 13$	84.3 ± 37.7	25.5 ± 12.6	3.3 ± 0.3	25.9 ± 3.9	8.9 ± 2.5	2.9 ± 0.4
African, $n = 3$	75.4 ± 30.5	22.3 ± 17.5	3.4 ± 0.4	$\rightarrow 0$	$\rightarrow 0$	–

with an increase in skin pigmentation and the statistical differences were confirmed by the Mann–Whitney U-test.

For an African skin-type volunteer (curve 2, Figure 1.4d), the fluorescence signal was not actually detected. The data obtained in an additional study in the same areas of the skin on a dark-skinned woman of 25 years shows that fluorescence is also absent at UV and green excitation wavelengths. However, using red wavelength allows you to excite small levels of fluorescence.

To describe and predict how melanin affects the fluorescence signal, a model of light propagation in biological tissue was proposed (Dremin and Dunaev, 2016).

The simultaneous presence of several fluorophores in tissues results in a complicated total fluorescence spectrum recorded from these substances, with a different number of maxima and minima. In the model, it is proposed to take into account the fluorescence signals from the main fluorophores of the tissue, NADH and collagen. The form of the total spectrum can vary depending on the fluorescence intensity of each of the fluorophores under consideration.

In the simulation, the blood content of the dermis was at a constant average level of 0.2% (Jacques, 2013).

As is well known, skin has a very complex structure, and therefore a simplified four-layer optical model of the skin was constructed for theoretical modeling. Incident radiation transmitted through the epidermis is absorbed to a greater extent by melanin and excites fluorescence in the NADH. The transmitted part is incident on the dermis, where it is absorbed predominantly by hemoglobin fractions and excites collagen fluorescence. The remaining probe radiation and secondary fluorescence radiation are diffusely reflected from the collagen fibers and again pass through the layers of skin being absorbed by hemoglobin and melanin.

The numerical modeling was carried out using the Monte Carlo method. This is currently one of the most commonly used methods to describe light propagation in biological tissues (Dremin et al., 2019). The possibilities of the TracePro software (Lambda Research Corp.), intended to analyze light propagation in optomechanical systems, were used as a modeling tool.

The absorption in the biological tissue is taken into account by the Beer–Lambert law:

$$\Phi = \Phi_0 \exp(-\mu_a t), \tag{1.9}$$

where Φ and Φ_0 are the transmitted and incident fluxes, respectively, μ_a is the absorption coefficient and t is the sample thickness.

Fresnel's law is used to take into account the refraction or reflection at the interface of two media. The Henyey–Greenstein function is most often chosen as the phase scattering function:

$$SDF = p(\theta) = \frac{1-g^2}{4\pi(1+g^2 - 2g\cos\theta)}, \tag{1.10}$$

where g is the anisotropy factor.

When a ray passes through a scattering medium, it propagates to a random distance x, determined by the probability distribution:

$$P(x)dx = \exp(-\mu_s x)dx, \tag{1.11}$$

where μ_s is the scattering coefficient.

The fluorescence is modeled in TracePro, taking into account the fluorescence properties in combination with the properties of the material of the object and using the laws given above. The specified parameters include the relative absorption $ab(\lambda)$ and the relative excitation $ex(\lambda)$, normalized to the molar extinction coefficient K_{peak} and the relative emission $em(\lambda)$. The concentration of fluorophores is determined by the molar concentration C_{molar}.

The absorption coefficient of fluorophores in a medium is defined as follows:

$$\mu_a(\lambda) = ab(\lambda)K_{peak}C_{molar}, \tag{1.12}$$

and the path length to the absorption event is equal to

$$d(\lambda) = -\log(x)/\mu_a(\lambda),$$
(1.13)

where x is a random number from 0 to 1.

The ratio of the number of photons that participate in the process to the number of photons that have been absorbed by the system is determined by specifying the quantum efficiency QE in the medium.

A family of model spectra was obtained as the melanin concentration varied in the range of 1%–43% (Figure 1.5a) was obtained from the results of the modeling. As can be seen, the melanin fluorescence signal is practically absent at concentrations above 15%.

It should be noted that the model spectra presented differ somewhat from those obtained experimentally (Figure 1.5b). A more intense experimental signal in the wavelength range of 500–570 nm can be caused by the fact that other fluorophores (FAD, pyridoxine, etc.), which are neglected during modeling, can contribute to the overall spectrum of skin fluorescence under real conditions. Other chromophores (bilirubin, porphyrins, caratinoids, etc.) that are not included in the simulation also affect the shape of the actual experimental spectrum in the range of 400–480 nm, and this leads to a difference between the model and experimental spectra.

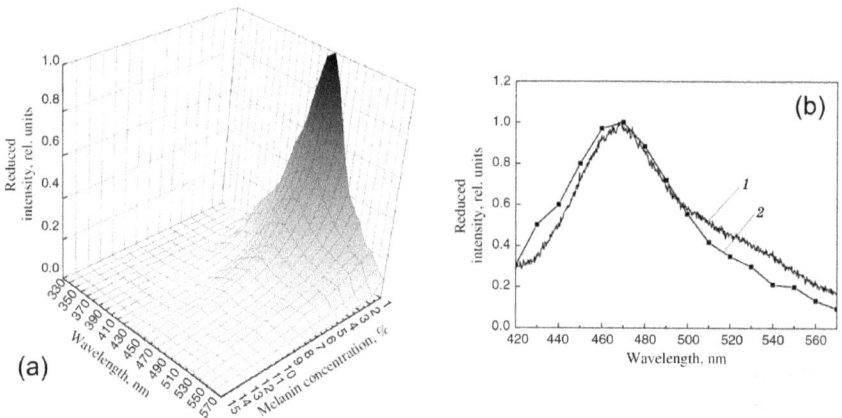

FIGURE 1.5   (a) Family of model spectra calculated by the Monte Carlo method and (b) comparison of experimental (1) and model (2) spectra in the case of European-type skin with 1% melanin concentration. (Reprinted with permission from Dremin and Dunaev (2016) © Optica.)

The influence of melanin should be taken into account both when calibrating FS devices and when developing electronic modules. For example, special requirements are required for the choice of a photodetector, since it must have high photometric sensitivity.

1.2.2 Effect of Blood Filling of Biological Tissue on the Recorded Signals

As you know, human skin (dermis) is permeated with arterioles, venules and capillaries. Consequently, blood contributes to the recorded fluorescence spectrum by absorbing probe radiation. Furthermore, depending on the percentage of oxyhemoglobin (HbO_2) in the total volume of hemoglobin contained in the blood, the blood has different absorption spectra. Thus, it is obvious that the level of blood supply in the study area makes a significant contribution to the fluorescence spectrum and does not allow to accurately assess the content of any biomarker in the skin.

To study the dependence of the signal on blood supply, studies were conducted at the site of biotissue with subcutaneous hematoma. Here, the main absorber is blood hemoglobin, whose absorption maxima are in the range of 400–550 nm. This range falls into the detected fluorescence when it is excited by UV light. Along with the fluorescence of the skin with the hematoma, the fluorescence of the intact tissue was also measured at a distance of no more than 3 mm from the object. The recorded spectra are shown in Figure 1.6.

As can be seen from the graphs presented, over time and with a decrease in the size of the hematoma, the fluorescence signal increased. It can be concluded that not only the intensity of the backscattered radiation but

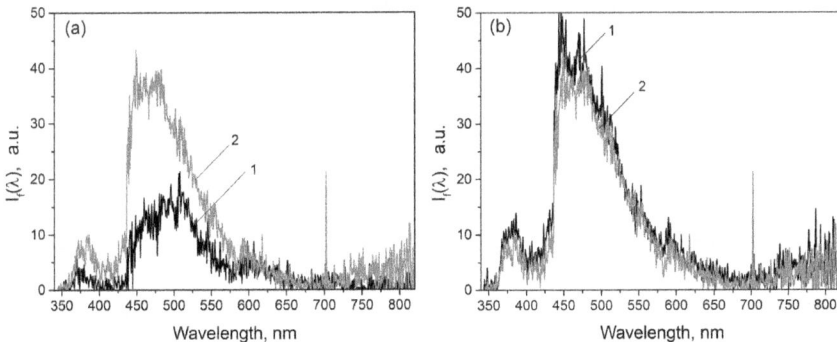

FIGURE 1.6 Examples of the fluorescence that registers the third day (a) and the eighth day (b). 1 – hematoma, 2 – intact tissue. (Reprinted with permission from Dunaev et al. (2015) © Elsevier.)

also the fluorescence signal itself depends on the blood supply of the biological tissue.

Various functional tests that are widely used in clinical practice can also affect the blood supply of biological tissues. One such test is the occlusion test. The test is carried out by clamping the examined limb with a tonometer cuff for 1–3 minutes in such a way as to create conditions for artificial tissue ischemia and subsequently monitor the restoration of blood flow.

Experimental studies were carried out with the participation of 19 conditionally healthy volunteers aged 18–22 years. Measurements were made on the right ring finger pad in the morning. Fluorescence spectra were recorded during the use of arterial brachial occlusion with a cuff pressure of 200–220 mmHg (3 minutes) and also for 3 minutes before and after occlusion. A total of 298 spectra were recorded. Endogenous fluorescence was excited at a wavelength of 450 nm.

On the basis of the Beer–Lambert law, the transmittance coefficients (T) were experimentally and theoretically determined. In general terms, the mentioned law can be represented as follows:

$$I = I_0 \cdot T, \tag{1.14}$$

where I_0 is the intensity of the incoming light beam and I is the intensity after the passage of the medium by light.

Experimentally, this coefficient was calculated by dividing the fluorescence spectrum before occlusion by the fluorescence spectrum during occlusion. During occlusion, the blood content of the studied area was significantly reduced, and therefore the effect of this attenuation on the intensity of the recorded fluorescence was excluded. The theoretical transmittance was calculated using the following formula:

$$T = 10^{-l\{C(HbO_2)\cdot 0.0054\varepsilon(HbO_2)+(1-C(HbO_2))\cdot 0.0054\varepsilon(Hb)\}}, \tag{1.15}$$

where $C(HbO_2)$ is an oxyhemoglobin concentration, $\varepsilon(HbO_2)$ and $\varepsilon(Hb)$ are extinction coefficients, and l is the depth of probing radiation.

When calculating the theoretical transmittance value, parameters such as the depth of the probing radiation and the percentage of hemoglobin related to oxygen were empirically chosen for each experiment. Thus, the maximum similarity of the theoretically calculated transmittance with the experimental value was achieved.

The fluorescence spectrum detected during the occlusion test was multiplied by the theoretically calculated transmittance. Thus, identical theoretically calculated and experimental fluorescence spectra were obtained which included two characteristic dips at wavelengths of 540 and 580 nm, respectively. Thus, we can conclude that blood has a significant effect on the recorded fluorescence spectrum of the skin when excited with a wavelength of 450 nm.

It is also known that the pressure exerted on an optical diagnostic probe is a significant factor that influences the measurement results. One of the main causes of this phenomenon is the influence of this pressure on local blood flow (Popov, 2017; Mizeva et al., 2019). In addition, pressure is a well-known technique for controlling the optical properties of biological tissue, which allows the depth and diagnostic volume to be increased, as well as the actual values of optical parameters of biological tissue in vivo (absorption, scattering, polarization, fluorescence, etc.), eliminating the effect of laser radiation absorption by the blood.

Quantitative studies of the effect of pressure on the results of measurements obtained using optical technologies were carried out (Zherebtsov et al., 2017). Experimental studies were carried out using the system described above. To change the pressure on the optical probe, a special tool attached to the optical fiber was designed and printed on a 3D printer. During experimental studies, the pressure gradually increased from 0 to 40 kPa and then again decreased to 0 kPa. The study area was the inner surface of the middle finger of the right hand, as well as the outer surface of the wrist. These areas were chosen as they are often used in studies with optical noninvasive diagnostic methods, as well as in wearable electronics.

The study involved seven conditionally healthy volunteers aged 24 ± 7 years. In the first series of measurements, the effect of pressure on the average level of the laser Doppler flowmetry (LDF) signal was investigated. The measurements performed allowed us to obtain the averaged curve of the recorded perfusion fall under pressure, and also to represent it in the form of an exponential approximation.

In the second series of measurements, the effect of pressure on the recorded fluorescence spectrum of the skin was investigated. Measurements were made at various levels of pressure with successive steps of increase and decrease in load. After the pressure was removed, the diffuse reflection spectrum was re-recorded. The measurements made it possible to obtain curves of increase in the recorded fluorescence intensity averaged over a group of volunteers with increasing pressure on the optical probe.

On average, with a maximum applied pressure of 40 kPa, the level of perfusion fell by 85% from the initial level. At the same time, at a pressure of 5 kPa, a decrease in perfusion was observed by 25%. With a maximum applied pressure of 40 kPa, the average fluorescence intensity increased when excited at wavelengths of 365 nm by 95%, at 450 nm by 105%, and at 532 nm by 40%. In this case, already at a pressure of 5 kPa, an increase in the fluorescence intensity was observed for 365 nm by 30%, for 450 nm by 25%, and for 532 nm by 22%. At a wavelength of 637 nm, no effect of pressure on the fluorescence intensity was detected.

The increase in recorded fluorescence intensity is due to the fact that with an increase in the load on the area under study, there is a decrease in the blood supply to the tissue due to the extrusion of blood from the diagnostic volume.

Thus, the pressure on the optical probe is a factor that has a significant effect on the microcirculation of blood in human skin, which in turn affects the resulting fluorescence intensity spectra.

1.3 IN VIVO FLUORESCENCE DIAGNOSTICS

1.3.1 Application of Fluorescence Spectroscopy to Assess Tissue Viability in Feet of Patients with Diabetes Mellitus

According to the International Diabetes Federation (IDF), early-stage diagnosis and monitoring of the effectiveness of treatment in diabetes are currently one of the highest priorities in modern health care. The medical, social and economic significance of diabetes is determined primarily by the high prevalence of this disease and the frequency of debilitating and quality of similar reducing effects suffered by affected individuals. The IDF report for 2021 indicated that there are 537 million diabetic patients worldwide, with this figure projected to increase to 783 million by 2045.

Over the last several years, multiple studies have indicated that timely diagnosis and treatment, including an increased level of patient monitoring, reduce the manifestation of various complications, potentially even reversing them at early preclinical stages (Schramm, 2006). To this effect, modern diagnosis of feet in patients with diabetes mellitus can be made using a variety of methodologies. These methodologies offer both unique advantages and disadvantages. Today, the use of various optical noninvasive methods is promising and informative for diagnosis of complications in diabetes (Zharkikh et al., 2020; Dunaev and Tuchin, 2022)). Thus, the aim of this part of the study was to attempt to experimentally study and analyze the potential of registering fluorophore autofluorescence to diagnose lower extremity disorders in patients with diabetes mellitus (Dremin et al., 2017a; Zherebtsova et al., 2019; Potapova et al., 2017).

To determine which fluorophores contribute to the resulting fluorescence signal, preliminary test experiments were conducted in the nail bed area. This area was chosen for visual control of blood flow parameters and gas exchange zones (perivascular zones) using the videocapillaroscopy method (Dremin et al., 2017b).

In this evaluation study, the area of the middle finger nail bed of the hand was illuminated by a LED radiation source with a wavelength of 365 nm (power ~2–3 mW) and a broadband halogen radiation source HL-2000 (Ocean Optics, USA, 360–2400 nm, ~5–7 mW). The high-aperture micro lens with an aperture of 0.12 and a projection long-focus lens formed an image on a monochrome CCD video camera. The fluorescence image was filtered using a long-wavelength cut filter.

For dynamic observation of changes in fluorescence, an occlusion test was chosen as a provocative effect (cuff placement in the brachial artery). Thus, a state of artificial ischemia was created. Depending on oxygen availability, the NADH molecules formed in the sixth glycolysis reaction have two ways of their further transformation: either stay in the cytosol and enter the eleventh glycolysis reaction (anaerobic conditions) or penetrate into the mitochondria and oxidize in the Krebs cycle respiratory chain (aerobic conditions). When hypoxia occurs, the oxidation of NADH in mitochondria slows down, and the glycolysis (anaerobic) pathway of NADH formation is also activated. In this regard, it can be assumed that the recorded level of fluorescence during such an experiment should increase (Mayevsky and Chance, 2007).

The study included occlusion with a cuff pressure of 220 mm Hg in 1.5 minutes. A pair of images (fluorescence and diffuse reflection) was recorded before and at the end of the occlusion test. Further stabilization and imposition of frames were performed.

As a result of experimental studies, images of fluorescence of the precapillary zones normalized to diffuse reflection images were obtained (Figure 1.7).

As can be seen from the data obtained, by the end of the occlusion test an increase in fluorescence occurs. This is especially pronounced in the precapillary zones, which may indicate the accumulation of NADH due to tissue hypoxia. Therefore, fluorescence measurements can be used to study the dynamics of changes in NADH concentrations.

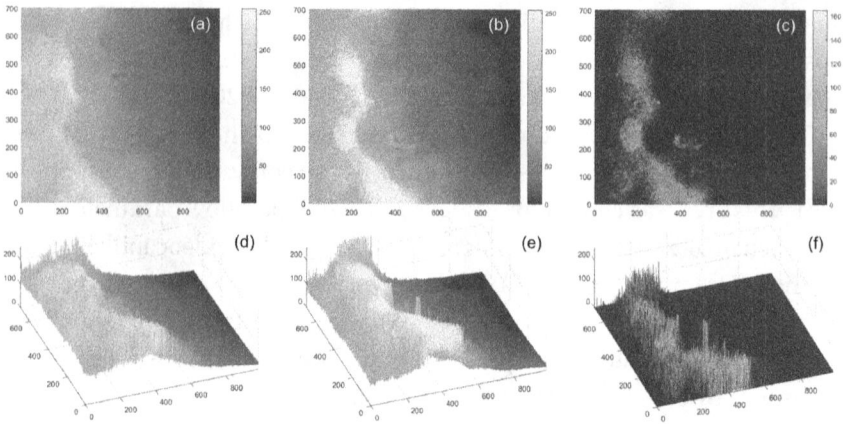

FIGURE 1.7 Fluorescent images before (a, d) and at the end (b, e) of the occlusion test; difference of images (c, f). (Reprinted with permission from Dremin et al. (2017b) © SPIE.)

The experimental study then involved 76 patients with type 1 and type 2 diabetes mellitus. Laboratory parameters were measured according to standard laboratory procedures. Fourteen people in the patients group were considered to have a more severe course of the disease. The decision on the degree of severity in each case was taken individually. This was based on a combination of elevated laboratory parameters, the presence of trophic disorders in the form of ulcers and consultation with the attending physician. The control group consisted of 48 healthy volunteers.

The registered auto fluorescence amplitudes of the coenzymes were evaluated using a LAZMA-D system (LAZMA Ltd, Russia). A 365 and 450 nm radiation sources were used for fluorescence excitation. A multi-optical fiber probe was used for delivery of probing radiation and registration of back-reflected secondary radiation from the tissue. The probe was secured to the dorsal surface of the foot to a point located on a plateau between the first and second metatarsal bones.

Experimental studies have shown that diabetic patients have elevated values of normalized fluorescence amplitudes (AF_{365} and AF_{450} – normalized to the intensity of the backscattered excitation radiation). At the same time, in the group of diabetics with additional complications, these parameters also differ significantly from the control and diabetes only groups (Figure 1.8).

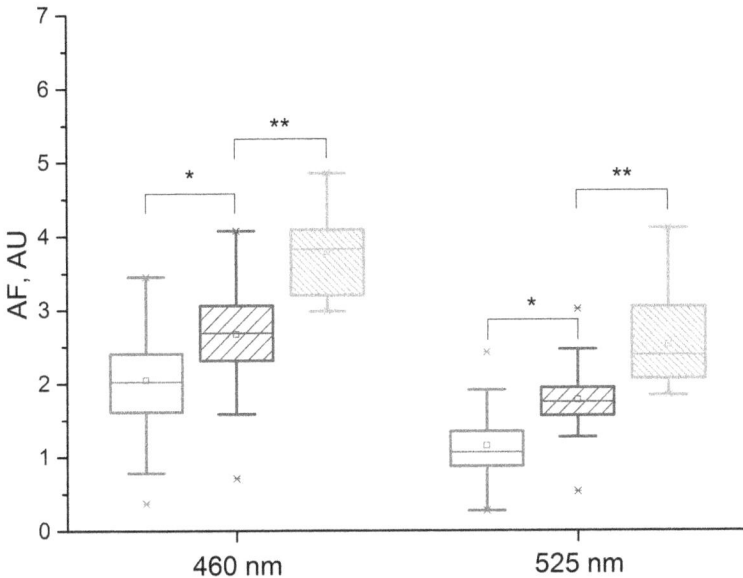

FIGURE 1.8   Comparison of the normalized fluorescence amplitude between the control groups (empty bars), diabetic groups (loose shading), and diabetic with ulcers groups (tight shading) groups. In each box, the central line is the median of the group, while the edges are the 25th and 75th percentiles. (Reprinted with permission from Dremin et al. (2017a) © SPIE.)

Recently, it has been established that long-existing diabetes with hyperglycemia results in an increase in protein glycation levels, which eventually leads to accumulation of so-called advanced glycation end products (AGE) (Gkogkolou and Bohm, 2012; Tan et al., 2002). AGEs become pathogenic when excessively their high levels are reached in tissues and circulation. In particular, AGEs contribute to the mechanisms responsible for the development of diabetic complications (Brownlee, 2005).

AGEs can induce cross-linking of collagen, which can cause vascular stiffening. AGEs can also bind to RAGE (receptor for AGE products) and cause oxidative stress and activation of inflammatory pathways in vascular endothelial cells (Giacco, 2010; Medzhitov, 2008).

The level of skin fluorescence observed in our studies is related to the degree of conventional glycation marker HbA1c determined in vitro. It is important to note, however, that the standard measure of glycation using HbA1c characterizes the glycation processes that occur only in the short term (around 3 months).

1.3.2 The Study of Epithelial Tissue Fluorescence in the Example of the Bladder Cancer

The high rates of recurrence and progression associated with bladder cancer (BC) make it the single most expensive cancer to treat per patient. It is among the ten most prevalent and expensive cancers in the world. Cases of aggressive muscle invasive and metastatic disease exhibit high fatality figures (Jemal et al., 2009; Sievert et al., 2009). Even non-muscle-invasive disease (accounting for around 70% of cases), which is generally non-fatal, experiences high rates of recurrence and progression, resulting in considerable patient morbidity (Ahmad et al., 2012).

A pig bladder was chosen as the object of preliminary experimental studies to assess the potential of the FS method in studying the metabolism of epithelial tissues. BC is of particular interest because of its position as one of the ten most common types of cancers in the world. Cases of muscle invasion and metastasis show high mortality rates. The percentage of relapses after treatment is 50%–95%. Therefore, there is a continuing need to improve diagnostic accuracy and predict response to treatment.

The porcine fresh bladder sections provided by the supplier (Wetlab, UK) were examined (Rafailov et al., 2016). The optical properties of the whole bladder wall were studied in the spectral range of 350–1800 nm on a Lambda 1050 spectrophotometer (PerkinElmer, USA) with an integrating sphere representing a two-channel double diffraction monochromator with an integrated control and recording system. The main advantage of the integrating sphere is that it can be used to collect almost all the light reflected or transmitted through the sample. The light is redirected and assembled by the detector. Its exact amount depends on the geometrical parameters of the sphere and the reflectivity of its walls and the sample.

In addition to spectrophotometric analysis, the samples were also subjected to fluorescence analysis. The fiber-optic probe of the device was installed close to the bladder tissue. The tissue was scanned sequentially using two excitation sources (365 and 450 nm). The resulting tissue fluorescence was recorded in the 300–800 nm wavelength range. The whole procedure was carried out at room temperature in a dark room without windows to limit the error of exposure to noise.

To process the results of experiments and determine optical parameters, we used the inverse adding-doubling method (IAD), which is widely used in biological tissue optics for processing spectrophotometric data using integrating spheres (Prahl, 1993). The IAD method allows one to determine the absorption coefficient μ_a and the transport scattering coefficient μ_s of the biotissue using the values of diffuse reflectance and total transmittance. During the calculations, the anisotropy factor g was recorded. In this case, g was assumed to be equal to 0.9, since this value is most typical for most biological tissues in the visible and near-infrared (NIR) spectral ranges.

To correct the light loss at the edges of the sample, a Monte Carlo calculation was used. The lost light was taken into account in the next iteration of the optical properties evaluation by the IAD method. This process was repeated until the optical properties stabilized.

Figure 1.9 shows the absorption coefficient (1.9a) and the transport scattering coefficient (1.9b) obtained using IAD modeling.

It can be seen that they agree quite well with those obtained in this study. Some inconsistencies are due to the use of different experimental data processing methods, as well as the difference in properties of specific biotissue samples. In Figure 1.9b, the absorption bands of hemoglobin (420, 540 and 580 nm) and water (1195 nm) are clearly visible. Water absorption peaks at 975 and 1195 nm are less pronounced.

For the scattering coefficient, it can be seen that it decreases with increasing wavelength, which is consistent with the general behavior of the biotissue scattering characteristics. The deviation from monotony is due to the effect of strong absorption in these areas.

It should be noted that the obtained dependence for the transport scattering coefficient in the considered range can be approximated with greater accuracy ($R^2 = 0.97$) using the Gunari power function.

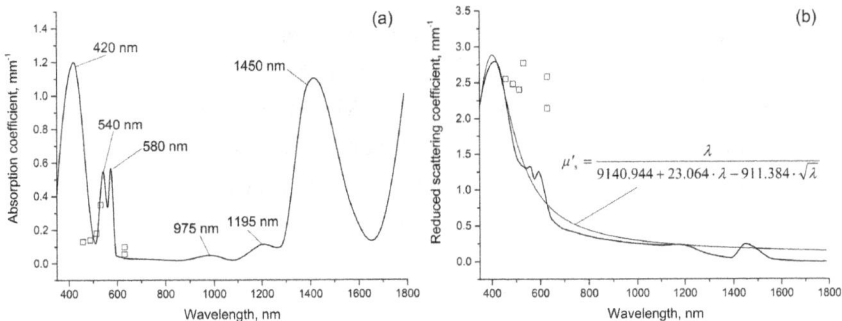

FIGURE 1.9 The absorption coefficient (a) and transport scattering coefficient (b) of a pig bladder sample. (Reprinted with permission from Rafailov et al. (2016) © SPIE.)

The light penetration depth is one of the most important characteristics for determining the capabilities of various optical noninvasive diagnostics methods, including fluorescence spectroscopy. Evaluation of penetration of the depth of light into the biological tissue was carried out using the following equation:

$$\delta = \frac{1}{\sqrt{3\mu_a(\mu_a + \mu'_s)}}. \tag{1.16}$$

In the spectral region of interest for fluorescence spectroscopy (350–600 nm), the radiation penetration depth is 0.5–2 mm, which allows one to excite the fluorescence of the main biomarkers (NADH, FAD, collagen, etc.).

Furthermore, the obtained coefficients were used when building the model in the TracePro software. Monte Carlo numerical simulations were performed. For the interesting wavelength range (360–610 nm), the refractive index n, the scattering μ_s and absorption μ_a coefficients, and the anisotropy factor g were specified for the tissue. The bladder tissue has a complex structure and, therefore, for theoretical modeling, a simplified two-layer optical model was constructed.

Theoretically, the incident radiation, passing through the mucous membrane, is partially absorbed and excites, depending on the wavelength, the fluorescence of NADH or FAD. The part that passes through enters the muscle layer, where it is also absorbed, excites collagen fluorescence, diffusely reflects from various structural components, and again passes through the layers, being absorbed and reaching the detector. The resulting model is shown in Figure 1.10.

The distance between the emitter and receiver (the so-called measurement base) was chosen $r = 1$ mm. The diameter of the receiver is $d = 0.06$ mm (analog of the receiving fiber of the LAKK-M system). From the simulation results, it can be seen that the diagnostic depth reaches 1 mm.

A comparison of the fluorescence spectra obtained from the simulation results with the experimentally obtained ones is presented in Figure 1.11.

There is good agreement between the model and the experimental spectra. Some differences may be due to the presence of fluorescence of other fluorophores in real tissue, which was not taken into account in the simulation. Furthermore, various other chromophores-absorbers can contribute to the modification of the real experimental spectrum.

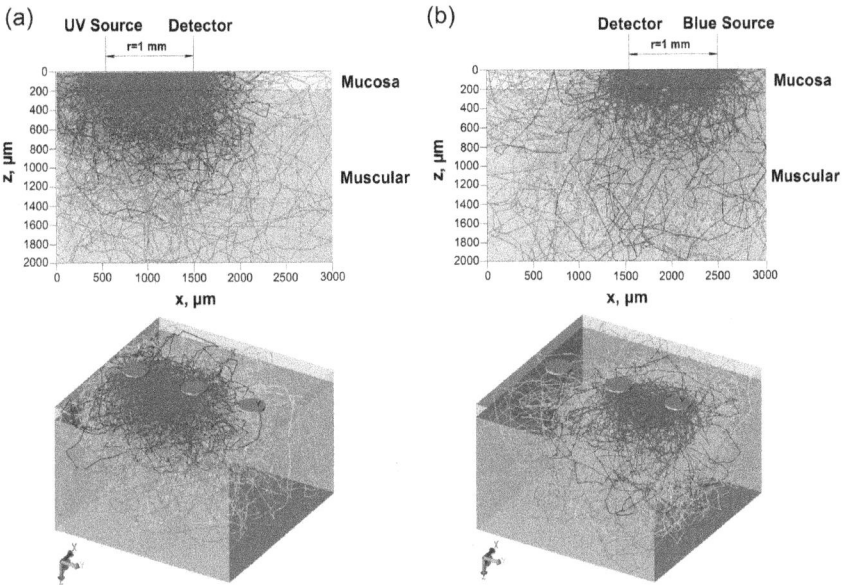

FIGURE 1.10 A side view and a full view of a 3D model imitating the passage of fluorescence radiation into tissue at excitations of 365 nm (a) and 450 nm (b). (Reprinted with permission from Rafailov et al. (2016) © SPIE.)

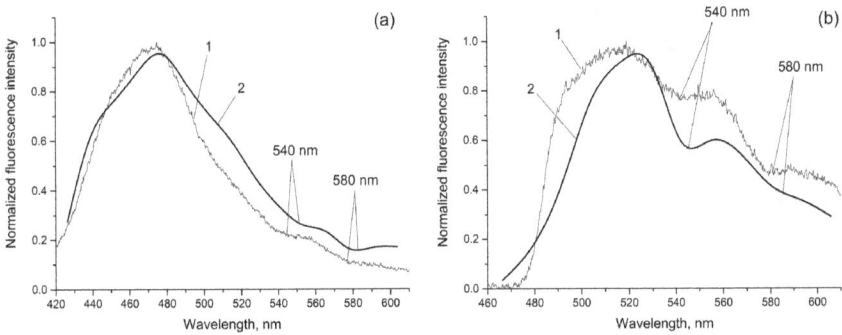

FIGURE 1.11 Comparison of experimental spectra (1) and model (2), calculated using the Monte-Carlo method. The model mimics the presence of NADH+collagen (a) and FAD+collagen (b). (Reprinted with permission from Rafailov et al. (2016) © SPIE.)

Furthermore, it can be concluded that the shape of the experimental fluorescence spectrum of bladder tissues is largely dependent on the fluorescence of NADH and collagen (at excitation 365 nm) or FAD and collagen (at excitation 450 nm). Studies indicate that mitochondrial NADH and FAD, as well as stromal collagen, are dominated by fluorescence of biological tissues.

The next stage of the study was a comparison of bladder fluorescence in the presence of BC with the control (Palmer et al., 2016). BC cell line 5637 was applied to purchased porcine bladders from freshly slaughtered pigs. The attachment of cancer cells to the scaffold in organoids on day 2 and the T1 transitional cell carcinoma phenotype on day 12 were confirmed by an experienced pathologist. Fluorescence spectroscopy measurements were performed using the LAKK-M system. At the time of registration, the optical fiber touched exactly the center of the mucous tissue without applying any pressure.

Measurements were carried out at the 0, 1, 4, 7, 11, 14, 18 and 21 days of study in the dark room to prevent interference from background noise. The fluorescence intensity upon excitation with light of 365 and 450 nm was recorded and, based on the data obtained, the RR was calculated using Eq. (1.1).

In the described experiment, the study of the fluorescence intensity of individual fluorophores seems to be unreliable because of the influence that day-to-day changes in laser power and changes occurring in tissues can have. Instead, we looked at ratios of particular fluorophores relative to one another.

A gradual decrease in the RR was demonstrated during the 21-day study. Organoids values were significantly lower compared to the control ($p < 0.05$). At the same time, the measurement data on day 0 of the study (before the addition of cancer cells) were not statistically different for the two samples. Figure 1.12 shows the average dynamics of the values of the RR during the study for the control and organoid groups.

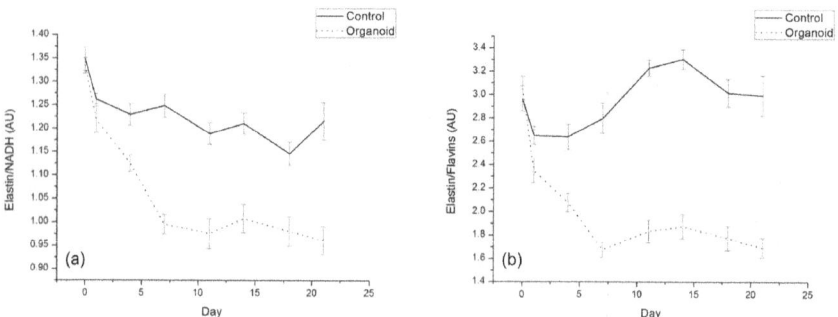

FIGURE 1.12 Average (a) elastin/NADH and (b) elastin/flavins ratios for control (solid line) and cancer organoids (dashed line) throughout the 21-day study. (Reprinted with permission from Palmer et al. (2016) © Optica.)

The ratios of elastin fluorescence to those of coenzymes NADH and FAD were also measured. The measured parameters showed a relative decrease in elastin content compared to other biotissue fluorophores during the study. The obtained dependencies are presented in Figure 1.12. We assume that such a dynamics of coenzyme concentrations may indicate adherence, epithelialization and invasion of tissue by cancer cells.

The next stage of the study was to evaluate the fluorescence of biopsy specimens from BC patients and to compare the data with the control group (Palmer et al., 2017). Based on a previous study (Palmer et al., 2016), we hypothesized that BC tissues taken from patient biopsy samples will demonstrate a reduced RR, an increased level of endogenous porphyrin fluorescence and a reduced NADH/porphyrin ratio compared to the control sample.

Twenty patients aged 16–90 years with suspected bladder tumors undergoing cystoscopic examination by white-light cystoscopy, with transuresthral resection of the bladder tumor (TURBT) participated in this study. The tissue removed from the patient was positioned, as far as possible, with the mucous side up in a black matte cuvette with known optical properties. Measurements were carried out on each sample under irradiation with light of wavelengths of 365 and 635 nm. A total of 122 measurements were taken, including 89 from cancer samples and 33 from healthy ones.

Analysis of the area under spectral curves revealed that there were no statistically significant differences in total fluorescence intensity (reflected by spectral amplitude) under 365 nm excitation ($p = 0.519$). This result can be accounted for the fact that there was a statistically significant difference in total fluorescence intensity under 635 nm excitation ($p = 0.00265$). This difference is attributable to the nonnormal distribution of tissue fluorescence intensity, which may be more exaggerated at UV wavelengths where blood and other tissue scatterers have a greater effect on measured autofluorescence.

The optical redox ratio (ORR) values for each sample were calculated and compared for statistically significant differences. A statistically significant decrease in the ORR of cancer tissue compared to healthy tissue can be observed ($p = 0.00891$). The amplitude of fluorescence of porphyrins was recorded and analyzed for statistically significant differences. Porphyrin levels in cancer samples are greatly increased compared to healthy samples. This difference was found to be extremely statistically significant ($p = 0.00241$). At the same time, values for the NADH/porphyrin ratios for cancer samples are greatly decreased. The difference between samples was found to be extremely statistically significant ($p = 0.00624$).

Tumors were shown to exhibit reduced ORR compared to healthy tissue. This is in correspondence with our previous findings in an organoid model of BC (Palmer et al., 2016). The most contemporary focus on ORR (Palmer et al., 2015) suggests that the metabolic alterations that occur during cancer development skew the degree to which cancer cells use their electron transport chain, thus causing accumulation of the primary electron donor NADH in cancer cells. However, there are not many data on ORR in human bladder tissue.

The statistically significant increase in porphyrin levels in cancer tissue suggests a selective accumulation similar to that observed in photodynamic diagnosis but without the need for photosensitizers administration (Datta et al., 1998). Previously, chronic hypoxia has been suggested to be an underlying factor of increased porphyrin levels in oral mucosa; therefore, the elevated porphyrin level and, more importantly, the reduced NADH/porphyrin values observed in BC may reflect an effect of tissue hypoxia on the reduction of cell metabolic activity.

1.4 FLUORESCENCE PHANTOMS

1.4.1 FAD Fluorescence Phantom

Development, calibration measurements, verification, and standardization of an optical diagnostic techniques require their comprehensive testing using biological tissue phantoms with known and quantitatively confirmed optomechanical properties, including structural geometric features and shape. Using phantoms as test objects allows for high-accuracy calibration of measurement systems, adjustment of measurement technique for obtaining a useful signal/image from a certain depth, and localization of measured volume, as well as for standardization of the measurement results obtained by devices from different manufacturers.

Phantoms of skin based on PVC presented above have demonstrated their effectiveness and stability when verifying measurements by various techniques, including hyperspectral imaging, OCT, laser speckle contrast imaging, etc. However, such phantoms have significant limitations in mimicking the fluorescent properties of biotissues. The conditions of the polymerization processes (increased temperature, use of chemically active polymerizing substances) lead to destruction or significant variation in the properties of fluorescence dyes, especially in the properties of such endogenous fluorescent substances as nicotinamide adenine nucleotide (NADH) and flavin adenine nucleotide (FAD).

Here, the manufacturing technique and the main optical properties of a new type of human skin phantom based on polymerizable polyacrylamide (PAA), collagen and an aqueous solution of FAD are presented (Shupletsov et al., 2021). PAA is an optically transparent elastic material with good temporal photostability, and it is actively used in biomedical practice. To simulate the base level of the fluorescence of the connective tissue of the skin, the collagen contained in gelatin was used. For the developed approach, moderate polymerization modes are typical, which do not affect FAD fluorescence. To design a denser elastic structure that was not subject to mold, we used the PAA gel as a bounding material with stable thermal and chemical properties. An important feature of the developed fluorescent phantoms is the lack of pronounced fluorescence of PAA in the UV and visible ranges. An aqueous FAD solution was used as the fluorophore, which is one of the main skin fluorophores upon excitation at a wavelength of 450 nm. In the human body, FAD plays a key role in cellular respiration and cell death processes, as well as in the continuous use of endogenous catecholamines (such as dopamine, adrenaline, and norepinephrine), being a cofactor of two known varieties of FAD-dependent monoamine oxidases that are primarily responsible for deamination processes in most cells in the organism.

The preliminary preparation of an elastic matrix base of human skin phantoms was carried out by mixing and homogenizing powdered gelatin (0.2 g) with 20 mL of distilled water until a homogeneous structure is obtained when heating at 40°C for 15 minutes. Subsequent homogenization of the obtained solution was carried out by mixing acrylamide (AA) (6 g) and bisacrylamide (BAA) (0.16 g) at room temperature for 15 minutes. To reproduce scattering properties, 0.03 g of zinc oxide (ZnO) was added to the manufactured polymer structure. To reproduce the fluorescence properties, FAD (which concentration normally varies in human body from several units up to several tens of mmoles per 100 g of tissue) was added to the obtained mixture, and they were mixed for 10 minutes. Five skin phantoms were fabricated: without FAD and with FAD concentrations of 5, 15, 20, and 25 mmoles per 100 g of material. Subsequent polymerization was performed until elastic light scattering structure was achieved by adding 15 mL of ammonium persulfate [$(NH4)2S2O8$] and 2.4 mL of tetramethylethylenediamine (TEMED).

Diffuse reflectance, diffuse, and collimated transmittance of the manufactured plastic composite base, as well as the base with the addition of 15 mM FAD, were measured with a spectrophotometer equipped with

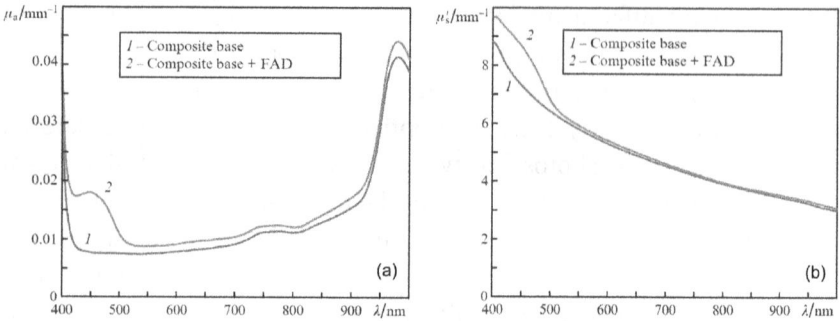

FIGURE 1.13   Spectral dependences of (a) absorption coefficients and (b) reduced scattering coefficients of the fabricated composite base without FAD and with the addition of 15 mM FAD. (Reprinted with permission from Shupletsov et al. (2021) © Turpion.)

an integrating sphere (Gooch & Housego, USA). The absorption coefficient (μ_a) and the reduced scattering coefficient (μ_s') were calculated by the inverse add-doubling technique in the range of 400–1000 nm (Figure 1.13).

The absorption spectra clearly show water absorption bands (760 and 975 nm) and an FAD absorption band (450 nm). Since the main aim of this work is mimicking fluorescence, no additional absorption components were added to achieve absorption equivalent to that of skin tissues in the course of phantom manufacturing. The refractive indices n of the phantoms were measured using an Abbe multiwave refractometer (Atago, Japan) at different wavelengths: $n = 1.358$ (450 nm), 1.350 (589 nm), 1.348 (632 nm), and 1.343 (930 nm).

Fluorescence parameters were measured using a setup that included a hyperspectral camera and a CCD spectrometer (Figure 1.14).

Radiation from a M450LP1 LED at a wavelength of 450 nm (Thorlabs, USA) passes through a bandpass filter MF445-45 (Thorlabs, USA). The transmitted radiation band goes to a dichroic filter MD416 (Thorlabs, USA) and is then directed to a skin MP for FAD fluorescence excitation. The back-reflected LED radiation is removed from the light flux with a dichroic filter and a light filter FELH0500 with a cutoff wavelength of 500 nm (Thorlabs, USA). Remaining sample fluorescence emission is recorded by a Specim hyperspectral camera (SPECIM Spectral Imaging Ltd., Finland) in the spectral range of 400–1000 nm. In the fluorescence spectroscopy channel, the spectra are registered with a FLAME-T-VIS-NIR-ES CCD spectrometer (Ocean Optics, USA) in the spectral range of 350–820 nm using optical fiber.

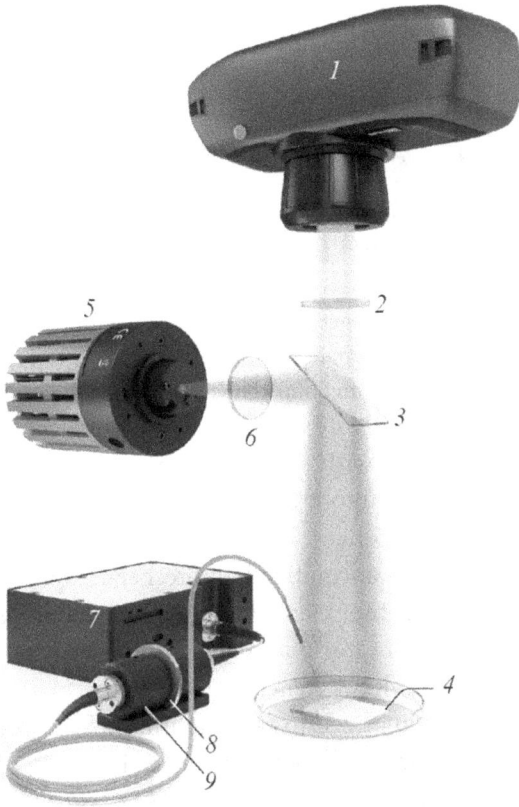

FIGURE 1.14 Setup for hyperspectral fluorescence imaging and fluorescence spectroscopy: (1) hyperspectral camera; (2, 8) long-wavelength emission filter; (3) dichroic filter; (4) test object; (5) LED source; (6) bandpass filter; (7) CCD spectrometer; and (9) filter holder. (Reprinted with permission from Shupletsov et al. (2021) © Turpion.)

The acquired hyperspectral fluorescence images of five skin phantoms with different concentrations of FAD are shown in Figure 1.15a. The images were registered with a camera exposition time of 500 ms and an average irradiance of $0.5\,mW/cm^2$. For further analysis, the fluorescence intensity values were averaged within the region of interest (ROI) boundaries, similar to those marked with a square in Figure 1.15a. For comparison of the fluorescence properties of elastic phantoms with a real biological object, fluorescence images of the human finger skin and forearm skin of a healthy volunteer were acquired (Figure 1.15b and c). Data from the selected ROIs after spatial averaging were used for the construction and analysis of the fluorescence intensity spectra. The maximum

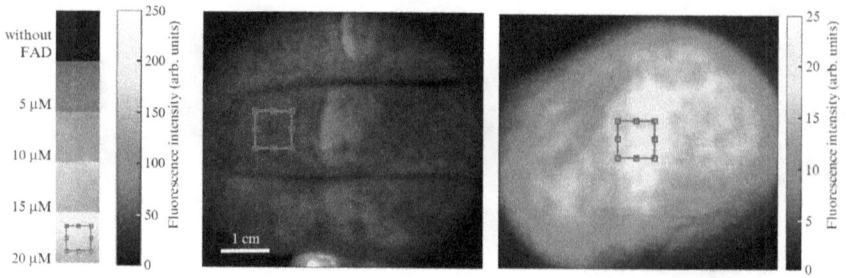

FIGURE 1.15   Fluorescence images of (a) phantoms, (b) finger skin, and (c) forearm skin, obtained using a hyperspectral camera at a wavelength of 530 nm. (Reprinted with permission from Shupletsov et al. (2021) © Turpion.)

intensity values measured with a CCD spectrometer were averaged over three spectra for each phantom and compared with the data obtained using a hyperspectral camera.

Figure 1.16a–c shows normalized fluorescence spectra and curves for the dependence of the maximum phantom fluorescence intensity versus FAD concentration obtained by hyperspectral imaging and CCD spectroscopy. The fluorescence spectra of the phantoms and skin (Figure 1.16d) were normalized to the maximum fluorescence value for a concentration of 25 mM and the fluorescence intensity of the forearm, respectively. The fluorescence intensity of FAD registered in the fluorescence imaging channel with a hyperspectral camera varies in proportion to the fluorophore concentration, which was also confirmed by the CCD spectrometer measurements (Figure 1.16c). Furthermore, the highest intensity variation rate with a change in FAD concentration is observed in the range of 5–10 mM, which is of the greatest interest to mimic the properties of healthy tissues. The obtained fluorescence intensity values for phantoms have a high correlation with FAD concentration (Pearson's correlation coefficient between measurements with two techniques is $r = 0.99$, $p < 0.001$). The variation of the fluorescence intensity signal to the fluorophore concentration ratio is a non-linear function resulting from absorption of the excitation radiation by a fluorophore and variations in the useful phantom/tissue volume, the signal from which is measured. In the general case, determination of this dependence is a nontrivial problem, the final decision of which is affected by fluorophore concentration, object absorbing and scattering properties, as well as the parameters of the detection system. The phantom spectra and the skin spectra have similar fluorescence peaks corresponding to

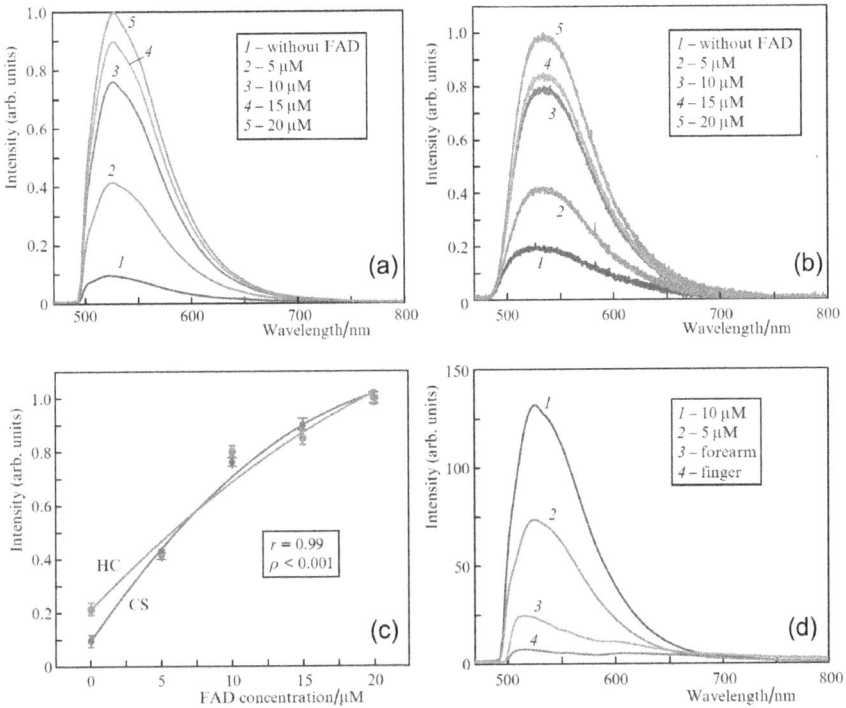

FIGURE 1.16 (a, b) Fluorescence spectra of skin phantoms obtained using (a) hyperspectral camera and (b) CCD spectrometer, (c) dependences of maximum phantom fluorescence intensity versus FAD concentration and (d) spectra of maximum phantom fluorescence for two FAD concentrations and maximum fluorescence of the finger and forearm skin obtained with a hyperspectral camera; CS, CCD spectrometer; HC, hyperspectral camera. (Reprinted with permission from Shupletsov et al. (2021) © Turpion.)

the FAD spectrum ($\lambda_{max} \approx 530$–$540$ nm) under excitation with blue light (450 nm). However, the shape of the skin fluorescence spectra, as well as the general signal intensity level, is different from those for phantoms, which is explained by the effect of blood on fluorescence absorption in skin. Moreover, the presented phantoms can be modified to account for absorbing properties at no significant cost.

A higher initial fluorescence level (Figure 1.16c) obtained during measurements with a fiber-optic CCD spectrometer without FAD is explained by the contribution of radiation to the measured signal from a greater depth of the phantom volume. A significant difference in the intensity of skin fluorescence for the finger and forearm (Figure 1.16d) is due to a sufficiently large number of capillaries and arteriovenular anastomoses in the skin of the hand palm, which significantly affects the absorption of fluorescence signals.

This part presents a technique for fabricating a new type human skin phantom based on PAA, collagen, zinc oxide, and FAD aqueous solution. The main advantage of the developed phantoms is that the conditions for PAA polymerization do not affect the FAD fluorescence properties in the final phantoms. At the same time, fabricated polymeric phantoms with confirmed scattering and fluorescence properties allow the reproduction of skin fluorescence spectra in the specified wavelength range with a sufficiently high accuracy. The developed elastic phantom matrix satisfies the stationarity condition required for calibration measurements. Manufactured forms should be stored at a temperature of 4°C and air humidity at a level of 90%–95%.

Application of the developed phantom manufacturing technology will allow testing, standardizing and calibrating systems for fluorescence imaging, as well as instruments for fluorescence spectroscopy, coupled with fiber-optic detection of optical radiation.

1.4.2 Riboflavin and PPIX Fluorescence Phantom

The idea of the optical phantom designed in this part was to combine the solid base for modeling of background collagen fluorescence and the liquid part to mimic the various concentrations of FAD and porphyrin fluorescence in biological tissues (Shupletsov et al., 2020).

To produce optical phantoms that mimic collagen fluorescence, it is possible to use gelatin, which is its hydrolyzed form. In this work, a multilayer model was created consisting of sheets of gelatin with a thickness of less than 1 mm and a weight of less than 5 g. The optimal number of gelatin sheets was experimentally selected by comparing the fluorescence intensity levels of gelatin sheets and skin collagen. To simulate the FAD fluorescence spectrum, a 1% solution ($26.6 \, \mu M/g$) of riboflavin mononucleotide was used. This substance belongs to the flavin group and has a fluorescence spectrum similar to that of FAD. Riboflavin has a higher quantum yield, and, unlike FAD, its quantum yield within pH 4–8 does not depend on acidity. Four concentrations of riboflavin were selected close to the real concentrations of FAD in biological tissues. The solution of riboflavin mononucleotide was diluted with distilled water in the following ratios: 1:32, 1:64, 1:128 and 1:256. Thus, the solid base of the optical phantom was composed of two sheets of gelatin. The liquid part was made of solutions of four different concentrations (0.84;

0.42; 0.21; 0.1 µM/g) of riboflavin distributed in four different areas of the phantom.

Protoporphyrin IX (PPIX) was obtained chemically from the dark egg-shell. It is known that PPIX, an immediate precursor of heme, is the main pigment that creates the shell color. Before extraction, the eggshells were thoroughly washed of albumen and shell membranes and dried. 10 g of the eggshells were mixed with 150 mL of a 1 M hydrochloric acid solution. The reacting mixture was maintained until the release of carbon dioxide ceased. The undissolved residue was separated by filtration through a paper filter. The resulting emulsion was centrifuged to completely separate the layers. The top layer containing PPIX was transferred to a conical flask and 10 g of pre-calcined sodium sulfate was added to PPIX. The PPIX solution was separated from the salt by decantation and evaporated in a hot water bath until the solvent was completely removed. The residue was dissolved in 5 mL of dimethylsulfoxide. As a result, PPIX was obtained at a concentration of 0.3 µM/g which was applied to a two-sheet gelatin model similar to riboflavin.

Drops of the same volume (20 µL) with different concentrations of riboflavin or PPIX were applied to gelatin sheets using a micropipette. The resulting phantoms with riboflavin and PPIX were located on a non-fluorescent non-reflective surface.

As a result, the registered images of created optical phantom under halogen lamp illumination and LED illumination after preliminary processing are presented in Figure 1.17a–c. After that, the intensities were normalized to the maximum intensity to represent the obtained data in the range of 0–1. The fluorescence spectra for each concentration of riboflavin and PPIX are presented in Figure 1.18.

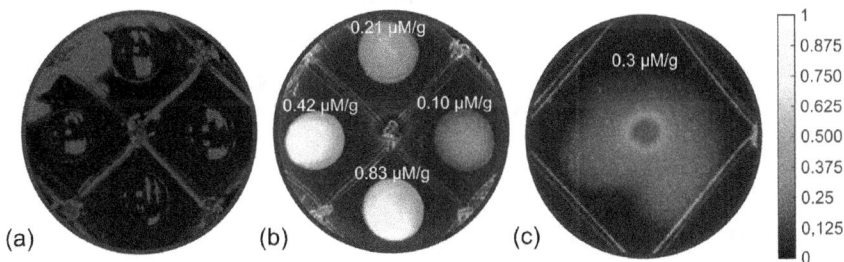

FIGURE 1.17 Obtained images of the optical phantom: (a) original image of the riboflavin phantom in white light, (b) fluorescence image of the riboflavin phantom, and (c) fluorescence image of the PPIX phantom. (Reprinted with permission from Shupletsov et al. (2020) © Turpion.)

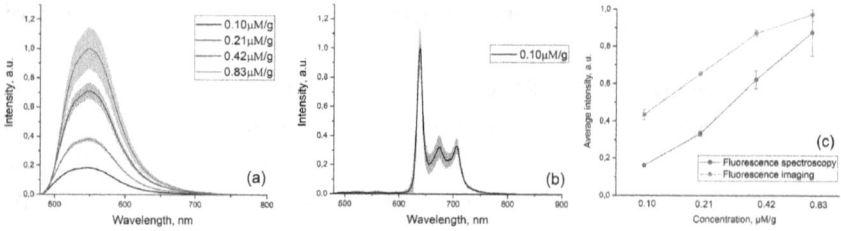

FIGURE 1.18   Average normalized fluorescence spectra of (a) riboflavin and (b) PPIX solutions. (c) Dependences of maximum phantom fluorescence intensity versus riboflavin concentration. (Reprinted with permission from Shupletsov et al. (2020) © Turpion.)

1.5 SUMMARY

Methods of fluorescence spectroscopy and imaging are considered to be promising modern methods of optical diagnostics. Noninvasive assessment of fluorescence of biological tissues allows us to draw conclusions about structural and metabolic changes that occur in various pathological processes. Fluorescence spectroscopy and imaging are widely used in various medical fields, including oncology and skin diagnostics. The data presented should be considered when developing new optical medical and biological techniques, as well as addressing specific diagnostic problems in clinical practice.

This chapter reviews the main problems that arise when analyzing the fluorescence of biological tissues, and also demonstrates some areas of application of fluorescence spectroscopy in the field of medical diagnostics. The possible application of this technology goes far beyond the scope of this chapter and covers the medical branches of minimally invasive and classical surgery, transplantology, diagnostics of brain metabolism, etc.

ACKNOWLEDGMENTS

The authors acknowledge the support of the Russian Science Foundation under projects No. 21-15-00325, 22-75-10088 and 23-25-00522.

REFERENCES

Ahmad, I., O.J. Sansom, and H.Y. Leung. 2012. "Exploring Molecular Genetics of Bladder Cancer: Lessons Learned from Mouse Models." *Disease Models & Mechanisms* 5 (3): 323–32.

Brownlee, M. 2005. "The Pathobiology of Diabetic Complications: A Unifying Mechanism." *Diabetes* 54 (6): 1615–25.

Datta, S.N., C.S. Loh, A.J. MacRobert, S.D. Whatley, and P.N. Matthews. 1998. "Quantitative Studies of the Kinetics of 5-Aminolaevulinic Acid-Induced Fluorescence in Bladder Transitional Cell Carcinoma." *British Journal of Cancer* 78 (8): 1113–18.

Dremin, V., E. Zherebtsov, A. Bykov, A. Popov, A. Doronin, and I. Meglinski. 2019. "Influence of Blood Pulsation on Diagnostic Volume in Pulse Oximetry and Photoplethysmography Measurements." *Applied Optics* 58 (34): 9398–405.

Dremin, V.V., and A.V. Dunaev. 2016. "How the Melanin Concentration in the Skin Affects the Fluorescence-Spectroscopy Signal Formation." *Journal of Optical Technology* 83 (1): 43–8.

Dremin, V.V., E.A. Zherebtsov, V.V. Sidorov, A.I. Krupatkin, I.N. Makovik, A.I. Zherebtsova, E.V. Zharkikh, et al. 2017a. "Multimodal Optical Measurement for Study of Lower Limb Tissue Viability in Patients with Diabetes Mellitus." *Journal of Biomedical Optics* 22 (8): 085003.

Dremin, V.V., N.B. Margaryants, M.V. Volkov, E.V. Zhukova, E.A. Zherebtsov, A.V. Dunaev, and E.U. Rafailov. 2017b. "Assessment of Tissue Ischemia of Nail Fold Precapillary Zones Using a Fluorescence Capillaroscopy." *Proc. SPIE* 10412: 104120W.

Dunaev, A.V., V.V. Dremin, E.A. Zherebtsov, I.E. Rafailov, K.S. Litvinova, S.G. Palmer, N.A. Stewart, S.G. Sokolovski, and E.U. Rafailov. 2015. "Individual Variability Analysis of Fluorescence Parameters Measured in Skin with Different Levels of Nutritive Blood Flow." *Medical Engineering and Physics* 37 (6): 574–83.

Dunaev, A.V., and V.V. Tuchin. 2022. *Biomedical Photonics for Diabetes Research.* Boca Raton, FL: Taylor & Francis.

Giacco, F., M. Brownlee, and A.M. Schmidt. 2010. "Oxidative Stress and Diabetic Complications." *Circulation Research* 107 (9): 1058–70.

Gkogkolou, P., and M. Bohm. 2012. "Advanced Glycation End Products: Key Players in Skin Aging?" *Dermatoendocrinol* 4 (3): 259–70.

Jacques, S.L. 2013. "Optical Properties of Biological Tissues: A Review." *Physics in Medicine & Biology* 58 (11): R37.

Jemal, A., R. Siegel, E. Ward, Y. Hao, J. Xu, and M.J. Thun. 2009. "Cancer Statistics, 2009." *CA: A Cancer Journal for Clinicians* 59 (4): 225–49.

Lakowicz, J.R. 2006. *Principles of Fluorescence Spectroscopy.* New York: Kluwer Academic Publishers.

Mayevsky, A., and B. Chance. 2007. "Oxidation-Reduction States of NADH in Vivo: From Animals to Clinical Use." *Mitochondrion* 7 (5): 330–39.

Medzhitov, R. 2008. "Origin and Physiological Roles of Inflammation." *Nature* 454 (7203): 428–35.

Mizeva, I.A, E.V. Potapova, V.V. Dremin, E.A. Zherebtsov, M.A. Mezentsev, V.V. Shupletsov, and A.V. Dunaev. 2019. "Optical Probe Pressure Effects on Cutaneous Blood Flow." *Clinical Hemorheology and Microcirculation* 72 (3): 259–67.

Mycek, M.A., and B.W. Pogue. 2003. *Handbook of Biomedical Fluorescence.* Boca Raton, FL: Taylor & Francis.

Palmer, S., K. Litvinova, A. Dunaev, J. Yubo, D. McGloin, and G. Nabi. 2017. "Optical Redox Ratio and Endogenous Porphyrins in the Detection of Urinary Bladder Cancer: A Patient Biopsy Analysis." *Journal of Biophotonics* 10 (8): 1062–73.

Palmer, S., K. Litvinova, A. Dunaev, S. Fleming, D. McGloin, and G. Nabi. 2016. "Changes in Autofluorescence Based Organoid Model of Muscle Invasive Urinary Bladder Cancer." *Biomedical Optics Express* 7 (4): 1193–1200.

Palmer, S., K. Litvinova, E. Rafailov, and G. Nabi. 2015. "Detection of Urinary Bladder Cancer Cells Using Redox Ratio and Double Excitation Wavelengths Autofluorescence." *Biomedical Optics Express* 6 (3): 977–86.

Petrov, G.I., A. Doronin, H.T. Whelan, I. Meglinski, and V.V. Yakovlev. 2012. "Human Tissue Color as Viewed in High Dynamic Range Optical Spectral Transmission Measurements." *Biomedical Optics Express* 3 (9): 2154–61.

Popov, A.P., A.V. Bykov, and I.V. Meglinski. 2017. "Influence of Probe Pressure on Diffuse Reflectance Spectra of Human Skin Measured *In Vivo.*" *Journal of Biomedical Optics* 22 (11): 110504.

Potapova, E.V., V.V. Dremin, E.A. Zherebtsov, I.N. Makovik, E.V. Zharkikh, A.V. Dunaev, O.V. Pilipenko, V.V. Sidorov, and A.I. Krupatkin. 2017. "A Complex Approach to Noninvasive Estimation of Microcirculatory Tissue Impairments in Feet of Patients with Diabetes Mellitus Using Spectroscopy." *Optics and Spectroscopy* 123 (6): 955–64.

Potapova, E., V. Dremin, E. Zherebtsov, A. Mamoshin, and A. Dunaev. 2020. "Multimodal optical diagnostic in minimally invasive surgery." in *Multimodal Optical Diagnostics of Cancer*, 397–424. Cham: Springer International Publishing.

Prahl, S.A., M.J.C. van Gemert, and A.J. Welch. 1993. "Determining the Optical Properties of Turbid Media by Using the Adding–Doubling Method." *Applied Optics* 32 (4): 559–68.

Rafailov, I.E., V.V. Dremin, K.S. Litvinova, A.V. Dunaev, S.G. Sokolovski, and E.U. Rafailov. 2016. "Computational Model of Bladder Tissue Based on Its Measured Optical Properties." *Journal of Biomedical Optics* 21 (2): 025006.

Schramm, J.C., T. Dinh, and A. Veves. 2006. "Microvascular Changes in the Diabetic Foot." *The International Journal of Lower Extremity Wounds* 5 (3): 149–59.

Shupletsov, V., K. Kandurova, V. Dremin, E. Potapova, M. Apanaykin, U. Legchenko, and A. Dunaev. 2020. "Fluorescence Imaging System for Biological Tissues Diagnosis: Phantom and Animal Studies." *Journal of Biomedical Photonics & Engineering* 6 (1): 010303.

Shupletsov, V.V, E.A. Zherebtsov, V.V. Dremin, A.P. Popov, A.V. Bykov, E.V. Potapova, A.V. Dunaev, and I.V. Meglinski. 2021. "Polyacrylamide-Based Phantoms of Human Skin for Hyperspectral Fluorescence Imaging and Spectroscopy." *Quantum Electronics* 51 (2): 118–23.

Sievert, K.D., B. Amend, U. Nagele, D. Schilling, J. Bedke, M. Horstmann, J. Hennenlotter, S. Kruck, and A. Stenzl. 2009. "Economic Aspects of Bladder Cancer: What Are the Benefits and Costs?" *World Journal of Urology* 27 (3): 295–300.

Tan, K.C., W.S. Chow, V.H. Ai, C. Metz, R. Bucala, and K.S. Lam. 2002. "Advanced Glycation End Products and Endothelial Dysfunction in Type 2 Diabetes." *Diabetes Care* 25 (6): 1055–59.

Zharkikh, E., V. Dremin, E. Zherebtsov, A. Dunaev, and I. Meglinski. 2020. "Biophotonics Methods for Functional Monitoring of Complications of Diabetes Mellitus." *Journal of Biophotonics* 13 (10): 202000203.

Zherebtsov, E., V. Dremin, A. Popov, A. Doronin, D. Kurakina, M. Kirillin, I. Meglinski, and A. Bykov. 2019. "Hyperspectral Imaging of Human Skin Aided by Artificial Neural Networks." *Biomedical Optics Express* 10 (7): 3545–59.

Zherebtsov, E.A., K.Y. Kandurova, E.S. Seryogina, I.O. Kozlov, V.V. Dremin, A.I. Zherebtsova, A.V. Dunaev, and I. Meglinski. 2017. "The Influence of Local Pressure on Evaluation Parameters of Skin Blood Perfusion and Fluorescence." *Proc. SPIE* 10336: 1033608.

Zherebtsova, A.I., V.V. Dremin, I.N. Makovik, E.A. Zherebtsov, A.V. Dunaev, A. Goltsov, S.G. Sokolovski, and E.U. Rafailov. 2019. "Multimodal Optical Diagnostics of the Microhaemodynamics in Upper and Lower Limbs." *Frontiers in Physiology* 10: 416.

Zherebtsov E., M. Zajnulina, K. Kandurova, E. Potapova, V. Dremin, A. Mamoshin, S. Sokolovski, A. Dunaev, and E. Rafailov. 2020. "Machine learning aided photonic diagnostic system for minimally invasive optically guided surgery in the hepatoduodenal area." *Diagnostics* 10 (11): 873.

Zherebtsov E., E. Potapova, A. Mamoshin, V. Shupletsov, K. Kandurova, V. Dremin, A. Abramov, and A. Dunaev. 2022. "Fluorescence lifetime needle optical biopsy discriminates hepatocellular carcinoma." *Biomedical Optics Express* 13 (2): 633–46.

CHAPTER 2

The Discrete Analysis of the Tissue Biopsy Images with Metamaterial Formalisation

Tatjana Gric

Aston University

CONTENTS

DOI: 10.1201/9781003228950-2

2.1 INTRODUCTION

Cancer is one of the leading causes of death worldwide. In this regard, its early diagnosis is crucial to start therapies [1]. The apoptosis of cancer cells plays a pivotal role in the shaping of organs in tandem with cell proliferation, regulation, and the removal of defective as well as excessive cells in immune system [2–4]. Consequently, it is important to create precise recognition technologies that can confirm if a biological tissue is cancerous. This chapter aims to refine the fundamental ideas used in electrodynamics and some optical problems and apply them for biological systems. We aim to correct a common practice if effective medium models are applied for biological systems.

Accurate prediction of the effective permittivity and permeability is one of the most basic requirements for electromagnetic (EM) composite performance design and EM-scattering characteristics analysis. Ever since J. C. Maxwell first studied the conductivity of composites consisting of conducting particles and non-conducting matrix medium, many formulae had been proposed for predicting the effective permittivity and permeability of composites. The most classic formulae are the Maxwell-Garnett formula and the Bruggeman formula, based on which most of the other formulae were proposed.

However, it is difficult to accurately predict the effective permittivity and permeability of composites in engineering using the existing formulae. One reason is that these formulae are derived under certain assumptions such as low particle concentration; another reason is that some necessary elements that have a significant effect on the calculated results cannot be obtained in engineering such as the permittivity and permeability of particles, particle geometric distribution, morphological distribution, and so on.

Topology is the branch of mathematics dedicated to studying the properties of geometric objects that are unchanged under continuous deformation. Herein, we consider a cancerous biological tissue as an anisotropic composite. Recent advances in 3D-printed metamaterials provide new insight to the challenge. Metamaterials were first introduced as novel EM materials and their characteristic structural length is one or more orders smaller than EM wavelengths. Since then, the concept of metamaterials has been extended to include any materials whose effective properties are delivered by its structure rather than the bulk behaviour of the base materials that compose it. In other words, the geometry, size, orientation, and arrangement of the unit cells of metamaterials grant them the desired properties. In the context of tissue-mimicking phantom, the key value of the "metamaterial" concept is the idea of constructing artificial models of tissue with heterogeneous microstructures that, although difficult to do conventionally, can be easily rendered by 3D printing. With multi-material 3D-printing technologies, the feasibility of designing the mechanical properties of metamaterials has been proven. Similarly, if a micro-structure material is embedded into a soft polymer, the mechanical properties of the combined material should be tunable by adjusting the structural parameters. With this principle, we consider a cancerous biological tissue as an anisotropic composite. It should be mentioned that machine-learning techniques can be widely applied to automate the process of modelling the phantom tissues.

The key feature of a cancer-affected tissue is the presence of the glioma cells in the sample. Current approaches in distinguishing healthy-tumour areas mainly focus on fluorescent, immunological, and morphological differences highlighted by different staining, intrinsic autofluorescence, and decretive microscopy methods rather than the "metamaterial formalism (MMF)" of the diseases. Fluorescence microscopy and immunofluorescence methods are the main approaches that identify and analyse tumour cells by imaging specific markers that depend on the phenotypes of the tumour cells [5]. Nevertheless, the former is quite challenging. Specifically, manual calculations and assessment by qualified specialists are required. This is prone to develop biased criteria and fatigue over time, which may lead to erroneous conclusions based on data. An implemented framework that can handle high data throughput in both the hardware and software is needed for reliable reproducibility and deterministic interpretation. Thus, a drastic minimisation of the human intervention has to be achieved [6]. MMF is an enhanced tool providing a fertile ground for the design of the entirely computerised system. It is worth mentioning that in this case human involvement is not needed. Thus, the biological tissue is treated as a disordered metamaterial model. Moreover, the former approach allows to significantly reduce the possibility of errors that are possible at the tissue-digitising stage. MMF allows to calculate the critical minimum of the glioma cells in the biopsy sample, thus recognising a developing tumour that might help to identify early-stage cancer. It is becoming possible to "see the metamaterial features" in the biological tissue samples with the development of effective medium approximation techniques. The advantage of this approach lies in its ability to define the biological tissue as the meta-material structure.

A large knowledge base has been created thanks to the recent studies of metamaterials [7–9]. Thus, the significance of MMF in dealing with biological challenges [10–12] is clearly observed. Sensing, chemical and biomedical applications are possible thanks to the recent studies on EM radiation in the Terahertz (THz) frequency range. THz metamaterials are composed of periodically arranged sub-wavelength metal structures. It should be stressed that biological tissue can be treated from the perspectives of the disordered metamaterial [13–15] theory in terms of the distribution of the cells composing the structures. Doing so, the MMF is widely applicable to treat the biological processes.

During the past years, the calculation of the effective permittivity of biological tissue non-linear characteristics in frequency domain being a serious challenge received tremendous attention [16,17]. To the best of our knowledge, there is no study that proposes the application of MMF to conclude if a sample is cancerous. This work evaluates the effective per-mittivity of biological tissue giving full credit to MMF. Here we imply a theoretical study of effective permittivity in biomaterials deliberately for mouse models. Recognition of cancerous tissues is possible because of the precise determination of the effective permittivity of the tissue samples.

The rapid development of machine learning and especially deep learn-ing allows for significant improvement of the accuracy of cancer screening [18]. Machine-learning algorithms can assist in analysing large amounts of data and solving complicated problems in a precise and fast way [19,20]. It can extensively assist physicians to improve the accuracy and efficiency in diagnosing cancer, choosing appropriate therapeutic approaches, and pre-dicting long-term outcomes. Artificial intelligence (AI) [21] usually deploys a subset of machine-learning techniques that identify patterns in data and train a machine how to learn [22]. Giving full credit to all the advantages possessed by the developed methodologies, their main drawback should be considered, which is the tremendous amount of computer resources needed to deal with challenges. The application of MMF will allow for a more effi-cient detection and identification of cancerous samples with lesser computer resources due to the applied effective medium approximation techniques.

For the first time to our knowledge, here we manage to formalise the biological tissues as a metamaterial helping in discriminating non- and cancerous areas in the brain tissues. The obtained effective permittiv-ity values were dependent on various factors, including the amount of different cell types in the sample and their distribution. Moreover, the recognition of the cancerous areas will be proposed based on their effective medium properties. MMF can have a dramatic impact on the development of methodological approaches seeking for a precise identification of pathological tissues and would allow for more effective detection of cancer-related changes.

To the best of our knowledge, there is no study applying MMF for recognising cancerous tissues. In the research we will deploy a theoretical analysis of the effective permittivity of materials aiming to explore the acceptability of the models [23] to treat biological tissues by providing a significant enhancement at the tissue digitisation stage.

2.2 THEORETICAL BACKGROUND

Effective medium theories are a perfect tool aiming to define an effective dielectric function for a composite material taking into account the dielectric function of its components and their geometrical distribution [24–27]. Let us now assume that inclusions are embedded into the host medium. Moreover, the implants are made of different materials with permittivities ε_n ($n = 1, 2, ..., N$). Then Maxwell-Garnett equation is generalised as

$$\frac{\varepsilon_{MG} - \varepsilon_h}{\varepsilon_{MG} + 2\varepsilon_h} = \sum_{n=1}^{N} f_n \frac{\varepsilon_n - \varepsilon_h}{\varepsilon_n + 2\varepsilon_h}, \tag{2.1}$$

where f_n is the volume fraction of the n-th component.

The random sequential addition (RSA) method can be used to generate the random point distribution for low-filling fractions. In the frame of this methodology, random particle positions are generated sequentially. Moreover, new random particle (satisfying uniform distribution) is accepted if it is not overlapping with existing particles. As this acceptance and rejection process continues, it will become more time consuming to find a new region to place a new particle. In this relation, there is a saturation limit (for equal-sized circular particle, 55% filling fraction) above which no further addition is possible. For higher filling fractions, random particle distributions can be generated using the molecular dynamic hard sphere packing method. As the filling fraction goes higher, it imposes more constraints on the particle distribution pattern, and the composite becomes wavy crystalline and then crystalline from disordered; thus in this study, the highest filling fraction for random composites is 80%.

$$\frac{\varepsilon_{MG} - \varepsilon_h}{\varepsilon_{MG} + 2\varepsilon_h} = f_1 \frac{\varepsilon_1 - \varepsilon_h}{\varepsilon_1 + 2\varepsilon_h} + f_2 \frac{\varepsilon_2 - \varepsilon_h}{\varepsilon_2 + 2\varepsilon_h} + f_3 \frac{\varepsilon_3 - \varepsilon_h}{\varepsilon_3 + 2(1)\varepsilon_h} \qquad (2.2)$$

One may derive from Eq. (2.2), that

$$\varepsilon_{MG} = -\frac{\varepsilon_h + \varepsilon_h(C + B + A)2}{C + B + A - 1}, \qquad (2.3)$$

where $A = \dfrac{f_3(\varepsilon_3 - \varepsilon_h)}{\varepsilon_3 + 2\varepsilon_h}$, $B = \dfrac{f_2(\varepsilon_2 - \varepsilon_h)}{\varepsilon_2 + 2\varepsilon_h}$, $C = \dfrac{f_1(\varepsilon_1 - \varepsilon_h)}{\varepsilon_1 + 2\varepsilon_h}$.

The spectrum of a tissue may be more appropriately described in terms of multiple Cole–Cole dispersion (Table 2.1)

$$\hat{\varepsilon}_h(\omega) = \varepsilon_\infty + \sum_n \frac{\Delta\varepsilon_n}{1 + (j\omega\tau_n)^{(1-\alpha_n)}} + \frac{\sigma_i}{j\omega\varepsilon_0} \qquad (2.4)$$

2.3 MODELLING OF THE PHANTOM TISSUE

The phantom tissue models are created based on the MMF approach. It is assumed that brain (grey matter) forms the host medium and cancerous cells are implanted in it. Following the former approach one may construct an anisotropic metamaterial (Figure 2.1) with the grey matter of the brain being the host material and the nanocylinders embedded in it possessing permittivity of the cancerous cells. Based on the presented approach, the obtained metamaterial media represents the disordered structure with the effective permittivity calculated by Eq. (2.3). It is assumed that the permittivity of the host medium is predicted by means of the Cole–Cole model (Eq. 2.4). Figure 2.2 demonstrates permittivity of the grey and white matter of the brain calculated by means of the Cole–Cole model (Eq. 2.4) along with the effective permittivity of the cancerous affected tissue. It was assumed that the biological tissue is highly affected by the cancerous cells. Herein, we will deal with the example of the glioblastoma cells embedded into the sample. Doing so, the filling ratio of the cancerous cells is $f_g = 0.95$.

TABLE 2.1   Parameters of Equation Used to Predict the Dielectric Properties of Tissues [28]

Tissue Type	ε_∞	$\Delta\varepsilon_1$	τ_1(ps)	α_1	$\Delta\varepsilon_2$	τ_2(ps)	α_2	$\Delta\varepsilon_3$	τ_3(ps)	α_3	$\Delta\varepsilon_4$	τ_4(ps)	α_4	σ
Brain (grey matter)	4	45	7.96	0.1	400	15.92	0.15	2×10^5	106.1	0.22	4.5×10^7	5.305	0	0.02
Brain (white matter)	4	32	7.96	0.1	100	7.96	0.1	4×10^4	53.05	0.3	3.5×10^7	7.958	0.02	0.02

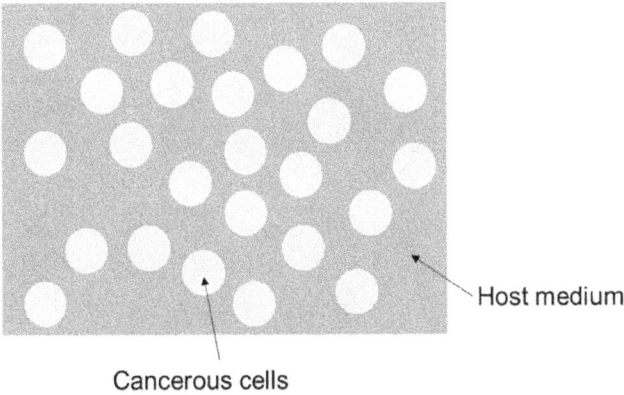

FIGURE 2.1   Biological tissue with the embedded cancerous cells.

It can be observed in Figure 2.2 that the effective permittivity of the cancerous media is larger than the values obtained for the healthy tissue case.

It is of particular interest to examine the effect of the amount of the cancerous cells on the material properties. Thus, Figure 2.3 depicts dependencies of the effective permittivities upon frequency for different filling ratios.

As it can be observed in Figure 2.3, presence of the cancerous cells in the sample makes a dramatic impact on the effective permittivity value. A significant increase in the permittivity is observed by the increasing amount of cancerous cells in the sample. The obtained results are in good agreement with those obtained in [28] for the cancerous tissue case. In this relation, one may conclude that presented metamaterial-based formalism approach stands for as a good tool to create the phantom tissue models needed for clinical practice. By comparing the results presented in Figure 2.2a and b, one may conclude that the presence of the cancerous cells is making a more dramatic impact in case of the white matter rather than the grey one. Figure 2.4 shows the effective dielectric function of a composite under consideration computed by means of Cole–Cole dispersion (Eq. 2.4). It is worth mentioning that effective permittivity value increases with the increase in the amount of the cancerous cells in the sample. Figure 2.4 clearly demonstrates that the value of the effective permittivity in case of the white matter is smaller in comparison with the grey matter.

2.4 MMF APPROACH

The structure of the fully automated MMF approach is in the form of several steps, i.e. digitisation of the biopsy image, digitised image analysis, and modelling of the disordered metamaterial (Figure 2.5). For understanding

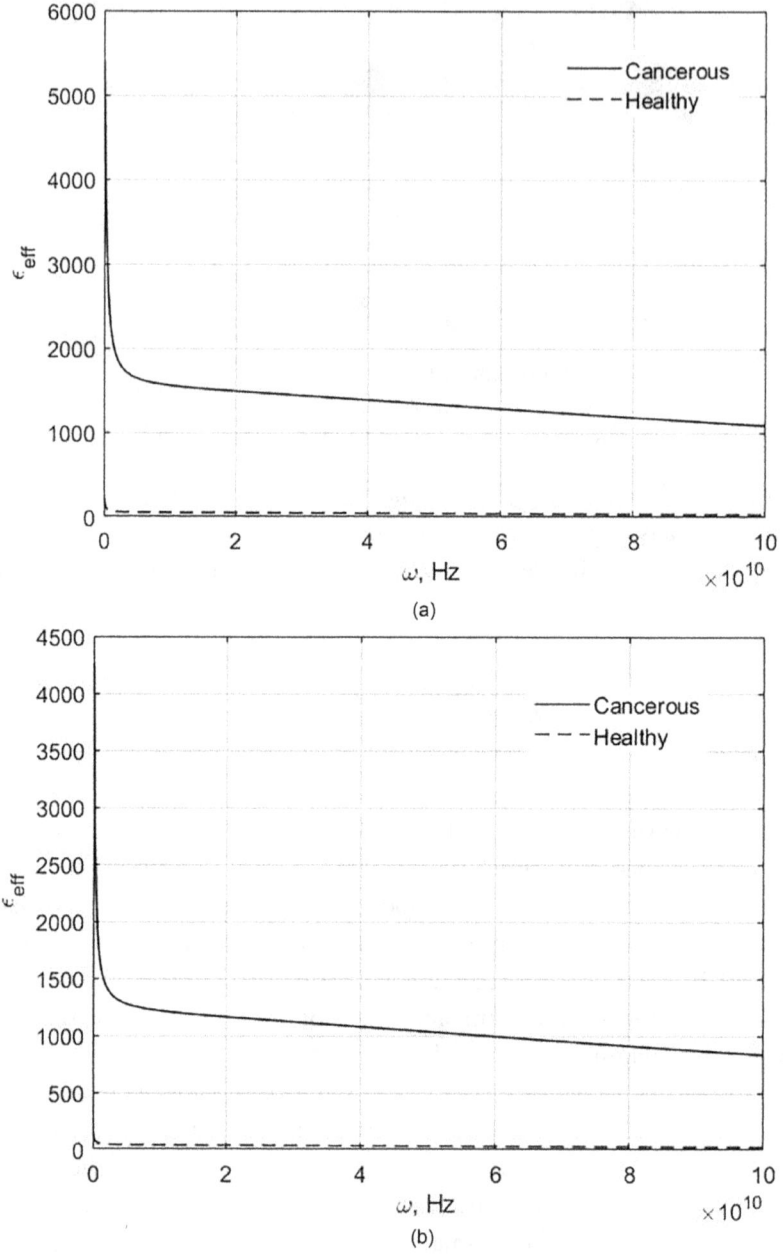

FIGURE 2.2   Dependence of the effective permittivity versus frequency. $f_g=0.95$ (a) grey matter; (b) white matter.

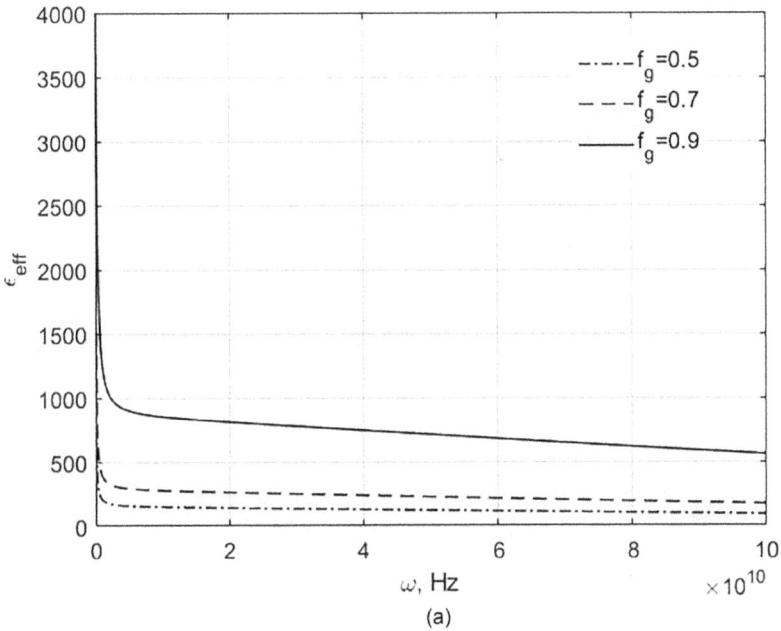

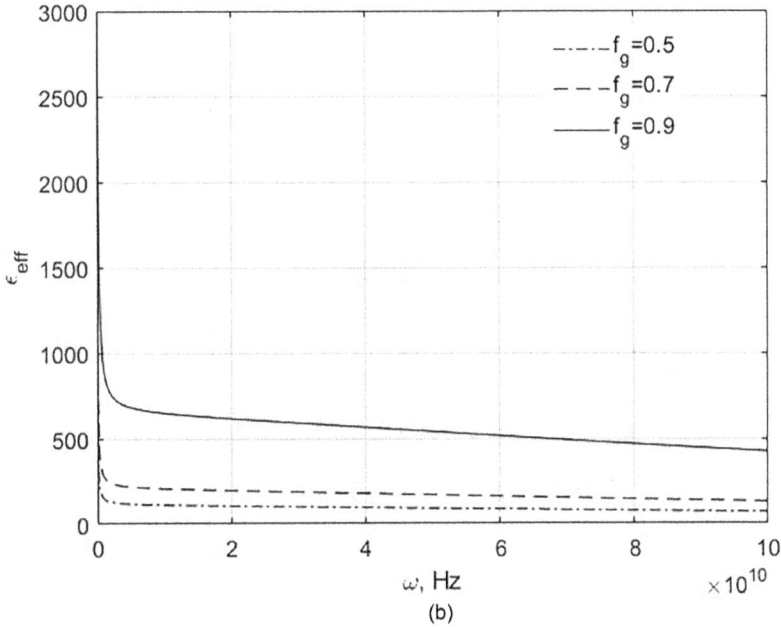

FIGURE 2.3 Dependence of the effective permittivity versus frequency for different filling factors of the cancerous cells. (a) grey matter; (b) white matter.

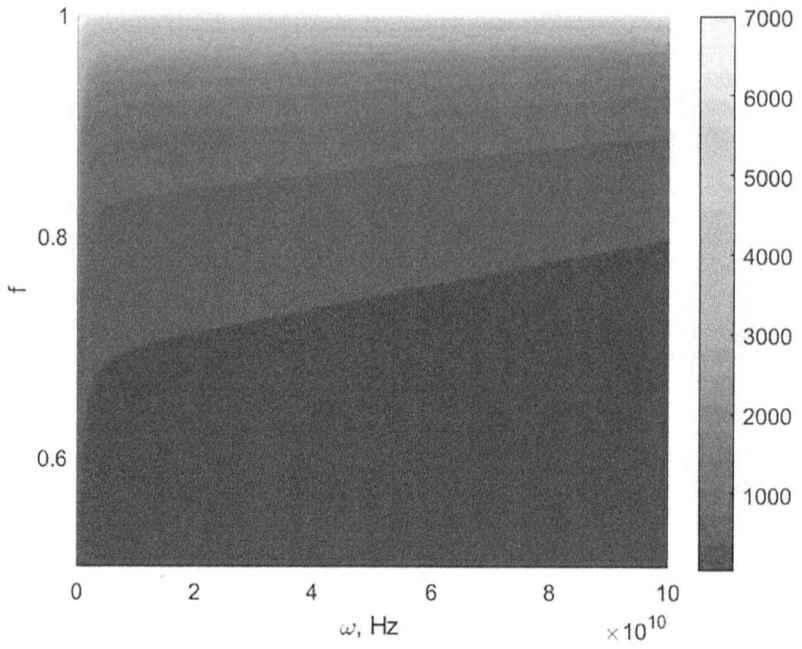

(a)

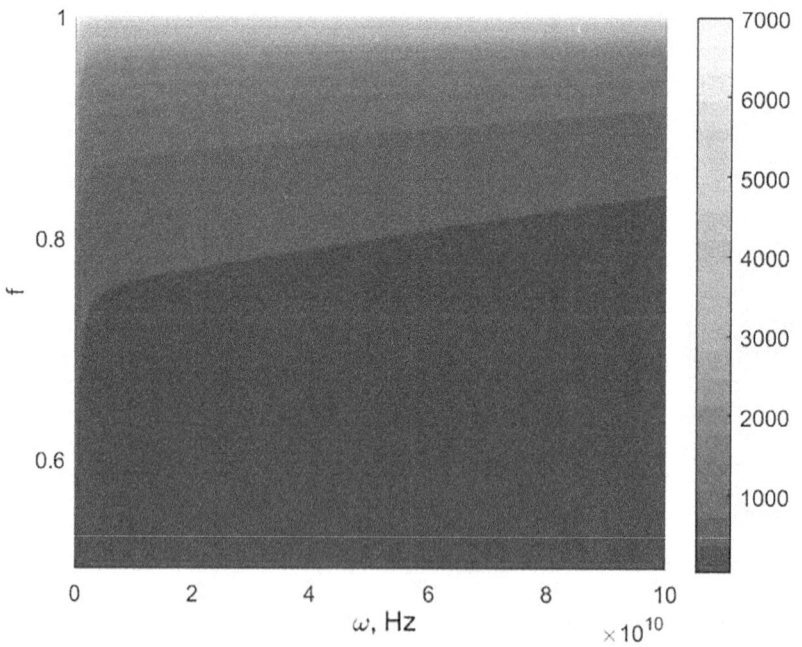

(b)

FIGURE 2.4 Dependence of the effective permittivity versus frequency and filling factor of the cancerous cells. (a) grey matter; (b) white matter.

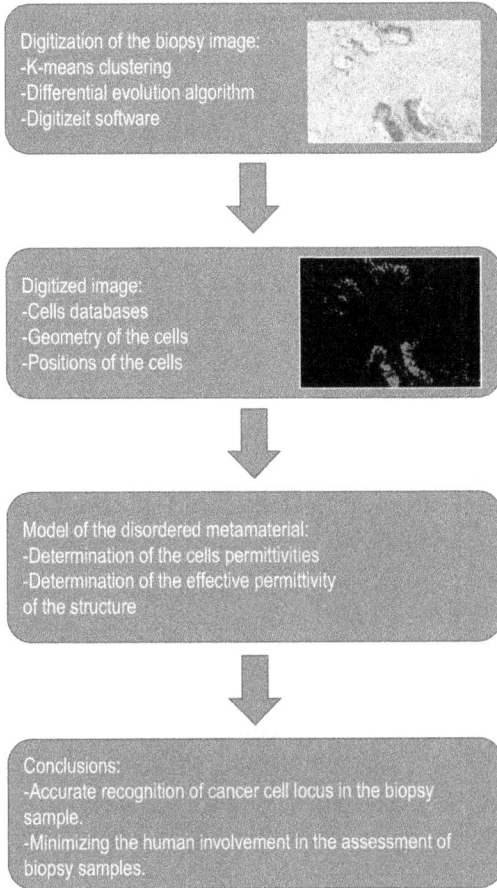

FIGURE 2.5   A scheme of the metamaterial-based algorithm approach in distinguishing precise location of the tumour locus.

whether the examined biological sample is non-cancerous, it is required to analyse it in terms of the effective medium approximation [29]. The applicability of the MMF becomes feasible when the distribution of the cells is clearly identified in the sample under investigation. Consequently, we will apply image digitiser techniques to identify all the morphological and functional cell types and their exact positions. Thus, the coordinates of the mouse brain biological tissue cells will be clearly depicted in samples. It is of particular importance to have a deep insight into the filling ratio of each type of the cells identified in the histograms that treat the obtained biological tissue image from the perspective of MMF. Furthermore, the optical properties of the cells should be described by Debye and Cole–Cole models [30].

Thus, the complex dielectric spectrum of all cell types is provided in $\varepsilon(\omega)$ space. A schematic illustration of the MMF-based approach is presented in Figure 2.5. The biopsy image is to be digitised at the initial stage of the data processing. It might be performed by choosing one of three approaches: i. e. K-means clustering, differential evolution algorithm, or Digitizeit software. At the next algorithmic step the obtained information is analysed in creating defined cell databases. Moreover, further proceeding with the application of the disordered metamaterial model, cell distribution within biopsy images should be accurately positioned. Particularly, we are interested in assessing the cell geometry, their shapes and sizes and cell location coordinates in the sample. These parameters used in full can finally create the disordered metamaterial model. Aiming to proceed further with the accomplished model, cell permittivities are identified seeking for a homogenisation of the structure in use by means of the effective medium approximation. All the presented steps might be fully automated by employing the AI approach.

2.4.1 Digitizeit Software

For identifying the position of cells comprising the tissue sample, segmentation algorithms are needed to locate the anticipated region boundaries and label all cells within a single continuous boundary as belonging to one region. Datasets of the cell types are designed based on the geometry, colour and size of the cells. Doing so, various measurements can be made using established methods [31]. One may take an advantage from this approach because of the reduced analysis time [32]. We apply https://www.digitizeit.de/ software to recognise the cell sets forming the considered tissue. Doing so, one may benefit from the faster operation time in comparison with OpenCV [33] for C# in Microsoft Visual Studio. On the contrary, the identification algorithm based on Otsu thresholding will require significant computer resources. The former is known as a threshold algorithm for image segmentation [34]. To conclude, our applied technique has a faster run time and requires less computer resources than cancer cell detection methods implemented with OpenCV [33] for C# in Microsoft Visual Studio. It is a perfect tool to obtain a digitised view of the biopsy sample under consideration, which will be treated as a disordered metamaterial media at the later stages of consideration. It is worth noting that fluorescence microscopy and immunofluorescence methods are used as the conventional techniques for tumour cell detection and assessment. Aiming to fulfil these procedures, imaging of specific markers that are dramatically affected by the phenotypes of the tumour cells is needed

[5]. Nevertheless, application of such approaches is quite challenging and complicated. Seeking for the reliable reproducibility and deterministic interpretation of a framework that can handle high data throughput in both, the hardware and software is of particular importance. Thus, human intervention can be significantly reduced [6].

2.4.2 Calculation of the Effective Permittivity of the Disordered Metamaterial Model

The MMF is a perfect tool to create an entirely computerised system. It is worth mentioning that in this case human involvement is not needed. The techniques created allow to calculate the critical limit of the glioma cells which allow to delimitate the tumour boundaries that in turn give opportunity to identify cancer at the early stages [23]. To confirm whether the biological tissue is non-cancerous, biopsy sample image is to be analysed using effective medium approximation [29]. One may apply the MMF method if the distribution of cells in the considered medium is clearly identified in terms of the distribution of the cells in the sample. Doing so, image digitiser techniques are applied to have a deep insight into the exact coordinates of the cell sets combining the sample. It should be mentioned that the coordinates of the glioma, glia and neuronal cells were clearly demonstrated in [23]. Aiming to apply the MMF approach, the optical properties of the cells should be characterised by Debye and Cole–Cole models [30]. In this relation, the complex dielectric spectrum for all cell types is shown in $\varepsilon(\omega)$ space.

To have a deep insight into the nature of the biopsy sample under investigation, creation of the permittivity model for brain tissue biopsies is of particular importance. A typical theory attained on the basis of empirical formula [30] is the Debye model. Other widely applied permittivity models based on binary mixtures do not account for the frequency domain, for instance, the Bottcher–Bordewijk model [35], Maxwell-Garnett formula [36], Bruggeman formula [37] and Hanai formula [38]. It should be mentioned that the Bottcher–Bordewijk model allows for a feasible prediction of the permittivity of the medium [35], i. e. effective permittivity of the biological tissue sample. The model is described as follows:

$$\frac{3\varepsilon_1}{2\varepsilon_{eff} + \varepsilon_1} f_1 + \frac{3\varepsilon_2}{2\varepsilon_{eff} + \varepsilon_2} f_2 = 1 \tag{2.5}$$

In this case cell structure is of a random nature possessing some predictable average properties such as cell size and cell distribution density. It can be modelled by an aggregation of randomly distributed spherical shells. This model can be applied to describe the two constituent materials. Another famous model put forward by Skipetrov [39] can be applied to the two-phase system. The former is found by solving Eq. (2.5) with respect to ε_{eff}, i.e.

$$\varepsilon_{eff} = \frac{3\varepsilon_1 f_1}{4} - \frac{\varepsilon_2}{4} - \frac{\varepsilon_1}{4} + \frac{3\varepsilon_2 f_2}{4} - A, \qquad (2.6)$$

Here $\quad A = \dfrac{\sqrt{9\varepsilon_1^2 f_1^2 - 6\varepsilon_1^2 f_1 + \varepsilon_1^2 + 18\varepsilon_1\varepsilon_2 f_1 f_2 + 6\varepsilon_1\varepsilon_2 f_1 + 6\varepsilon_1\varepsilon_2 f_2 - 2\varepsilon_1\varepsilon_2 +}}{4}$

$A = \dfrac{\sqrt{9\varepsilon_2^2 f_2^2 - 6\varepsilon_2^2 f_2 + \varepsilon_2^2}}{4}$, ε_1 denotes the permittivity of the neuron cells, ε_2

of the glioma cells, and f_1 and f_2 are the volume fractions of each cell type accordingly. Furthermore, ε_{eff} is the effective permittivity characterising effective properties of the medium. The dielectric properties $\varepsilon_k(\omega)$, $k = 1, 2$, are obtained by means of the Cole–Cole spectral function [40].

$$\varepsilon_k = \varepsilon_k(\infty) + \frac{\varepsilon_k(0) - \varepsilon_k(\infty)}{1 + (i\omega\tau_k)^{1-\alpha_k}} + \frac{\sigma_k}{i\varepsilon_0\omega} \qquad (2.7)$$

where $\varepsilon_k(0)$ – static dielectric permittivity, $\varepsilon_k(\infty)$ – high-frequency dielectric permittivity, τ_k – relaxation time, α_k – distribution parameter and σ_k – DC conductivity. On the basis of the described methodology, the dependencies of the effective permittivity upon frequency for different cases (differences in the volume fraction f, permittivities of the building blocks (cells)) have been attained. It should be mentioned that the effective permittivity was obtained theoretically by means of the Skipetrov model (Eq. 2.6). The spatially dependent volume fraction has been extracted from the digitised images and included into the effective medium model (Eq. 2.6). The former assumes the prior knowledge of the frequency-dependent permittivity of the building block (cells) characterised by (Eq. 2.7). An outstanding feature of the described model is the possibility of the extraordinary nature of the effective permittivity. This is illustrated by the peak of the effective permittivity curve in a certain case at the frequency range (0–10 THz) [23] if the total amount of the glioma cells in the sample exceeds 5%.

As it was discovered in [23] (Figure 2.6), effective permittivity values are negative. The former takes place due to the characterisation of the cells by means of the Cole–Cole spectral function (Eq. 2.7). It should be

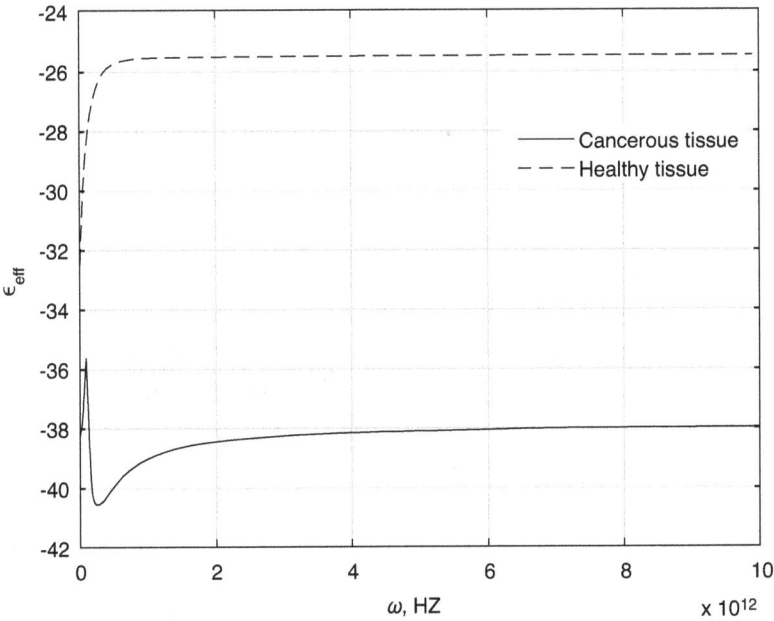

FIGURE 2.6 Example of the dependence of the effective permittivity upon frequency for the case of mouse brain cancer and healthy tissue [23].

mentioned that the biological sample described by the metamaterial [23] experiences extraordinary behaviour. This is due to certain amount of glioma cells exceeding a certain limit, i.e. 5%. It is worth mentioning that the minimum detectable tumour area is 0.3 μm². It can be concluded that the tissue is cancerous because of the extraordinary behaviour of the effective permittivity curve. It is clearly observed that there is a certain peak at the frequency around 0.1 THz. Consequently, the extraordinary behaviour occurs when the amount of unhealthy specimen(s) in the sample exceeds a certain limit. Based on the obtained results, a high amplitude peak is found in the case of 154 M [23] sample. This serves as the evidence for the presence of highly cancerous tissue zones [23] in the sample. A higher amplitude of ε_{eff} corresponds to later-stage cancer. Here, stage refers to the extent of cancer and is based on factors such as dimensions of the tumour and possibility for it to spread. In order to approbate created algorithm, randomly chosen tissue samples (25 instances) were considered. The described metamaterial approach allows for a precise recognition of the healthy and cancerous tissues. The obtained results have been approved by histological analysis with 100% success rate [23].

2.5 INVESTIGATION OF THE MOUSE BRAIN TISSUE SAMPLES BY MEANS OF MMF APPROACH

Mouse brain tissue samples presented in Figure 2.7 were used for investigations to find out if the tissue is healthy. It is worth noting that 100 samples were considered. Herein, we present only four of them. Histological sections were stained with standard haematoxylin and eosin dyes [41].

A popular method for measuring image features is the use of algorithms that automatically partition an image into a set of regions of interest. This process is commonly called Segmentation [42]. To identify the location of different types of the cells composing the tissue sample, segmentation algorithms can be designed to locate the anticipated region boundaries and label all cells within a single continuous boundary as belonging to one region. Datasets of the cell types are created by taking into account geometrical shape, colour and size of the cells. From this segmentation, various measurements can be made using established methods [31]. A key benefit of this approach is in analysis time [32], which is much faster. Measurement by a predetermined software algorithm also allows the results to be repeated without any inter-operator variation. We apply https://www.digitizeit.de/ software to distinguish all the cell types comprising the tissue under the consideration. The samples are saved by firstly providing examples of each cell type. Once the examples are provided, the software searches for identical cells in the selected area of the tissue sample. It is worth noting that the geometrical size of the glioma cells is larger in comparison with other types. In other words, it is larger than 50 conventional units. On the contrary, glia cells are small; the most prominent feature of the neuron cells in the images is the blurred colour. In other words, we implemented automated cell recognition and counting routine using *Digitizeit*, which is capable of distinguishing glioma cells from a background by training a software to recognise it. Human contribution is needed at early stages of the cell database creation. The main advantage of this approach is the faster operation time in comparison with OpenCV [33] for C# in Microsoft Visual Studio. The recognition algorithm based on Otsu thresholding, which is a threshold algorithm for picture segmentation that automatically selects the optimum value to separate two classes in a grey-level image [34], and colour detection from processed images for the cell size and position will require significant computer resources. It should be noted that outputs are presented by the sets of x and y coordinates. In other words, finally we get the sets of the coordinates and each set corresponds to each cell group. The results were exported as .csv files.

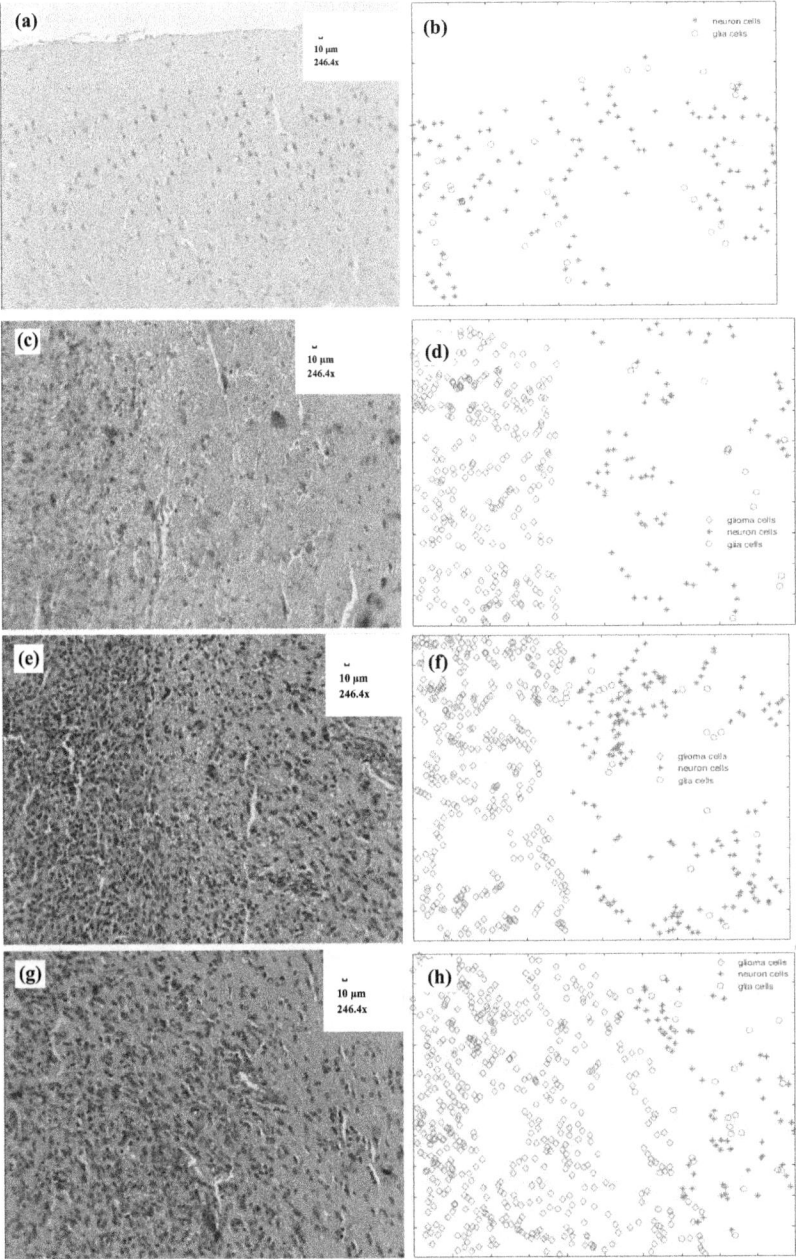

FIGURE 2.7   Images of cancerous and non-cancerous mice brain biopsies (a, b – 39M; c, d – 138M; e, f – 153M; g, h – 154M). Glioma cells are marked with hexagons, neuron cells with asterisks and glia cells with circles. Tissue biopsies are presented in a, c, e, and g figures, digitised images made with "Digitizeit" software (www.digitizeit.de/) in b, d, f, and h.

A Matlab.m file is used to read the .csv file and to extract the information. The described technique allows us to plot datasets by using information about the coordinates. Moreover, the obtained data fully allows the application of MMF. The chosen approach has a faster run time and requires less computer resources than cancer cell recognition techniques performed with OpenCV [33] for C# in Microsoft Visual Studio. Fluorescence microscopy and immunofluorescence techniques are employed as the typical methods for tumour cell identification and analysis by imaging specific markers that depend on the phenotypes of the tumour cells [5]. However, application of such approaches is quite challenging and complicated as it requires manual counting and analysis by trained technicians. It is prone to develop biased criteria and fatigue over time, which can lead to mistaken conclusions based on data. To achieve reliable reproducibility and deterministic interpretation, one needs to implement a framework that can handle high data throughput in both the hardware and software. Doing so, human intervention can be drastically minimised [6]. MMF is a perfect tool for the creation of a fully automated system without the need for human intervention. Moreover, it prevents the errors that might occur at the tissue-digitising stage. It is worth mentioning that the created techniques allow for calculating the critical limit of the glioma cells thus allowing to control tumour development and even to prevent cancer at the early stages. Although this limit has attracted particular research interest, the majority of past studies could only probe this limit by applying biological tissue digitisation techniques. The iterative aspect of machine learning is important. They are capable of learning from previous computations to produce reliable, repeatable results, and based on them trustful conclusions in diagnostics minimising the human subjectivism can be arrived at.

To figure out whether a biological tissue is healthy, one needs to analyse it from the perspective of the effective medium approximation [29]. The application of the mentioned formalism is possible in case the geometry of the considered medium is clearly identified. Thus, we have applied image digitiser techniques aiming to identify the exact positions of all the cell types that the tissue consists of. Doing so, the coordinates of the glioma, glia and neuron cells were clearly depicted in samples presented in Figure 2.7a, c, e, g. It is of particular interest to examine the filling ratio of each type of the cells identified in the histograms. Moreover, the optical properties of each type of the cells should be described by applying Debye and Cole–Cole models [29]. Doing so, the complex dielectric spectrum for all cell types is provided in $\varepsilon(\omega)$ space.

The cell shape and shape of the intracellular structures are evaluated using effective medium approximation. Establishment of the tissue permittivity model for brain tissue biopsies would help us to simplify its complex structure. A typical theory is the Debye model. It is very famous and explains many compositions well. Moreover, it was obtained on the basis of empirical formula [35]. It is a widely used model for studying the dielectric properties of biological tissues in frequency domain. The model of binary mixtures is usually used for investigating effective permittivity of a mixture system because of its significance in understanding the intermolecular interactions. There are many well-known permittivity models based on binary mixtures. However, they do not account for the frequency domain, for instance, the Bottcher–Bordewijk model [35], Maxwell-Garnett formula [36], Bruggeman formula [37] and Hanai formula [38]. Each theory can only be successfully applied to a certain type of composition. It is worth noting that the Bottcher–Bordewijk model allows for a feasible prediction of the permittivity of a mixture [35], i.e. effective permittivity of the biological tissue sample.

Doing so, the dependences of the effective permittivity upon frequency for different cases (differences in the volume fraction f, permittivities of the building blocks (cells)) have been obtained. The crucial result is the ability of the effective permittivity to behave in an extraordinary way characterised by the peak of effective permittivity curve in a certain case at the frequency range (0–10 THz) (Figure 2.8) if the total amount of the glioma cells in the sample is greater than 5%. It is worth noting that one may experimentally determine the complex permittivity of material using a split ring resonator (SRR) metamaterial structure. A single SRR unit fabricated on a substrate arranged between transmitting and receiving probes acts as a test probe.

As shown in Figure 2.8a, effective permittivity values are negative. The tissue sample (with high likeness to the metamaterial) under consideration is not experiencing extraordinary behaviour. The former feature represents the description of a healthy tissue sample. It is worth noting that the biological tissue represented by the metamaterial (Figure 2.8b, 153 M) experiences extraordinary behaviour due to certain amount of glioma cells in the sample being greater than a certain limit, i.e. 5%. We may conclude that the tissue is unhealthy due to the extraordinary behaviour of the effective permittivity curves, i. e. there is a certain peak at the frequency around 0.1 THz. Therefore, extraordinary behaviour appears when presence of the unhealthy specimen(s) in the sample is greater than a certain limit. A high amplitude peak is observed in the case of the 154 M sample. This feature

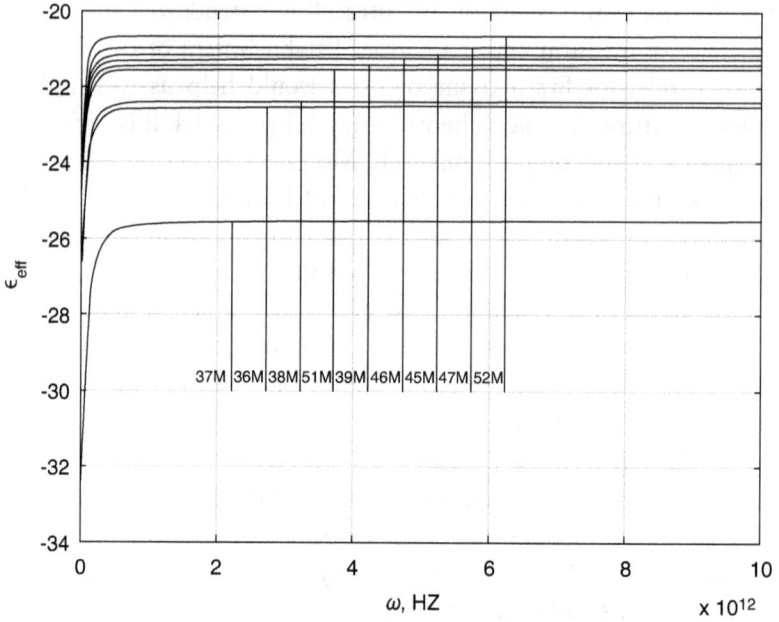

(a)

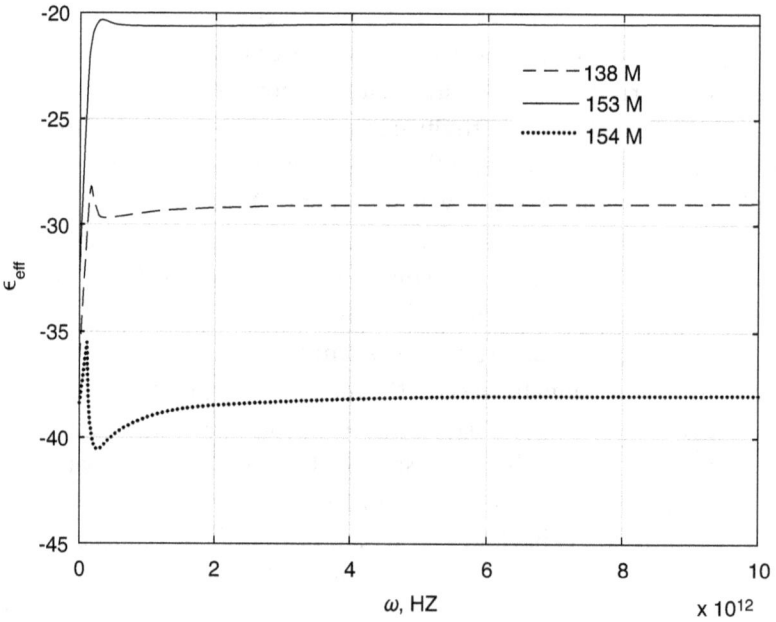

(b)

FIGURE 2.8   Dependencies of the effective permittivities upon frequency for healthy (a) and unhealthy (b) samples.

evidences the presence of highly cancerous tissue zones. To conclude, one may figure out the stage of cancer by data depicted in Figure 2.8b. A higher amplitude of ε_{eff} corresponds to late-stage cancer. Here, stage refers to the extent of cancer and is based on factors such as how large the tumour is and if it has spread. Once the stage of cancer is known, it is possible to suggest the treatment and to make the prognosis.

Going further with what was described above as the extraordinary regime shift it becomes possible to evaluate pathological, healthy and intermediate "blocks" in the brain tissue biopsies (Figure 2.9). Using this nomenclature 138M, 153M, 154M sample images were represented as the blocks of different colour (Figure 2.9b, d, f, h). It is worth noting that metamaterial experiences extraordinary behaviour for the intermediate case, and for the highly affected zones effective permittivity ε_{eff} is negatively characterised in a strong way by the jumps at the 0.1 THz frequencies.

2.6 INVESTIGATION OF THE LIVER SAMPLES BY MEANS OF MMF APPROACH

2.6.1 Dataset Composition

The study was carried out in accordance with the 2013 Declaration of Helsinki by the World Medical Association. Patients scheduled for a regular needle biopsy for a suspected liver malignancy were recruited for study participation. The lesions had to be safely accessible. Patients at increased risk of bleeding were excluded. After receiving the description of the protocol, the patients signed informed consent indicating their voluntary willingness to participate in the study. The experiments were conducted under established protocols. The measurements were performed during standard needle biopsy procedure in 15 patients (six male, nine female) with supposed liver cancer, and the median age was 66 years (range from 45 to 78 years).

The procedure was carried after proper skin disinfection and injection of a local anaesthetic (2% lidocaine hydrochloride solution). At each selected site, the surgeon inserted a 17.5G needle 1.3 mm into the liver tissue. We followed the standard procedure of biopsy sampling and histological examination. The tumour tissue samples were fixed with 10% neutral-buffered formalin, dehydrated, and embedded in paraffin. Approximately 5-μm-thick sections were stained by haematoxylin and eosin method according to standard procedures. The histological specimen was examined using a Leica DM2000 microscope at a magnification of ×100, ×200, and ×400. The resulting tissue slices were examined by light

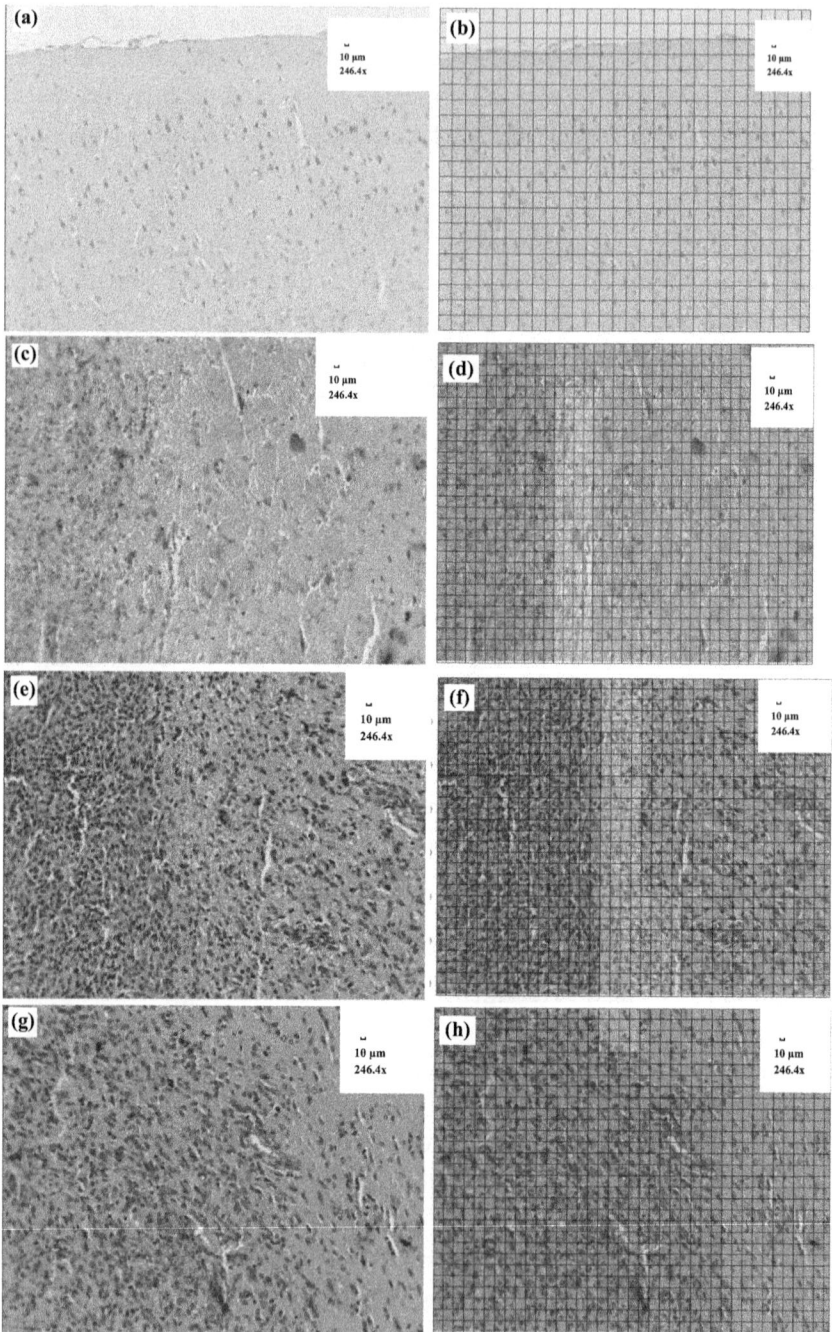

FIGURE 2.9   Images of cancerous and non-cancerous mice brain tissue biopsies
(a, b – 39M; c, d – 138M; e, f – 153M; g, h – 154M). Division of the tissue samples
by the building blocks of different conditions is demonstrated. Tissue photos are
presented in a, c, e, and g figures, and analysed images are shown in b, d, f, and h.

microscopy by an experienced pathologist. Digital images of various fields of view were obtained using a Leica DFC295 camera, four micrographs at each magnification.

2.6.2 K-Means Clustering

K-means is an extensively applied clustering approach to partition data into k clusters [43,44]. Clustering is an approach which is based on collecting two types of data points, with analogous feature vectors into a single cluster and with different feature vectors into other clusters. Basically, feature space selection is a key point in K-means clustering segmentation. An RGB colour map comprises R, G, and B values for each item. The RGB colour space is further converted to a CIELab colour model (L*a*b*) [45] aiming to extract significant features aiming to benefit from the clustering approach. The L*a*b* space involves a luminosity layer L*, a chromaticity-layer a*, which indicates where colour falls along the red–green axis, and chromaticity-layer b*, which indicates where the colour falls along the blue–yellow axis. Both the a* and b* layers comprise all mandatory colour information. This way allows to classify the colours in the a*b* space by means of K-means clustering. When the clustering process is fulfilled, the cluster comprising an area of interest is designated as the primary segment. To remove the pixels which are not related to the selected cluster, histogram clustering may be applied by luminosity feature L* to derive the final segmented result.

2.6.3 Differential Evolution Algorithm

The automatic detection of cancer cells is still an unresolved problem in medical imaging. The examination of the obtained images has stimulated an unprecedented interest for researchers from the areas of medicine and computer vision. It is worth noting that cancer cells can be approximated by an ellipsoid form. Doing so, one may successfully apply an ellipse detector algorithm to identify such elements. We have applied the automatic recognition of the cancerous cells implanted into complex and cluttered smear images. Thus, the complete process is treated as a multi-ellipse detection task. The detection task is transformed into an optimisation issue that represents candidate ellipses. The former procedures are dictated by the approach, which is based on the DE algorithm. An objective function allows to evaluate if such candidate ellipses are present in the edge map of smear image. Guided by the values of such function, a set of encoded candidate ellipses (individuals) are evolved using the DE algorithm so that they can fit into the WBC which are enclosed within the edge map of the smear image.

2.7 CNN-BASED ANALYSIS OF LIVER BIOPSY IMAGES AFTER APPLICATION OF MMF

The digitised images of the mouse liver biopsies are shown in Figure 2.10. The staining procedure for histological preparations was carried out under standard conditions. The sections were of the same thickness, certified dyes were used, and the same staining time and temperature were applied. The internal quality control process was handled by the histologist and pathologist independently. Some visual discrepancy in colour is due to different increases in preparations. Figure 2.10a shows the liver tissue. The degree of staining of the cytoplasm here is somewhat different from Figure 2.10d, but fully corresponds to the picture that the researcher sees in the microscope, which is important. Figure 2.10d shows more eosinophilic staining in areas of connective tissue (between tumour cells), whereas there are no such areas in Figure 2.10a.

All the types of the cells have been recognised by K-means clustering approach. The segmentation aims to classify the cells into different groups. By calculating effective permittivity plots after careful investigation of the

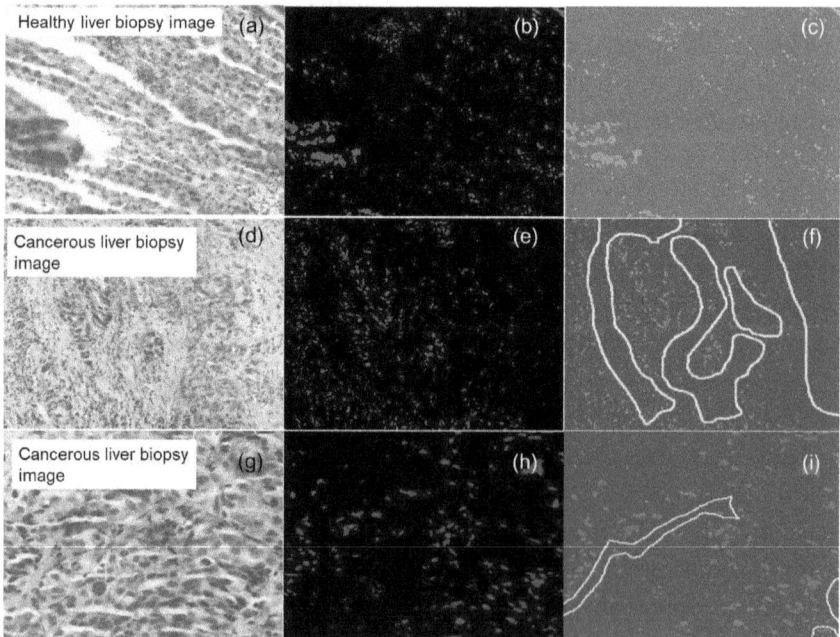

FIGURE 2.10   Representative images of liver biopsy samples: a, d, g – original images of Haematoxylin- and Eosin-stained biopsies; b, e, h – images obtained by K-means clustering approach; c, f, i – images with the highlighted cancerous/non-cancerous areas (lines depict cancerous regions detected by MMF).

cell permittivities (Eq. 2.3), MMF approach [23] allows to detect cancerous locus within the biopsy images.

In the proposed K-means clustering method, a liver biopsy image consists of regions that represent cancer cells, the background and the connective tissue. In these data sources, visual judgements suggest three primary clusters, when $k = 3$. Figure 2.10b–h shows the image labelled by cluster index from the K-means process for different kinds of feature vectors. Using index labels, we can separate objects in the liver image by three colours: white, blue, and pink. The final segmentation results generated by histogram clustering are shown in Figure 2.10b–h.

As can be observed in Figure 2.10f, i, the applied metamaterial approach allows to perform a precise segmentation and classification of the cells composing the biopsy. Doing so, the errors occurred at the image digitisation stage fulfilled by applying the K-means clustering approach can be easily detected by the MMF. The healthy areas in Figure 2.10f, i are marked by the areas created by the lines.

2.8 CONCLUSIONS

It was concluded that cancerous tissues can be treated from the perspectives of the highly disordered metamaterial medium. In this relation, effective permittivity of the biological tissue under consideration can be considered. It has been shown that a cancerous composite with effective dielectric function described in the framework of classical effective medium theories provides larger values of the effective permittivity in comparison to the calculated properties of the healthy, undamaged medium case. The presented approach may serve as a perfect tool to create phantom tissue models for the clinical applications. Here we used the MMF approach for automated and comprehensive cancer cell detection in biopsy images with high proximity to be used further for clinical diagnostics. This advanced approach allows to simplify the image digitisation procedures since there is no need for the precise recognition of the cancerous cells at early stages of the data analysis. Then cancer cell recognition itself is performed by estimation of the cells permittivity with consequently applied effective medium approximation which considers properties of the whole image as a disordered metamaterial model. The main advantage of the proposed technique is its capability to detect the scale of the tumour development giving a powerful diagnostic tool to clinicians for fighting cancer. The described formalism can identify tumour locus, helping in decision making on cancer propagation level in the sample.

REFERENCES

1. R. L. Siegel, K. D. Miller, and A. Jemal, "Cancer statistics, 2015," *CA: A Cancer Journal for Clinicians*, vol. 65(1), pp. 5–29, 2015.
2. A. Kaczmarek, P. Vandenabeele, and D. V. Krysko, "Necroptosis: The release of damage-associated molecular patterns and its physiological relevance," *Immunity*, vol. 38(2), pp. 209–223, 2013.
3. A. Kamal, S. Faazil, and M. S. Malik, "Apoptosis-inducing agents: A patent review (2010–2013)," *Expert Opinion on Therapeutic Patents*, vol. 24(3), pp. 339–354, 2014.
4. B. Levine and J. Yuan, "Autophagy in cell death: An innocent convict?" *The Journal of Clinical Investigation*, vol. 115(10), pp. 2679–2688, 2005.
5. S. Bhakdi, P. Thaicharoen, "Easy employment and crosstalk-free detection of seven fluorophores in a widefield fluorescence microscope," *Methods and Protocols*, vol. 1, p. 20, 2018.
6. E. Meijering, A. E. Carpenter, H. Peng, F. A. Hamprecht, J.-C. Olivo-Marin, "Imagining the future of bioimage analysis," *Nature Biotechnology*, vol. 34, pp. 1250–1255, 2016.
7. T. Gric, M. Cada, "Analytic solution to field distribution in one-dimensional inhomogeneous media," *Optics Communications*, vol. 322, pp. 183–187, 2014.
8. T. Gric, O. Hess, "Controlling hybrid-polarization surface plasmon polaritons in dielectric-transparent conducting oxides metamaterials via their effective properties," *Journal of Applied Physics*, vol. 122, p. 193105, 2017.
9. T. Gric, O. Hess, "Tunable surface waves at the interface separating different graphene-dielectric composite hyperbolic metamaterials," *Optics Express*, vol. 25, pp. 11466–11476, 2017.
10. Z. Zhang, H. Ding, X. Yan, L. Liang, D. Wei, M. Wang, Q. Yang, and J. Yao, "Sensitive detection of cancer cell apoptosis based on the non-bianisotropic metamaterials biosensors in terahertz frequency," *Optical Materials Express*, vol. 8, pp. 659–667, 2018.
11. M. Zhu, L. Zhang, S. Ma, J. Wang, J. Su and A. Liu, "Terahertz metamaterial designs for capturing and detecting circulating tumor cells," *Materials Research Express*, vol. 6, p. 045805, 2019.
12. A. Khokhlova, I. Zolotovskii, S. Sokolovski, Y. Saenko, E. Rafailov, D. Stoliarov, E. Pogodina, V. Svetukhin, V. Sibirny, A. Fotiadi, "The light-oxygen effect in biological cells enhanced by highly localized surface plasmon-polaritons," *Scientific Reports*, vol. 9, p. 18435, 2019.
13. J. Gollub, "Characterizing the effects of disorder in metamaterial structures," *Applied Physics Letters*, vol. 91, p. 162907, 2007.
14. M. V. Gorkunov, S. A. Grdeskul, I. V. Shadrivov, Y. S. Kivshar, "Effect of microscopic disorder on magnetic properties of metamaterials," *Physical Review E*, vol. 73(5 Pt 2), p. 056605, 2006.
15. C. Helgert, C. Rockstuhl, C. Etrich, E.-B. Kley, A. Tünnermann, F. Lederer, T. Pertsch, "Effects of anisotropic disorder in an optical metamaterial," *Applied Physics A*, vol. 103, pp. 591–595, 2011.

16. J. Leroy, C. Dalmay, A. Landoulsi, F. Hjeij, C. Mélin, B. Bessette, C. Bounaix Morand du Puch, S. Giraud, C. Lautrette, S. Battu, F. Lalloué, M. O. Jauberteau, A. Bessaudou, P. Blondy, A. Pothier, "Microfluidic biosensors for microwave dielectric spectroscopy," *Sensors and Actuators, A: Physical*, vol. 229, pp. 172–181, 2015.
17. G. Li and X.-F. Pang, "Effects of electromagnetic field exposure on electromagnetic properties of biological tissues," *Progress in Biochemistry and Biophysics*, vol. 38(7), pp. 604–610, 2011.
18. L. Shen, L. R. Margolies, J. H. Rothstein, E. Fluder, R. McBride, W. Sieh, "Deep learning to improve breast cancer detection on screening mammography," *Scientific Reports*, vol. 9, p. 12495, 2019.
19. E. Callaway, D. Castelvecchi, D. Cyranoski, E. Gibney, H. Ledford, J. J. Lee, L. Morello, N. Phillips, Q. Schiermeier, J. Tollefson, A. Witze, "2017 in news: The science events that shaped the year," *Nature*, vol. 552, pp. 304–307, 2017.
20. A. E. Fetit, J. Novak, D. Rodriguez, D. P. Auer, C. A. Clark, R. G. Grundy, A. C. Peet, T. N. Arvanitis, "Radiomics in paediatric neuro-oncology: A multicentre study on MRI texture analysis," *NMR Biomedicine*, vol. 31, pp. 1–13, 2018.
21. S. Goldenberg, G. Nir, S. E. Salcudean, "A new era: Artificial intelligence and machine learning in prostate cancer," *Nature Reviews Urology*, vol. 16, pp. 391–403, 2019.
22. I. Banerjee, A. Crawley, M. Bhethanabotla, H. E. Daldrup-Link, D. L. Rubin, "Transfer learning on fused multiparametric MR images for classifying histopathological subtypes of rhabdomyosarcoma," *Computerized Medical Imaging and Graphics*, vol. 65, pp. 167–175, 2018.
23. T. Gric, S. G. Sokolovski, N. Navolokin, O. Glushkobskaya, and E. U. Rafailov, "Metamaterial formalism approach for advancing the recognition of glioma areas in brain tissue biopsies," *Optical Materials Express*, vol. 10, pp. 1607–1615, 2020.
24. V. M. Shalaev, *Nonlinear Optics of Random Media: Fractal Composites and Metal-Dielectric Films*, Springer, Berlin, 2000.
25. S. Bosch, J. Ferré-Borrull, N. Leinfellner, and A. Canillas, "Effective dielectric function of mixtures of three or more materials: A numerical procedure for computations," *Surface Science*, vol. 453(1–3), pp. 9–17, 2000.
26. T. Gric, S. G. Sokolovski, N. Navolokin, O. Semyachkina-Glushkovskaya, and E. U. Rafailov, "Metamaterial formalism approach for advancing the recognition of glioma areas in brain tissue biopsies," *Optical Materials Express*, vol. 10, pp. 1607–1615, 2020.
27. T. Gric, S. G. Sokolovski, A. G. Alekseev, A. V. Mamoshin, A. Dunaev and E. U. Rafailov, "The discrete analysis of the tissue biopsy images with metamaterial formalization: Identifying tumor locus," *IEEE Journal of Selected Topics in Quantum Electronics*, vol. 27(5), pp. 1–8 (2021).
28. S. Gabriel, R. W. Lau and C. Gabriel, "The dielectric properties of biological tissues: III. Parametric models for the dielectric spectrum of tissues," *Physics in Medicine & Biology*, vol. 41, p. 2271 (1996).

29. O. Kidwai, S. V. Zhukovsky, and J. E. Sipe, "Effective-medium approach to planar multilayer hyperbolic metamaterials: Strengths and limitations," *Physical Review A*, vol. 85, p. 053842, 2012.

30. P. Zakharov, F. Dewarrat, A. Caduff, and M. S. Talary, "The effect of blood content on the optical and dielectric skin properties," *Physiological Measurement*, vol. 32(1), pp. 131–149, 2011.

31. P. Salembier, J. Serra, "Flat zones filtering, connected operators, and filters by reconstruction," *IEEE Transactions on Image Processing*, vol. 4(8), pp. 1153–1160, 1995.

32. H. Sun, J. Yang, M. Ren, "A fast watershed algorithm based on chain code and its application in image segmentation," *Pattern Recognition Letters*, vol. 26(9), pp. 1266–1274, 2005.

33. G. Bradski, The OpenCV Library. Dr. Dobb's J. Softw. Tools, 2000.

34. N. Otsu, "A threshold selection method from gray-level histograms," *IEEE Transactions on Systems, Man, Cybernetics*, vol. 9, pp. 62–66, 1979.

35. T. H. Tjia, P. Bordewijk, and C. J. F. Böttcher, "On the notion of dielectric friction in the theory of dielectric relaxation," *Advances in Molecular Relaxation Processes*, vol. 6(1), pp. 19–28, 1974.

36. J. C. Maxwell-Garnett, "Colours in metal glasses and films," *Philosophical Transactions of the Royal Society A Mathematical Physical & Engineering Sciences*, vol. 203, pp. 385–420 (1904).

37. M. Bruggerman, W. Kalkner, A. Campus, and A. Smedberg, "Electrochemical effects at the conductor/dielectric interface-a description of the mechanism," *IEEE International Conference on Solid Dielectrics*, vol. 1, pp. 383–386, 2004.

38. T. Hanai, "A remark on theory of dielectric dispersion due to interfacial polarization," *Colloid Polymer Science*, vol. 175(1), pp. 61–62, 1961.

39. S. E. Skipetrov, "Effective dielectric function of a random medium," *Physical Review B-Condensed Matter and Materials Physics*, vol. 60(18), pp. 12705–12709, 1999.

40. C. J. F. Böttcher, P. Bordeweijk, *Theory of Electric Polarisation*, Elsevier, Amsterdam, 1978.

41. N. A. Navolokin, D. A. Mudrak, A. B. Bucharskaya, O. V. Matveeva, S. A. Tychina, N. V. Polukonova, G. N. Maslyakova, "Effect of flavonoid-containing extracts on the growth of transplanted sarcoma 45, peripheral blood and bone marrow condition after oral and intramuscular administration in rats," *Russian Open Medical Journal*, 6(3), 304 (2017).

42. C. R. Gonzalez, R. Woods, *Digital Image Processing*, New Jersey: Pearson Education, 2002.

43. M.-N. Wu, C.-C. Lin, C.-C. Chang, "Brain tumor detection using color-based K-means clustering segmentation," *IIH-MSP '07: Proceedings of the Third International Conference on International Information Hiding and Multimedia Signal Processing (IIH-MSP 2007)*, vol. 2, pp. 245–250, 2007.

44. M. Rakesh, T. Ravi, "Image segmentation and detection of tumor objects in MR brain images using FUZZY C-MEANS (FCM) algorithm," *IJERA*, vol. 2(3), pp. 2088–2094, 2012.

45. C. Christine, F. Thomas, "A study of efficiency and accuracy in the transformation from RGB to CIELAB color space," *IEEE Transactions on Image Processing*, vol. 6(7), pp. 1046–1048, 1997.

CHAPTER 3

Biomedical Applications of Terahertz Radiation

Amit Yadav
Aston University

Andrei Gorodetsky
University of Birmingham

CONTENTS

DOI: 10.1201/9781003228950-3

3.1 INTRODUCTION

Terahertz (THz) frequency band, despite its modest location between well-known microwave (MW) and broadly studied infrared (IR) ranges (Figure 3.1), has been relatively unexplored due to the lack of controlled natural sources and detectors. Until about 30 years ago, these frequencies were usually referred to as sub-mm or far-IR radiation, depending on which side of the

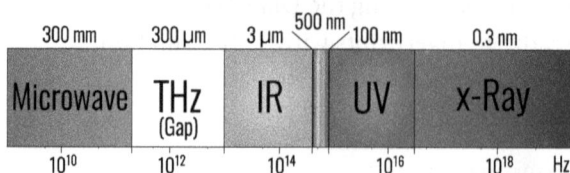

FIGURE 3.1 Part of electromagnetic spectrum with frequency ranges outlined.

electromagnetic spectrum the narrator was working, and for the next 20 years frequencies between 100 GHz and 10–20 THz were referred to as THz 'Gap'!

Extensive research in the past 30 years and development of compact ultra-fast lasers, as well as ultrafast semiconductor technology, has transformed THz into a separate field of research, with its own sections at well-known international summits and special THz-only conferences gathering hundreds of researchers from all around the globe. The key properties of THz radiation related to biological science is its sensitivity to water content and photon energies in the large molecular vibrations range. On the other hand, sensitivity to water is the main limitation, not allowing for deep tissue remote sensing.

After the first pioneering experiments in the early 2000s, because of the low signal-to-noise ratios of the living tissue samples, and limited availability of the setups, as most of them were homebuilt at the THz labs, THz biomedical research found itself almost in limbo for the next 15 years to face its renaissance after the maturation of the pulsed THz technology and establishment of the THz device market, when THz setups appeared even at non-photonic laboratories. The vast majority of papers used here were published after 2018.

The main directions of THz biomedical research can be put into the mind map shown in Figure 3.2. A thumping majority of applications make

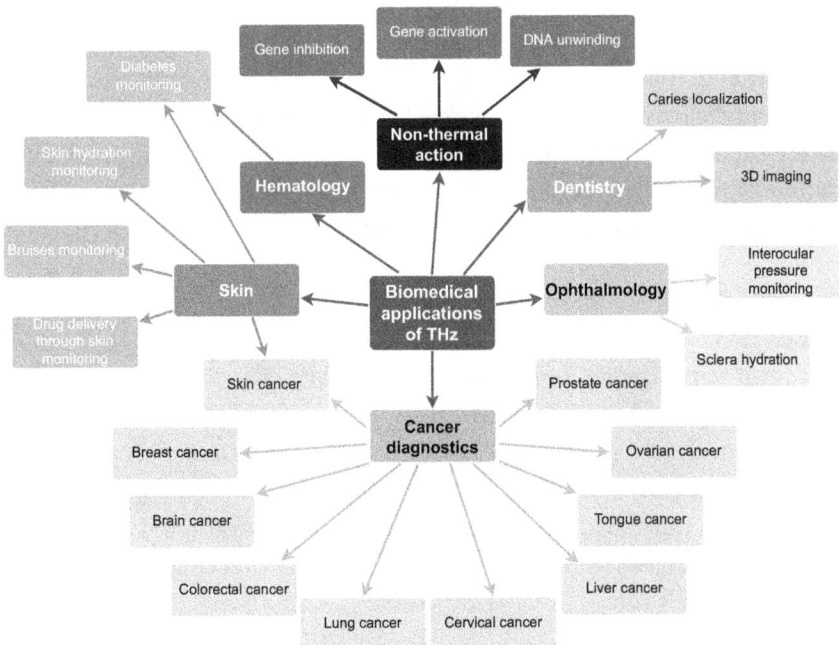

FIGURE 3.2 Biomedical applications of THz radiation.

use of the THz sensitivity to water to not only study water content in cells and tissues and dynamics of tissue moisturizing but also differentiate healthy and cancerous tissues.

In this chapter, we will provide some general knowledge about THz technology, necessary for the understanding of the chapter's body; however, we do encourage every reader to turn to one of the numerous existing reviews on either development of THz research and methods – see [1–6] to name a few – or certain aspects of biomedical THz applications: early results [7–9], cancer diagnostics with THz [10–16], general reviews written 2–5 years ago [17–22], biomolecular studies [23,24], effect of THz radiation on living biological systems [25,26], THz biomedical imaging [27–29], skin studies with THz radiation [30], and the newest reviews on bioaspects of THz radiation [31,32].

THz is still a young technology, and the most amount of research has appeared within the past 7 years. We anticipate its further growth and bright achievements in future and without further ado proceed to the body of the chapter.

3.2 TERAHERTZ SPECTROSCOPIC AND IMAGING SYSTEMS

Pioneered in early 1990s, THz technology has established into a developed research direction [1], bringing in several unique characterization techniques applicable for biological and medical studies among many others. We will briefly introduce here the main experimental techniques used for biomedical THz studies. The most used approaches include terahertz time-domain spectroscopy (THz-TDS), terahertz pulsed imaging (TPI), terahertz pulse time-domain holography (PTDH), and THz continuous wave imaging, holography, and microscopy.

3.2.1 Pulsed THz Components and Setups

Pulsed THz technology, due to relative compactness and the amount of data it can provide, is mostly used for both spectroscopy and imaging nowadays, including biomedical applications. Further in this chapter, probably over 90% of research reported here uses pulsed THz radiation. THz pulses are generated through non-linear downconversion of near-IR femtosecond pulses from ultrafast lasers. There are four main approaches to such downconversion, and we will very briefly overview them all, and outline their advantages and weaknesses.

3.2.1.1 *Photoconductive Antennas and Principles of THz Time-Domain Spectroscopy*

Photoconductive antennas (PCAs) are used as pulsed THz sources in a vast majority of commercially available setups due to their efficiency, ability to work with rather low pump powers, and robustness of the antenna-based setups. Similar antennas with slightly different electrode topology can be used as detectors. Nonlinear crystals possessing the electro-optic linear Kerr effect can show better detection performance due to lower noise and higher sensitivity. Nonlinear crystals can also be used as THz generators, but due to their nonlinear nature they require higher pulse energies for efficient operation and hence are used only in high-power setups.

The general construction and principle of PCA is shown in Figure 3.3.

The antenna consists of the semiconductor substrate, biased electrodes, and in most cases a silicon hemispherical or hyperhemispherical lens. Once the substrate is illuminated by a pulse from the pump laser (pulse envelope is shown in the top plot of Figure 3.3b), photocarriers are generated in the surface layer of the semiconductor. Under action of the electric field created by the biased electrodes, the carriers move across the gap, creating a spike of the current (middle plot of Figure 3.3b), that decays with time, as carriers relax. Fast alternating current generates a single oscillation picosecond pulse in the far field (bottom plot of Figure 3.3b). Spectrum of such pulse lies in the THz range, with maximum being around 0.7-1 THz. The silicon lens on th reduces the Fresnel losses and enhances the directivity of

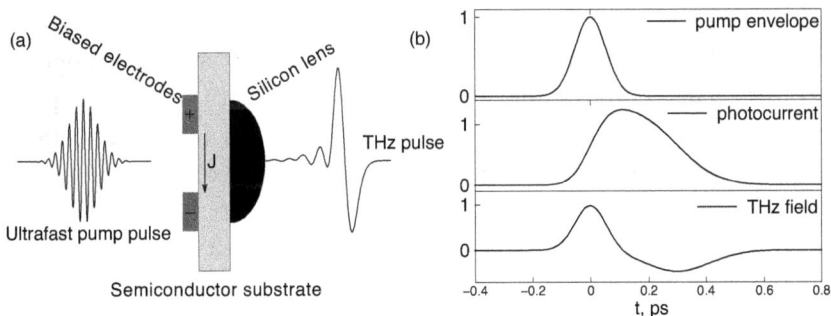

FIGURE 3.3 (a) PCA layout and principle of operation and (b) time traces of pump radiation envelope, pump photocurrent in the PCA gap, and the generated THz field.

the PCA. The key properties of the substrate material are ultrashort carrier lifetime, high optoelectronic efficiency, and decent carrier mobility. Short carrier lifetimes are necessary for providing an ultrashort current spike, as THz field value is proportional to the photocurrent time derivative. Optoelectronic efficiency (providing higher carrier concentration) and mobility (resulting in faster carrier movement and, hence, higher current and current derivative values) serve the same purpose. Depending on the pump wavelength, typical PCA substrate materials are as follows: For ≤800 nm wavelength (Ti:Sapphire lasers and second harmonic of Er-doped ultrafast fiber lasers) low temperature grown GaAs is used [33,34]. It provides shortest carrier lifetimes, slightly sacrificing the mobility. These setups are common for lab use as Ti:Sapphire lasers are expensive and bulky [35]. Most commercially available setups use 1550 nm telecom wavelength erbium-based ultrafast fiber lasers as pump source and PCAs on low temperature grown InGaAs substrates with various doping [36]. PCAs are fiber coupled to the pump laser thus such setups do not require user alignment, allow for turn-key operation, and take up reasonable space. Such setups do not require user alignment, allow for turn-key operation, and take up reasonable space. Ytterbium-based ultrafast fiber lasers can serve as pump sources for GaBiAs [37] and low temperature grown InGaAs-based [38] PCAs. Another perspective approach suggests using InAs/GaAs heterostructures in conjunction with semiconductor ultrafast lasers based on the same materials and operating at wavelengths of around 1200 nm as even more efficient and compact THz transceivers [39,40]. Efficiency of PCAs can be further enhanced by addition of anti-reflection coating, or introduction of optical nanoantennas into the PCA gap, or both [41,42].

THz radiation detection in the PCA occurs pretty much the opposite way to its generation. An unbiased PCA is pumped with an ultrafast pulse from the pump laser (referred to as 'probe pulse', as it is used for detection), thus creating photocarriers, which are dragged by the overlapping part of the THz pulse across the PCA gap, resulting in a current proportional to the THz field. By changing the time delay between the optical probe and pump pulses, it is possible to strobe the full profile of the THz pulse and thus record the temporal dependence of its electric field. For higher signal-to-noise ratio, PCA-generator bias is chopped at a kHz frequency, and this frequency is locked to the lock-in current amplifier at the detector. The possible result of such measurement is shown in Figure 3.4.

Spectral information can be retrieved with Fourier transform of the measured data. To obtain the sample transmission in the THz range, its transmission spectrum is normalized to the reference THz signal, which,

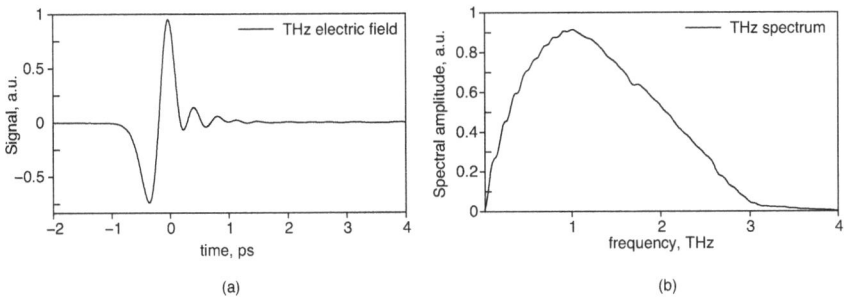

FIGURE 3.4   (a) Typical THz pulse and (b) its spectrum.

depending on the sample, is either the bare spectrometer signal or the transmission spectrum of the substrate. Similar detection and processing principles are used for all THz-pulsed setups, and we would like to note that being a coherent field measurement technique, THz-TDS allows for retrieval of not only the transmission coefficient but also the refractive index of the sample [43].

3.2.1.2 Nonlinear Crystals and Laser Filaments as THz Sources

Non-linear crystals are the second most popular approach of ultrafast laser pulse downconversion into THz radiation. They possess certain advantages over the PCAs, often offering broader spectrum and working with higher pump powers; however, due to their non-linearity they are efficient only at higher pump pulse energies, achievable only by the amplified laser setups [4]. Another requirement for efficient operation of such converter is the phase matching between the optical and THz radiation upon their propagation inside the crystal. Usually it is achieved by selection of the crystal that possesses the required refractive indices in IR and THz regions, for example, ZnTe for an 800 nm pump, or other crystals [44], or by non-collinear phase matching, when a wave front of the pump laser pulse is tilted by a diffractive element, thus equalizing the group velocity of the IR pulse with phase velocity of the THz inside the crystal. Such layout is usually used in LiNbO$_3$-based setups [4].

Non-linear crystals are rarely used in commercial THz spectroscopic setups as sources of THz radiation; however, they often replace the PCA at the detection stage. For THz detection in such crystals, linear Kerr effect is used, when polarization of the optical probe pulse is modulated proportionally to the electric field applied to the crystal by the THz pulse. The approach is shown in Figure 3.5.

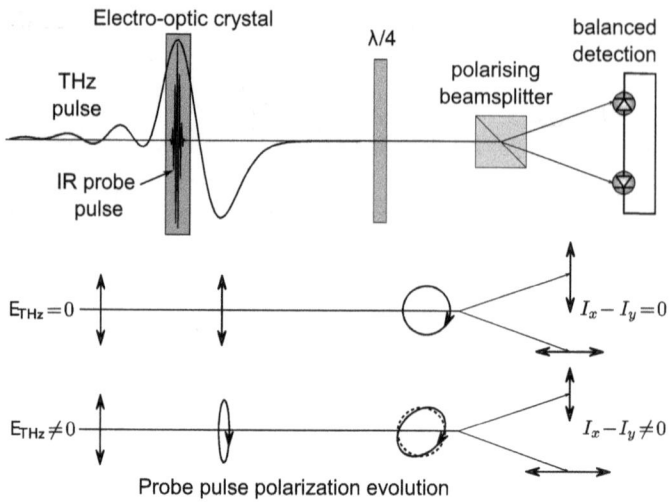

FIGURE 3.5   Electro-optic detection.

If an external field of a THz pulse is present in the electro-optic crystal, it induces birefringence, resulting in the change of initially linear polarization of the probe beam into elliptical. Unlike precisely circular polarization that comes out of the quarter wave plate in the case of linearly polarized input, elliptical polarization observed in the case of the elliptical input does not equalize the signal on balanced detector, thus providing the voltage proportional to the electric field applied. Similar to the PCA setup, the profile of the electric field is recorded by changing the mutual delay between the THz and probe pulse. Sensitivity of detection will depend on the electro-optic coefficient of the crystal and its thickness. However, thick crystals may result in poorer phase matching and, hence, narrower bandwidth. Thus, the crystal is selected depending on the wavelength (GaP or ZnTe for 800 nm, CdTe for 1040 nm), and its thickness is chosen with respect to the application.

Laser filaments happen naturally if high-energy ultrafast laser pulses are focused in the air or other gas. Plasma electrons act similar to the carriers in semiconductors, and cubic plasma non-linearity adds to higher frequency THz signal generation [4]. Most efficient converters were shown for two-color plasma filaments when the second harmonic of pump radiation breaks the symmetry of the electric field in plasma [45]. Even higher efficiencies were obtained for 3000 nm amplified pumps [46]. Laser filaments can be produced with high energy pulses from amplified systems and are rarely available in commercial setups. Similar to PCAs and crystals, filaments can detect THz radiation [47].

3.2.1.3 Spintronic Emitters

Spintronic emitters are the last but not least emitters of THz radiation we would like to mention here. Having appeared relatively recently [48], these emitters offer unprecedented spectral bandwidth, ultimate scalability, and relatively cheap production; they are already available on the market. Spintronic emitters rely on the inverse spin-hall effect in operation: they consist of at least two (usually more) thin (3–10 nm thick) metal layers, ferromagnetic and antiferromagnetic. The ferromagnetic layer is magnetized by the external permanent magnetic field, and the spin oriented electrons excited by the femtosecond pump pulse move to the antiferromagnetic layer, generating the transverse current because the product of the density, band velocity, and lifetime of spin-up electrons in ferromagnetic metals is significantly higher than that of the spin-down electrons. The only drawback of such sources is the need of the magnetic field. They are rarely available in commercial setups only due to their novelty, and we believe they will share a bigger part of the THz transceivers market very soon.

3.2.1.4 Setups for Pulsed THz Spectroscopy and Imaging

We have already overviewed the general approaches to generation and detection of pulsed THz radiation in THz-TDS setups that are based on PCAs and electro-optic crystals. Laser filaments can be used as well, in pretty similar layout, and spintronic emitters can replace any emitter mentioned above. In this section, we will present the most general layouts for THz-TDS and TPI setups in transmission and reflection modes. Above, we tried to outline the most important components, regardless their nature – these setups can be based either on PCAs or non-linear crystals/filaments or use spintronic emitter as a source, with almost any 'mix and match' you can think of. Precise beam alignment will differ, and in most commercial setups optical beams will be fiber coupled, but the principle layout stays the same for any TDS/TPI setup. The beam from the ultrafast laser is split into two parts: the first part (usually more powerful) is used to generate the THz beam, and the second is used for detection. THz beam can be focused and collimated either by lenses, as shown in the illustrations – polymer lenses (TPX, teflon) are usually used – or by off-axis parabolic mirrors, seen more often in older and lab-based setups. Off axis parabolic mirrors provide slightly less losses and tighter focus spot, but are trickier in alignment. Optical delay line is used to scan the THz pulse with much shorter optical pulse. Mechanical motion of the mirrors on the delay changes the length of one of the arms without changing its position on the detector. In the illustration, the optical delay line is shown in the probe beam, but technically it does not matter which optical arm changes its length, as soon as the THz pulse is fully detected anyway. Detected THz pulse and its spectrum can be seen in Figure 3.4, Section 3.1.1.1. We outline three typical setup modes: THz-TDS in transmission (Figure 3.6a), THz-TDS for attenuated total reflection (ATR) measurement (Figure 3.6b), and THz-TDS in oblique

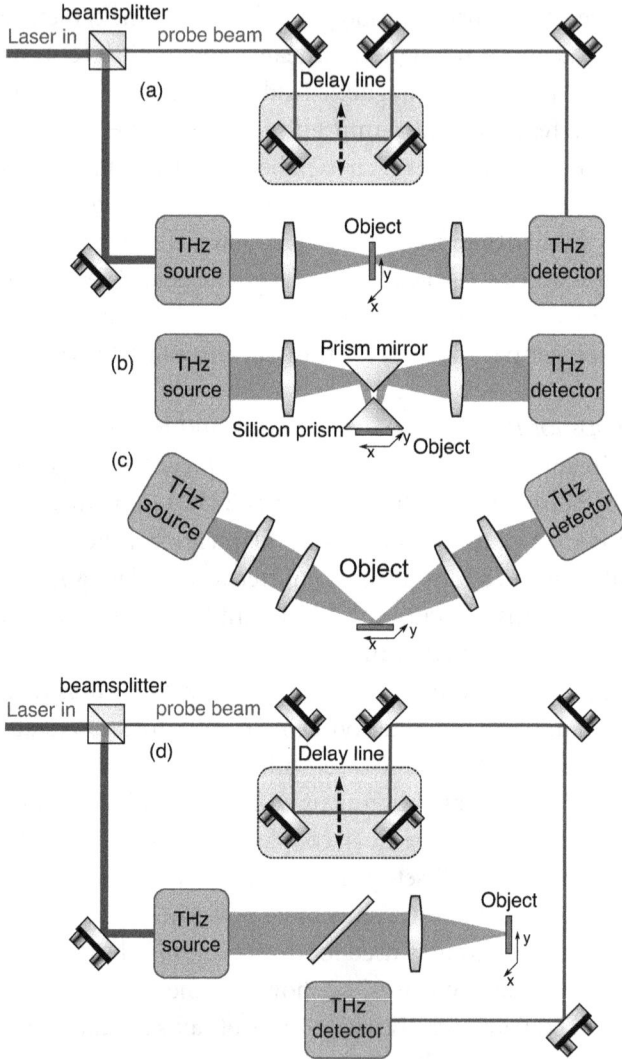

FIGURE 3.6 Setups for THz-TDS/TPI. (a) Setup for transmission measurement; (b) alteration of the setup for attenuated total reflection (ATR) measurement; (c) alteration of the setup for oblique reflection measurement. (d) Setup for normal reflection measurement. TPI is realized by moving the object in transverse to the THz beam directions.

(Figure 3.6c) and normal reflection mode (Figure 3.6d). Some setups may even combine transmission and reflection measurements using two detectors working simultaneously. All setups share the same operational principle: signal transmitted/reflected from the sample is focussed onto a detector for coherent detection provided by the probe pulse arriving there simultaneously. THz pulsed imaging (TPI) is performed by transverse scanning of the sample with the focussed beam.

3.2.1.5 Terahertz Pulse Time-Domain Holography

THz PTDH is a powerful tool for imaging in the THz domain. Unlike TPI, it uses a collimated (unfocused) beam to probe the sample, instead of point-by-point scanning, and the full wave front is detected afterward [49,50]. Numerical reconstruction allows for full 3D wave front retrieval at all spectral components. Matching the longitudinal resolution of the TPI, THz PTDH provides better transverse resolution (down to $\frac{\lambda}{\sqrt{2}}$) [51], which potentially can be numerically enhanced even further with iterative algorithms [52]. Moreover, as full wave front detection removes the need for point-by-point scanning, the acquisition process takes much less time. To allow for full wave front detection, because of the sensitivity limitations, this technique works better when implemented on amplified powerful setups.

3.2.2 CW Terahertz Components and Setups

Continuous-wave THz imaging (CW TI) can be a very useful tool as it provides real-time video rate image, as proper selection of wavelength narrows the acquired dataset to only essential values. The most popular sources of CW THz radiation are backward wave oscillators (BWO) [53–55], Impact Ionization Avalanche Transit Time (IMPATT) diodes [53,56], Gunn diodes, Schottky diodes [57] and other types of direct semiconductor sources [58], Quantum Cascaded Lasers (QCL) [59], and CO_2 laser pumped gas lasers [60]. While the former types operate at frequencies below 1 THz, the latter two cover the band between 2 and 6 THz.

There are several technologies for non-coherent THz sensing; some of them exist only as single pixel detectors, while other are scalable into linear or matrix arrays. A large group of detectors are heat-based and migrated from the IR domain. Among these, we'd like to mention opto-acoustic detector or Golay cell [61] which is a single pixel thermal detector, quite sensitive to THz radiation, and hardly scalable. They are still available on the market and are quite handy when it comes to setup alignment, even for very low power-pulsed THz systems; however, they are not too practical in measurements due to their instability and slow acquisition times. The second approach, bolometric detection, is the most sensitive and at the same time most expensive. This is also a heat-based approach, and it provides several orders of magnitude of magnitude higher sensitivity over the Golay cell, if liquid gas-cooled bolometers are used [62]. Recently, room-temperature hot electron bolometers allowed for sensitive 2D microbolometer arrays acting as real-time THz cameras [63], now available on the market. Pyroelectric detectors, also available as 2D matrix arrays and usually made for IR and FIR, are also sensitive and can be successfully applied to imaging THz beams [64]. They are well-established technology and can be purchased both as single-pixel sensor and cameras. Most of the heat transfer-based incoherent detectors are capable of measuring THz pulsed radiation and are often used for preliminary alignment.

Another approach uses semiconductor detectors that are more critical to the radiation frequency, but can be matched to the source. Among them we can mention ultrafast Schottky diodes and plasmonic linear and matrix array detectors [56]. CW THz technology offers more choice of components and physics behind them than pulsed, and there are not many face-to-face comparisons of the sources and detectors due to their price and practical availability of only one of a kind in the lab [65,66]. We will try to explicitly state the technology behind the result, where possible, within this chapter.

3.2.2.1 CW Terahertz Imaging

Both single-pixel and matrix detectors can be used for CW THz imaging (CWTI), and now we will turn to the main setups used in the experiments. We outline them in Figure 3.7. Single-pixel detector-based setups are shown in the left column, while THz camera-based setups are on the right.

In Figure 3.7a, we have put the simplest realization of point-by-point scanning CW THz imaging setup. It is pretty analogous to the TPI setup; however, it does not provide either spectral or phase information. However, fast acquisition makes it a simple and viable solution. Similar layouts for reflective imaging and ATR are shown in Figure 3.7b and c, respectively. Setup in reflection can be modified with beam splitter for normal incidence [67], similar to the THz-TDS setup shown in Figure 3.6d. Figure 3.7d shows a very different approach to single-pixel imaging that does not require point-by-point scanning of the object.

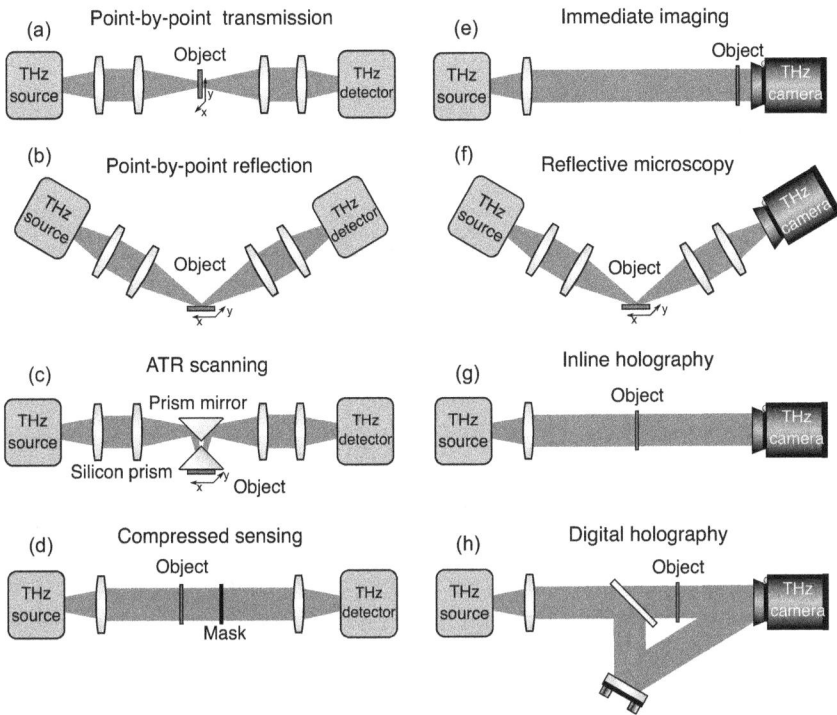

FIGURE 3.7   Setups for CW THz imaging.

Such approach is called compressed sensing, and it involves either mechanically [68] or optically tunable [69] masks. Masks cover certain part of wave front, and the set of intensities is used for image reconstruction. This method is significantly faster than point scanning, and still uses more affordable single-pixel detector.

The simplest camera-based layout for THz imaging uses the THz camera immediately after the object of interest as shown in Figure 3.7e. Although this method is simple in setting up and provides some general information of the object and reveals some hidden features inside dielectric objects is not very practical for biomedical applications, as most objects will be either strongly absorbing the THz radiation and require the reflection layout, or be equally transparent, with the data of interest hidden inside the phase of the measured radiation. Moreover, this approach has quite poor resolution due to diffraction.

Another approach, usually referred to as THz reflective microscopy [57], shown in Figure 3.7f, is similar to the one in Figure 3.7b, with the only difference being the use of the camera instead of the single pixel source. The camera allows for detection of a higher number of spatial frequencies of the point-spread function registration and thus higher image resolution.

THz inline holography [60] setup (Figure 3.7g) looks quite similar to the simplest imaging approach (Figure 3.7e); however, it uses the iterative procedure that enables not only reconstruction of the object amplitude with relatively high resolution but also object phase retrieval [70]. Unlike THz-TDS, the detection stage is incoherent; however, the iterative procedure with subsequent numerical wave front expansion provides excellent resolution even with relatively small detector. A similar approach with iterative reconstruction has been shown in reflection as well [71].

THz digital holography setup [72], shown in transmission mode in Figure 3.7h, is probably the most complicated, but at the same time it provides the most precise information about the object under study. A similar setup can be realized in reflection mode [73]. Like in classical optical holography, this approach uses reference beam for phase information retrieval, and object information is numerically reconstructed. We should note that although most approaches from holography in visible domain can be adapted for use in the THz range, a very different approach, where propagation distance and hologram/object size are only several tens of wavelengths in size, applies very different constraints onto algorithms and approximations.

Among other setups used for biomedical THz imaging that are not listed here, we could name THz computed tomography [74,75], which is an extension of the setup shown in Figure 3.7a with rotation stage. This setup allows for classical tomographic reconstruction of the 3D object profile; THz solid immersion microscopy [54], where a single-pixel reflection mode setup is upgraded with specially designed aspherical plastic lens, allows for resolution as low as 0.15λ [55].

Having described the THz apparatus usually used for biomedical THz studies, we will now turn to the main application directions and outline the most significant results demonstrated within biomedical THz photonics research.

3.3 THz STUDIES OF THE SKIN

Skin, as the most accessible tissue in the body, was the first one to be studied with THz radiation. These studies began in the early 2000s with newly homebuilt THz-TDS setups in reflection mode [76–78]. For the next

15 years, and this can be true for most biomedical THz research, there were very few papers issued [79,80] until approximately 2018. We associate this decline with complexity of the setups and the need to build them from scratch at the times, while most research was geared towards the development of new, more efficient, and cheaper ways to generate and detect THz radiation instead of its practical applications. During these years, several THz companies opened offering their products, and some well-established manufacturers introduced their THz components and THz-TDS setups. As a result, THz-TDS setups became more affordable and easier in operation, and even those labs that never worked with ultrafast lasers could easily get hands on the THz-TDS table-top fiber-based system. Needless to say, the specifications of the new devices on the market were outstanding, especially in comparison with older setups in terms of signal-to-noise, dynamic range, and acquisition time.

The result was not long in coming – a rising tide of papers from numerous groups, revisiting old results and offering new studies. Zaytsev et al. [81] performed a thorough research on THz-TDS in reflection (Figure 3.6d) of healthy human skin *in vivo*, providing the results for nearly all parts of the human body. Wang et al. [82] studied the effect of pressure on the sample from imaging window. Using the THz-TDS setup in reflection (Figure 3.6b), they report a drop in the reflected from the quartz-skin interface signal amplitude and rise in its refractive index value when the sample is subject to stronger pressure, and the measured difference in signal is over 10% of the amplitude for the pressure range between 1.5 and 3.5 N/cm². They associate such difference with higher water concentration in compressed tissue and confirm the experimental results with simulations, thus confirming previous results [83]. Later, the researchers of the group propose the experimental protocol for experimental *in vivo* skin studies [84].

Some of these results were confirmed later by Wang et al. [85] for the THz-TDS in ATR regime (Figure 3.6b), who found that reflection drops both with pressure increase and due to the duration of the contact between the skin and the substrate, also affecting water concentration.

Vilagosh et al. [86] compared previously published *in vivo* and *ex vivo* results and agreed that most data are consistent and declined the hypothesis that the change in THz properties of skin tissue are temperature related, but instead they can be explained with *postmortem* changes. Peralta et al. [87] looked into the THz properties of *ex vivo* human skin with different melanin content using THz-TDS in transmission (Figure 3.6a) and found, with the data collected being coherent with previous studies, no certain dependence of optical constants in the THz range for the skin samples with different melanin content.

In addition to general studies of human skin properties in the THz range, there are more specific skin-oriented applications of the THz radiation.

3.3.1 Skin Burns and Bruises Monitoring

Skin scars and their recovery were extensively studied since relatively early days of the THz-TDS system's involvement in biomedical photonics. Taylor et al. [79] investigated *in vitro* porcine skin burns with reflective THz-TDS setup (Figure 3.6c), including the measurements done through the ten layers of dry medical gauze. Burned and unburned skin had a drastic difference in their properties, the latter demonstrating significantly worse reflection due to the lack of water in burned skin areas. The study of Tewari et al. [77] was performed on burned rat skin *in vivo*. THz-TDS in reflection was used (Figure 3.6c), which found exactly the opposite to the *in vitro* result of hyper-reflectivity at the areas correlating to the area of most severe injury. Reflectivity enhancement in living skin is associated with natural local water concentration increase after injury. Reflection from the skin should not be confused with quartz–skin interface reflection often used in the most recent experiments, for example, on skin occlusion pressure studies [82–85].

Fan et al. [88] studied human scars *in vivo* with THz-TDS in reflection (Figure 3.6c) during their healing process and reported a distinguishable contrast between the scar and surrounding tissue refractive index, even for ones difficult to see with the naked eye. These differences persisted over months after the wound recovered and became optically indistinguishable. Figure 3.8 reprinted from [89] shows the THz reflectivity superimposed onto the optical image of the wound within several hours after the incident. Dynamics of water content are clearly visible. All studies in this section were performed in reflection mode, either with or without spectroscopic data [90,91], and demonstrated THz technology as a powerful tool for wound-healing monitoring, allowing for checking its state even through the dry medical gauze. Refractive index is shown to be a more useful characteristic for scar state monitoring.

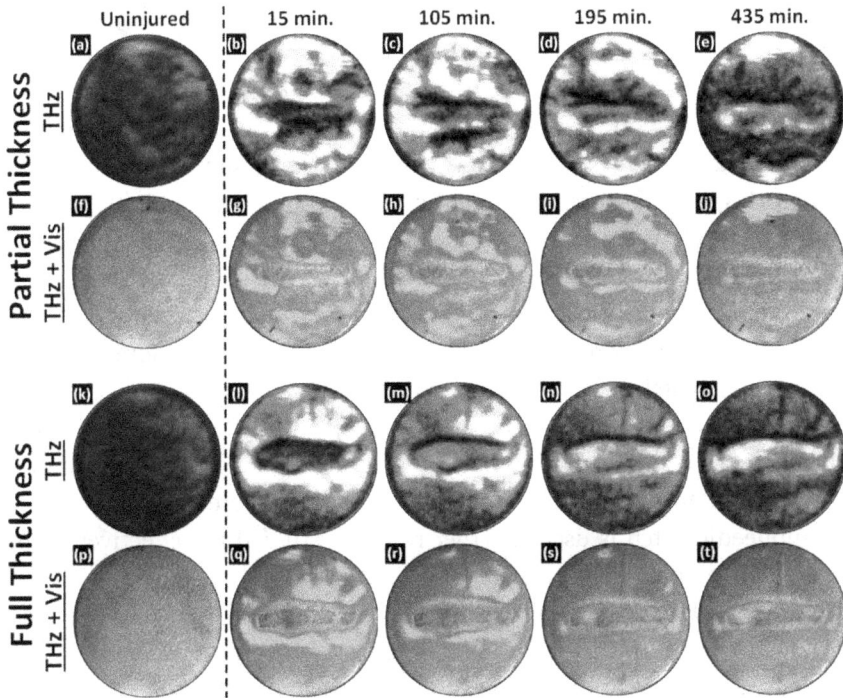

FIGURE 3.8 Burn wound time series imaging results. (a)–(e) THz images of a partial thickness burn. (f)–(j) Partial thickness THz images superimposed on the registered visible frame. (k)–(o) THz images of a full thickness burn. (p)–(t) Full thickness THz images superimposed on the registered visible frame. THz contrast is distinct for each burn wound severity. In time-series THz images of a partial thickness burn, the contact area shows a drop in tissue water content and an edematous front superior to the burn over time. In contrast to the partial thickness wound the contact area of a full thickness burn does not display a significant drop in tissue water content. Additionally, the contact area is surrounded by a ring of tissue water content which runs concentric and coincident with the burn contact zone. (Reprinted with permission from [89] © 2019 Optica Publishing Group under the terms of the Optica Open Access Publishing Agreement.)

3.3.2 Drug Delivery through Skin Monitoring

Another useful application of THz technology is found in monitoring of various substances, including medicaments and cosmetics penetration through the skin layers. As THz waves are extremely sensitive to water content, it can help to trace the penetration of cremes through the skin layers.

The first research on this subject was published by Kim et al. [80], penetration of dimethyl sulfoxide (DMSO), an organosulfur compound used for transdermal drug delivery (TDD), containing ketoprofen, through excised rat skin. THz-TDS in reflection (Figure 3.6c) was used. The study showed that THz radiation is sensitive to DMSO and can be successfully used for monitoring DMSO-based treatment penetrations. Wang et al. [92] used a similar setup layout and studied the approaches to TDD with a phantom drug, consisting of aspirin/alcohol/water/glycerin mixture. They compared the methods of TDD with THz radiation: a simple dripping of the drug onto skin was compared with cotton pad deposition, nanoneedle, and microneedle patch delivery. The reduced reflection of THz radiation due to displacement of water by the drug phantom in the skin was recorded. Spatial maps of the imaged reflection coefficient demonstrate the ability of THz-TDS to monitor the TDD and reveal the increased TDD rate if a nanoneedle patch is used. Further research studied the effectiveness of film vs woven patches for TDD [93] by a similar method. Sueda et al. [94] used THz-TDS in modified layout, with the sample being placed onto the THz source and immediately reflecting the generated pulses for monitoring the speed of liquid penetration into the skin. The shift of the THz time-domain peak position corresponds to the liquid penetration boundary. Other studies looked into the effect of cosmetic skin lotion [95,96] and nicotine-containing substance [97] on THz response of the skin.

3.3.3 Skin Hydration Monitoring

The hydration state of the skin may serve as a monitor for its health status. This is another opportunity for applying THz sensitivity to water content for non-invasive monitoring. Review of early results on this topic was published in 2011 [98]. As it has been outlined earlier in this chapter, a higher water content in the tissue during occlusion demonstrates lower reflectivity in THz frequency region [83,93]. The dynamics of this observation was further studied in order to examine water diffusivity during the skin occlusion [99]. Ellipsometric research made available by the two modified ATR setups (Figure 3.6b), adjusted for *s*- and *p*- polarization measurement, revealed the anisotropic properties of the *stratum corneum* (SC) [100]. This method proved its efficiency by comparison of the THz response of untreated skin and skin treated with aqueous, anhydrous, and a water–oil emulsion. The water–oil emulsion and aqueous samples turned out to be indistinguishable by THz-TDS in reflection [101].

You et al. used THz-TDS in normal reflection layout (Figure 3.6c) to determine the frequency-dependent property of skin penetration depth during water sorption–desorption. Penetration depths were determined to be 0.1–0.3 mm for most frequencies.

3.3.3.1 Monitoring the Diabetes

Fine monitoring of skin hydration can help with early detection of diabetes. Several publications of Hernandez-Cardoso et al. proved that THz-TDS of the foot in reflection (Figure 3.6c) was an efficient way to detect diabetes [102,103].

Smolyanskaya et al. studied the effect of diabetes on glycerol penetration through tissue layers and have shown that glycerol as a dehydration agent works better on healthy samples than diabetic tissues under study [104]. Further research revealed the possibility of non-invasive real-time glucose concentration monitoring with ATR setup (Figure 3.6b) [105].

Another approach to diabetes studies with THz radiation uses blood samples and spectral features of glucose in the THz frequency range. Blood samples from a specimen rat with diabetes have lower absorption coefficient and higher refractive index than those of healthy ones [106,107]. Blood plasma pellet samples were studied later and diabetic samples were shown to have larger refractive index and absorption coefficient [108].

Arguably the most convenient way of diabetes diagnostics was suggested by Kistenev et al. [109]. This method applies THz-TDS for breath analysis and reveals that acetone in breathed out air can be easily detected by the THz-TDS setup, and its concentration is strongly correlated with diabetes. Similar studies with CW THz setup allowed for smoker breath detection [110].

3.3.4 Reading Fingerprints with THz Radiation

Among other skin-related applications of THz, there is one rather unrelated to health. Being a high-resolution imaging approach, sub-THz CW [111] and THz-TDS [112] ATR imaging were suggested as methods for fingerprint reading.

3.4 CANCER CELL DETECTION BY THz RADIATION

Cancer screening cannot be underestimated as the most perspective approach to early-stage cancer detection [113]; however, there are certain financial burdens to direct countrywide screening implementation.

THz technology is known to be quite non-invasive, and proper instrumentation and methods could lead to more affordable and simple methods for non- or minimal-invasive population-wide cancer screening.

3.4.1 Skin Cancer

Skin cancer was the first one to be studied by THz spectroscopy and imaging [114–130]. Both melanoma and non-melanoma skin cancer have been studied for THz properties. Various THz techniques including reflectometry, time-domain spectroscopy, and 3D imaging have been employed to study human or mice skin samples. In addition, THz pulsed imaging has also been used to study inflammation and scarred skin tissues [131]. Woodward et al. [114] used TPI in reflection setting (Figure 3.6c) to study contrast between normal and diseased skin cells. Time post-pulse algorithm is used to study contrast, and differentiate among the skin tissues. *In vitro* basal cell carcinoma (BCC) samples imaged with TPI showed better contrast between normal and cancer part of the sample with many similarities in histology in comparison. At the same time, the *in vivo* THz imaging of human skin cells highlighted the ability of TPI to measure hydration and thickness of SC along with topographic features of the surface. They further used the reflection TPI to study relative THz absorption (relative change in THz absorption as compared to normal tissue) by the normal, inflamed, and cancerous skin tissues [115]. The *in vitro* samples showed higher absorption (see Figure 3.9 from [115]) of THz by normal tissue for frequencies up to 0.5 THz as compared with cancer and inflamed tissue samples. At the same time, frequency domain analysis showed almost no variation in relative absorption of THz for cancer and inflamed tissue and only very slight variation for frequencies <0.4THz. The same research group further applied TPI in reflection mode to study the 21 *ex vivo* samples [116]. The sample set had four control samples and were unknown during imaging. The authors published clear contrast in tumor and normal tissue parts of the samples investigated. Only the control samples showed no regions of contrast as expected. The tumor regions identified with THz (0.1–2.7 THz) imaging in each sample correlated well with histology and showed same or better demarcation of the tumor extent in comparison to visible light imaging (see Figure 3.10 from [116]). The authors suggest that the origin of contrast in THz images is due to increased THz absorption in the tumor tissue either due to increased interstitial water content or variation in vibrational modes of water.

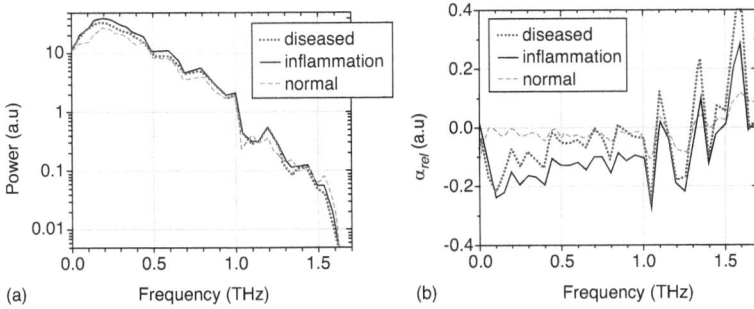

FIGURE 3.9   (a) The mean raw power spectrum and (b) the relative THz absorption α_{rel} of the selected regions of tissue [115] ©Kluwer Academic Publishers.

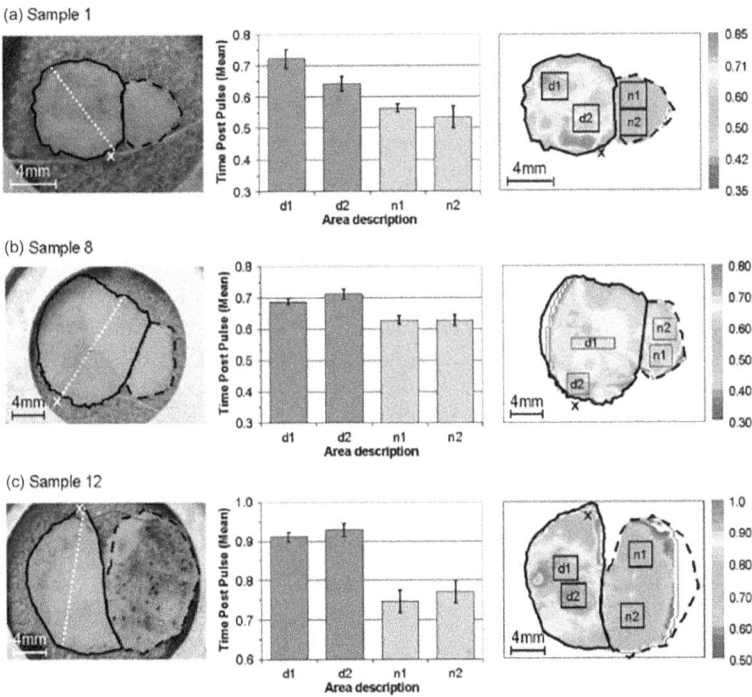

FIGURE 3.10   Visible and THz images. A comparison between the visible images, on the left, and the THz images, on the right, of samples 1, 8, and 12 (a, b, and c). The diseased tissue, on the left of the visible image, is marked by a solid boundary, and the normal tissue on the right by a dashed boundary. The dotted white line indicates the axis of the vertical histology section. The white 'x' marks the location of the suture. The histograms show the mean TPP value, and the error bars its resultant standard deviation in the areas highlighted by the boxes in the THz images, in which 'x' marks the location of the suture. Equal size areas d1 and d2 were located on the diseased tissue, and n1 and n2 on the normal tissue. ([116] ©The Society for Investigative Dermatology, Inc.)

These imaging observations generated interest in the scientific community to study THz interaction with normal human skin as well as cancerous skin. Wallace et al. [117] performed the first of such study using THz pulse spectroscopy to shed some light on the contrast observed in previously mentioned TPI images. THz parameters i.e. refractive index (n) and absorption coefficient (α) were extracted for the freshly excised skin samples, in a total of 23 samples of which 13 were diseased samples. They used THz frequency range from 0.2 THz to 2.0 THz to demonstrate that both α and n are different for cancerous samples and closer to THz response of water thus indicating increased water content in such tissue. It is also shown by the authors that the two properties find strong/maximal expression in different THz frequency range. While higher absorption for diseased tissue is evident for frequencies 1THz and above, greater difference in refractive index between two types of tissue samples is more evident at frequencies below 1 THz. At the same time by estimating the percentage difference between the THz properties of both sample types, 0.5 THz is seen to be the optimal frequency for observing both the absorption (see Figure 3.11 from [117]) and refractive index (see Figure 3.12 from [117]).

Imaging as a tool to assist/guide in accurate resection by improved delineation of cancer regions is one of the key goals for the non-invasive

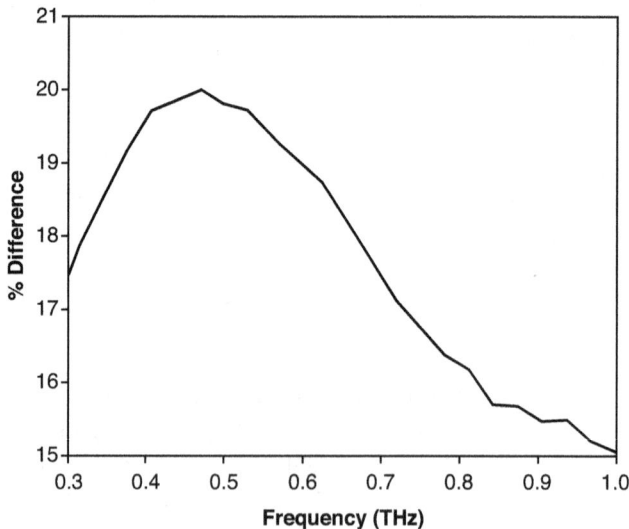

FIGURE 3.11   Normalized percentage difference in absorption between diseased and normal tissue. The maximum difference of 20% occurs at 0.5 THz. ([117] ©Society for Applied Spectroscopy.)

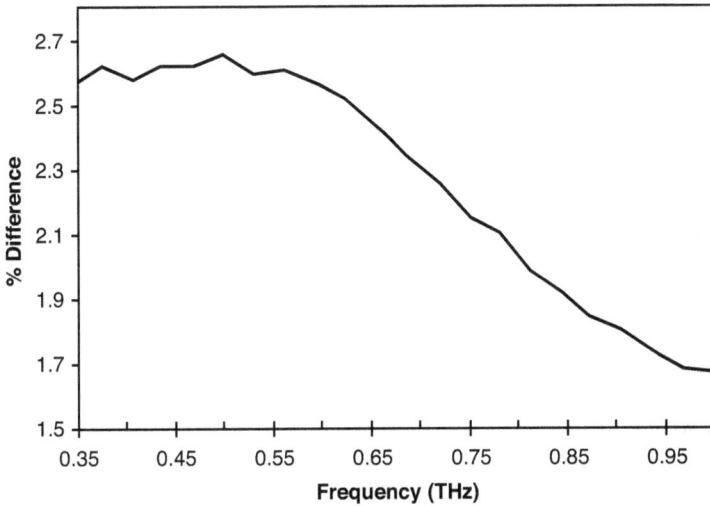

FIGURE 3.12 Normalized percentage difference in refractive index between diseased and healthy tissue. The maximum percentage difference of 2.6% lies between 0.35 and 0.55 THz. ([117] ©Society for Applied Spectroscopy.)

technologies under study including THz imaging. A study done by Joseph et al. [119] used a combination of optical (400 nm) and THz (CW, 0.584 THz, 10.23 mW average power) imaging to leverage the advantages of resolution and contrast, respectively, offered by the two technologies. Polarization-sensitive CW terahertz images and optical images were compared with histology for nine skin cancer samples (6 BCC and 3 SCC). The samples were images within 6 hours of Mohs micrographic surgeries. Dehydration is prevented using salination solution (pH 7.4). Reflected radiation of linearly polarized incident beams (for both THz and optical setups) from the sample is collected in cross-polarized and co-polarized regimes. Images generated with cross-polarized reflection, for THz, from the sample produced an image with better correlation with H & E histopathology for the regions of cancer and provided better contrast between normal and cancer regions (for more detail, see figure 3 in [119]). However, polarization difference images and cross-polarized images generated with optical imaging offered better morphological details due to better resolution (for more detail, see figure 4 in [119]). Thus, more accurately identifying the extent of cancer spread. The authors also reported lower THz reflectivity from cancer cells (for more detail, see figure 7 in [119]). Such observation is in contrast to other previous reports. Higher THz absorption due to increased water content and loss of skin structure (for cancerous region) reducing refractive index fluctuations for long THz wavelength.

At the same time, studies using terahertz pulsed spectroscopy (TPS) is done to differentiate between dysplastic and non-dysplastic skin nevi. Zaitsev et al. [120] proposed a method to extract dielectric parameters and permittivity from spectroscopic data *in vivo*. A comparison, using the said method, of dielectric complex permittivity for normal skin, dysplastic nevi, and non-dysplastic nevi revealed a difference in permittivity of the three types of skin at higher THz frequencies of 0.85–0.95 THz (see Figure 3.13) [120]. For frequencies >1 THz, scattering of THz due to skin inhomogeneity poses a restriction. Referring to double Debye model, which describes complex permittivity for skin [126], the origin of the observed difference is linked to different relaxation processes in the three type of skin under study [120]. Scattering of THz by Rskin cancer tissue can be useful for developing detection systems or algorithms for imaging in THz regime. A simple procedure to study such scattering using double Debye model is demonstrated by Huang et al. [126]. They used Born approximation and discrete complex image method to calculate scattered fields. Such fields are calculated with an understanding that in such simulations the skin organ can be treated as homogeneous

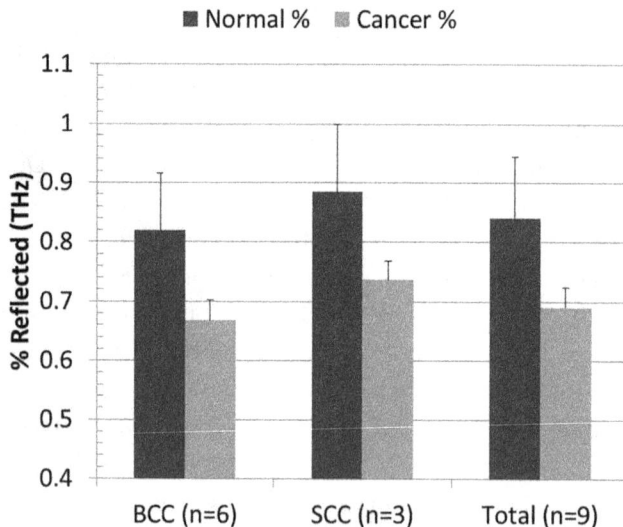

FIGURE 3.13 Normal and cancer mean terahertz reflectivity values (%), averaged over all BCC, SCC, and total samples. ([117] ©WILEY-VCH Verlag GmbH & Co. KGaA, Weinheim.)

layered media and any abnormalities like BCC on such a media can be seen as a slight change in complex permittivity.

THz-based technologies for early detection of cancer have shown signs of promise, and for them to be used as diagnostic tools still a substantial research is needed. In the case of skin cancer, Rahman et al. [121] tried to use THz reflectometry, 3D imaging, and TDS as a combination for early detection of BCC. A significant difference is observed between the normal and BCC skin samples when the thickness profile of these skin samples (up to 1.2 mm) is probed with THz scanning reflectometry. The diminished presence of multi-layer reflection (skin is a layered organ) and lower overall reflection from BCC as compared to normal skin indicate loss of regular pattern in BCC samples [121]. The lower reflectance values from BCC samples are attributed to increased absorption of THz frequencies. Next, using a transmission TDS system and Eigen frequency analysis characteristic absorption spectra for BCC and normal skin sample is revealed. It can be seen from Figures 3.14 and 3.15 [119] that a few of the peaks visible in the absorption spectra of normal skin are missing from BCC spectra. It is also of note that the time-domain spectrum of the transmitted pulse through the two samples are quite dissimilar (see figure 6 and 7 in [121]). The two measurements i.e. reflectometry and TDS provide complimentary information in terms of higher absorbance (by TDS) and low reflectance (by reflectometry) for BCC samples. THz 3D-reconstructed imaging is used by the authors to generate layer-by-layer images for both types of samples. The images, as expected, revealed a clear pattern for normal skin while the same was lacking for BCC samples. This study shows the promise of THz-based technologies in identifying BCC from normal skin; however, before it is to be used as a non-invasive diagnostic tool further investigations are needed to establish differences between, for example, a mole and melanoma and similar questions.

The 3D reconstructive reflectance imaging as discussed in [121] is used to demonstrate dissimilarity of structure and pattern among normal, BCC, and SCC skin samples [127]. An image of the sample structure from reflected THz is constructed using modified Beer–Lambert's law for 3D data matrix and "gridding with inverse distance to power equations". The generated images showed non-uniformity of pattern in BCC and SCC samples as compared to healthy skin. A uniform and linear pattern is observed from images of normal skin whereas images of BCC sample revealed lobular structures along the depth of the sample and non-uniformity in the linear pattern otherwise (see Figure 3.16 [127]). Moreover,

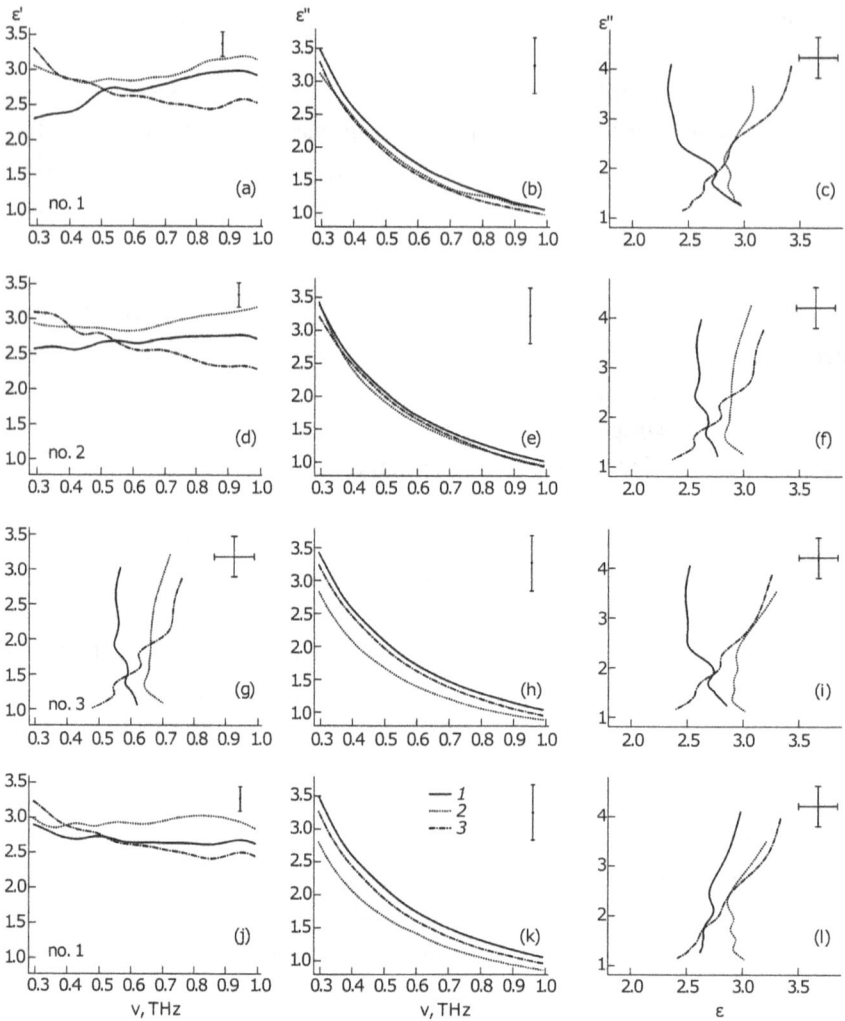

FIGURE 3.14 Spectral curves of permittivities of (solid lines) healthy skin $\tilde{\varepsilon}_S$, (dashed lines) dysplastic nevi $\tilde{\varepsilon}_D$, and (dashed-and-dotted lines) non-dysplastic nevi $\tilde{\varepsilon}_N$ for four patients: (a), (d), (g), and (j) real parts ε' and (b), (e), (h), and (k) imaginary parts ε'' of complex permittivity $\tilde{\varepsilon}$ and (c), (f), (i), and (l) Cole–Cole diagrams $\varepsilon''(\varepsilon')$ based on the THz dielectric characteristics of tissues. ([120] © Pleiades Publishing, Ltd., 2015.)

change in cellularity and epidermis is seen in BCC samples at higher magnification (50 μm × 50 μm), whereas corneocytes can be seen in normal skin at the same magnification. These observations with THz 3D reconstructive imaging shows its potential as an early diagnostic tool in future.

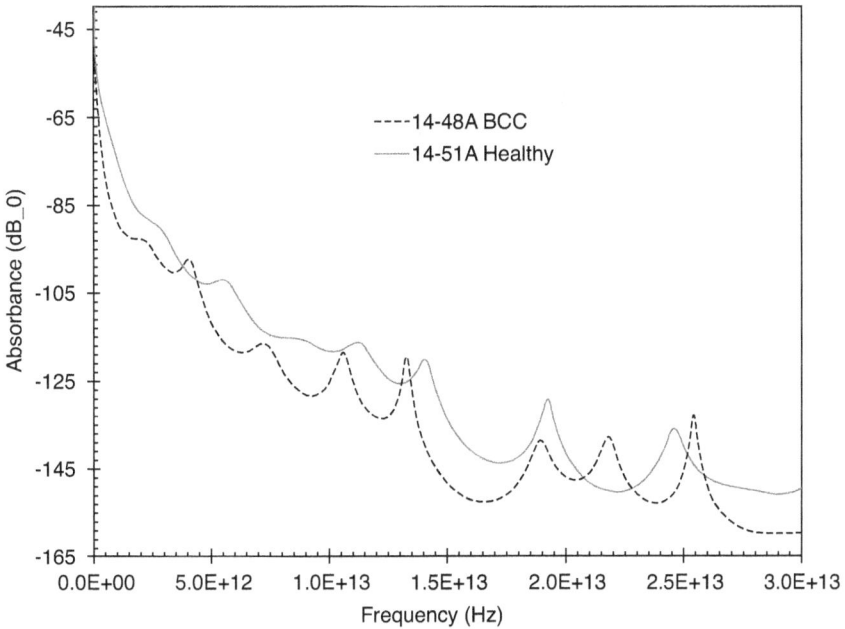

FIGURE 3.15 Eigen frequency absorbance spectra of healthy and cancerous skin samples. Healthy skin shows lower absorbance compared to the BCC skin. However, some of the peaks of the healthy skin sample are not present in the BCC sample. The thickness of the measured healthy skin samples is 1.2 mm and that of the BCC samples is 1.4mm. ([121] ©Elsevier B.V.)

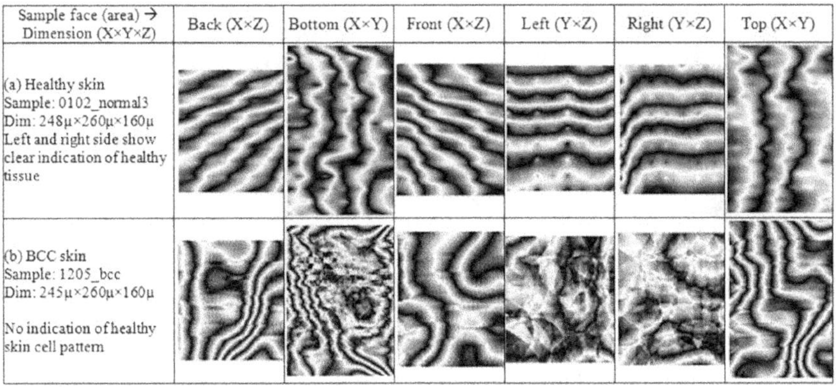

FIGURE 3.16 These images are the six faces of 3D reconstructions of (row-a) healthy skin and (row-b) basal cell carcinoma. Scanned volume is as shown for the respective specimen. ([127] ©.)

Similar to [119,121], the idea of using a combination of non-invasive technologies for investigation of skin cancer to obtain better, precise, and informative data or images is also adopted by Fan et al. [123]. They used TPI and optical imaging combined on eight BCC samples of residual cancer for better delineation between healthy and diseased skin. The images obtained using TPI and polarized reflectance optical imaging at 410 nm showed good correlation with histology. The TPI and optical images were obtained as explained in [123]. The TPI images were obtained at 0.47 THz and the choice of frequency was informed from [115]. The optical images were obtained in pairs of co- and cross-polarization. As can be seen in Figure 3.17 from [123] the TPI images, generated from power values of THz signal, are in good correlation with both histology and optical images in terms of location and dimensions of the affected areas. At the same time the limitation in resolution of TPI-generated images is evident from the

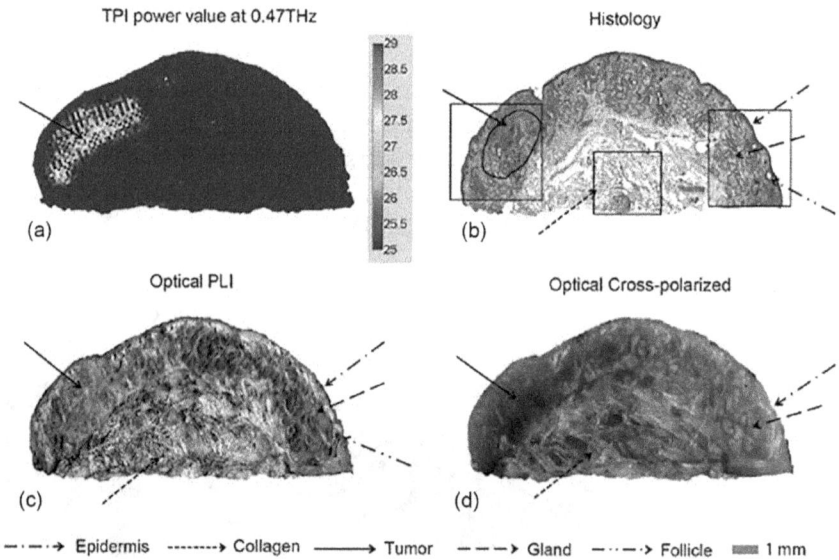

FIGURE 3.17 Images of a representative skin sample with basal cell carcinoma. (a) Terahertz power value image obtained at 0.47 THz. (b) H & E-stained histology image of a 5 mm thick section of the tissue. Tumor region is outlined with solid black line. The images of the areas outlined by the squares are presented in Figure 6. (c) Optical polarized light image (PLI). (d) Optical cross-polarized image. Solid arrow indicates tumor site, dash arrow indicates gland, dotted arrow indicates collagen, and dash-dot-dash arrow indicates epidermis. Scale bar is 1 mm. ([123] ©Wiley Periodicals, Inc.)

lack of morphological detail which can be clearly seen in optical images of both polarization. This contrast was even better highlighted in magnified images. It is also noted that optical images can complement THz-generated images in cases where a false positive of normal region as cancer region comes up with TPI. In studies by Fan et al. [123], they noted two occasions of false positives where TPI images highlighted more regions as affected than real. In such cases, optical images were useful to highlight the difference. The reason behind these false positives is speculated to be trapped water or inflammation; however, further studies are required to ascertain the correct reasons which can then inform on improved protocol for such imaging techniques. Nonetheless, this work highlights the capabilities and promise of THz technologies in isolation and in combination toward identification of skin cancer.

THz time-domain spectroscopy imaging has been used to generate THz images for identification of melanoma in BALB/c mouse skin samples infected with B16 melanoma [129]. This is verified with optical images and H&E stained images of the samples. Higher refractive index and absorption coefficient is referred to be the reason for the contrast observed between melanoma and normal skin in THz images. The same is confirmed by the authors by calculating both the refractive index and absorption coefficient for the samples using THz-TDS in transmission mode. The time-domain transmission spectra of melanoma tissue shows larger time delay as compared to normal tissue indicating higher refractive index. Next, using mass weighing method as explained in [129], the water content of adipose and melanoma tissue is calculated, and it is found that melanoma tissue has higher water content. From the H&E staining images it is also seen that the number of cell nuclei for melanoma is far more than normal adipose, thus increasing the cellular density in the affected region leading to higher refractive index. In summary, Li et al. [129], using accepted available different methodologies, deliberated on the causes/reasons for higher refractive index and absorption coefficient for melanoma tissue which provides contrast in THz images.

3.4.2 Breast Cancer

Breast cancer is the second most studied cancer type with THz radiation. First experimental data date back to 2006 when Fitzgerald et al. [132] studied 22 samples of excised human breast tissue specimens. The experiments were done in reflection and found that THz potentially can be used for discrimination between cancerous and healthy tissues by their refractive index. Ashworth et al. [133] studied freshly excised breast cancerous and healthy tissues with THz-TDS in transmission (Figure 3.6a) and noticed a pronounced difference between healthy and cancer tissues of around 10% in absorption coefficient (cancer tissue being less transparent) and 8% in refractive index.

Chen et al. [134,135] used a CW THz setup in transmission (Figure 3.7a) at 108 GHz, for imaging cancer tissue *in vivo*. YIG oscillator was used is the THz source, and Schottky diode detected the radiation. As shown in Figure 3.18, the tumor is clearly visible as it has about 50% larger absorption coefficient than surrounding tissue. St. Peter et al. [136] presented the results of CW THz imaging of excised human malignant and benign breast tissues in normal reflection layout with THz gas laser operating at 1.89 THz as a source. Refractive index of the tissues was extracted from the THz reflectivity of the sample Γ from Fresnel reflection as $|\Gamma|^2 = \left(\dfrac{n-1}{n+1}\right)$.

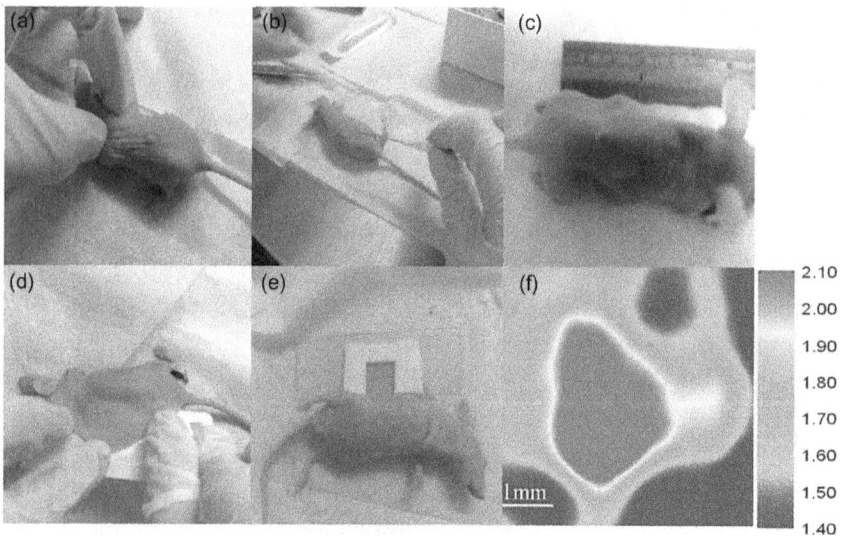

FIGURE 3.18 (a)–(e) Photos of a mouse taken during preparation: (a) A visible breast tumor with a size about 2.1 mm×3.2 mm×1.3 mm developed on the 46th day after the cancer cell implantation; (b)–(c) Fat implantation; (d)–(e) Stretched mouse dorsal skin with area 15 mm×10 mm and sandwiched by 2 mm cover glasses. (f) *In vivo* THz imaging of a visible cancer in mouse dorsal skin. The color bar is defined as α from 1.4 to 2.1 mm^{-1}. (Reprinted from [134] © 2011 Optical Society of America under the terms of the OSA Open Access Publishing Agreement.)

Since cancer is the most reflective among studied tissue types, a refractive index threshold value was selected to discriminate it automatically in post-processing. Further comparison with histological maps superimposed onto optical images of the tissue showed a very decent ability of the THz imaging to discriminate cancer tissues with automatic post-processing.

Bowman et al. [137–145] used THz-TDS in reflection (Figure 3.6c) to study dehydrated and freshly excised breast cancer tumors. Time-of-flight analysis of the reflected THz signal allowed for 3D reconstruction of the tumor volume, and authors developed an image-processing routine that enhances the distinguishability between cancer and healthy tissues by adding a dynamic range and further edge detection. Later, they applied a supervised regression approach for image classification.

Figure 3.19 shows results of such classification. Receiver operating characteristic (ROC) curves were obtained by pixel-by-pixel comparison, and a very high classification ability can be seen for formalin-fixed, paraffin-embedded (FFPE) tissues and for the first presented sample. Results from transgenic mice [139] demonstrated that only 50% of the 15 fresh tumors had reasonable correlation between THz images and pathology, which is consistent with earlier works of the group. Further works on larger number of samples [141] and separate spatial plots for refractive index and absorption coefficient showed even better consistency, having demonstrated that collagen areas had higher refractive index than fat, with cancer areas still showing the greatest refraction index among all tissues. Further studies involved a dimension reduction for low-dimensional ordered orthogonal projection-based machine-learning approach to tissue classification [143], supervised Bayesian-learning model [144], and an established protocol for THz imaging of freshly excised breast cancer tumors [142]. Rootendorst et al. [146] used a quartz prism-enhanced THz-TDS setup in reflection and developed two alternative approaches to classifications of the reflected impulse functions as malignant or benign – one using heuristic parameters in combination with support vector machine (SVM) classification and another based on Gaussian wavelet deconvolution with Bayesian classification. The results were quite comparable to the ones shown by Prof. El-Shenawee's group, with accuracy, sensitivity, and specificity of 75%, 86%, and 66% for the first method, and 69%, 87%, and 54% for the second method, respectively, but the apparatus used is more adjusted for *in vivo* THz imaging. Wavelet packet transform and machine learning-based classification of THz-TDS transmission data of paraffin-embedded tissue samples was proposed by Liu et al. [147]. Using index of energy to Shannon

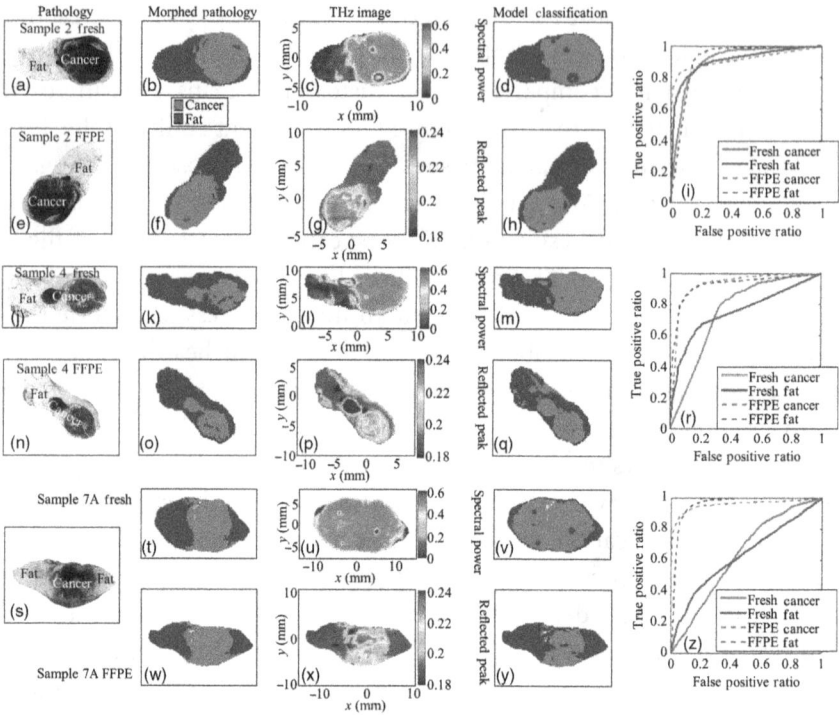

FIGURE 3.19   Correlation results for tumor samples 2, 4, and 7A. For tumor sample 2, images (b–d) for freshly excised tumor tissue and images (f–h) for formalin-fixed, paraffin-embedded (FFPE) tissue: (a) pathology image, (b) morphed pathology mask, (c) THz image, and (d) t-distribution model classification; (e) pathology image [same as in (a)], (f) morphed pathology mask, (g) THz image, and (h) t-distribution model classification; and (i) the receiver operating characteristic (ROC) curves. For tumor sample 4, images (k–m) for fresh tissue and images (o–q) for FFPE tissue: (j) pathology image, (k) morphed pathology mask, (l) THz image, and (m) t-distribution model classification; (n) pathology image, (o) morphed pathology mask, (p) THz image, and (q) t-distribution model classification; and (r) the ROC curves. For tumor sample 7A, images (t–v) for fresh tissue and images (w–y) for FFPE tissue: (s) pathology image, (t) morphed pathology mask, (u) THz image, and (v) t-distribution model classification; (w) morphed pathology mask, (x) THz image, and (y) t-distribution model classification; and (z) the ROC curves. (Reprinted from [138] © 2018 The Authors. Published by SPIE under a Creative Commons Attribution 3.0 Unported License.)

entropy ratio as the main parameter, they demonstrated accuracy, sensitivity, and specificity of 92.85%, 89.66%, and 96.67%, respectively. Morphological dilation combined with refractive index thresholding allowed Cassar et al. to classify the tissue regions with a sensitivity of around 80% and a specificity of 82% [148].

A very different approach to metastatic breast cancer cell detection was suggested by Hassan et al. [149]. It is called THz chemical microscopy (TCM) or scanning point terahertz source (SPoTS) microscopy, and is a variation of a THz-TDS setup with sample placed directly onto the unbiased THz emitter plate. Unprecedented resolution is achieved by scanning the emitter with a tightly focused IR pump. The authors proved that TCM using aptamers as ligands have a limit of detection as small as one breast cancer cell in 100 μL of sample. A similar system was used by Okada et al. [150], with minor difference in the emitter material, and simultaneous measurement of transmitted and reflected signals. They report visualization of micrometric (~250 μm) inhomogeneities of cancer cell density.

Nowadays, histologic verification of the surgical resection margin is done after the operation, and as a result 20%–70% of procedures must be repeated [136,146], THz imaging, providing the ability to discriminate malignant and benign tissues, can become a very helpful tool for operational real-time monitoring.

3.4.3 Brain Cancer

In the case of brain tumors the ability to distinguish and delineate normal tissue from tumor tissue is critical. Toward this, THz spectroscopy and imaging is being explored for brain gliomas [151–163]. The focus of these techniques is to make use of non-ionizing nature and response of tissue/cell components in the THz range. It is understood that the changes that occur in glioma tissues change their refractive index, absorption coefficient, and dielectric permittivity when compared to normal tissues. THz sources in the range of 0.1–4 THz have been used to study these changes with a goal of delineating healthy tissues from diseased.

THz absorption of water is well known and investigations are done to exploit this property to differentiate glioma tissues (and other cancer types) based on variation of water content [159]. At the same time, frozen tissues and dehydrated paraffin-embedded normal and glioma tissues are investigated to study the variation in refractive index ($n(\omega)$), absorption coefficient ($\alpha(\omega)$), and complex dielectric permittivity ($\varepsilon(\omega)$) by removing the effect of absorption by water (interstitial or otherwise) [152]. For such embedded samples, authors in [152] used transmission THz spectroscopy to extract the aforementioned three parameters (n, α, and ε) from 20 samples (both normal and glioma) of thickness in the range of 1–2.5 mm.

They observed that n and α for normal tissue samples is smaller than glioma samples, indicating that this difference in parameters for two types of tissues is due to cell morphology and cellular components. It is also noted by the authors that the real and imaginary part of ε showed a better contrast when relative rates of variation are considered. Based on this they proposed to use real part of ε for higher THz frequencies (1.5–2.0 THz) and imaginary part of ε for lower THz frequencies (<1.0 THz, especially 0.55 THz) for a THz-imaging system based on complex dielectric permittivity (see Figure 3.20b) [152].

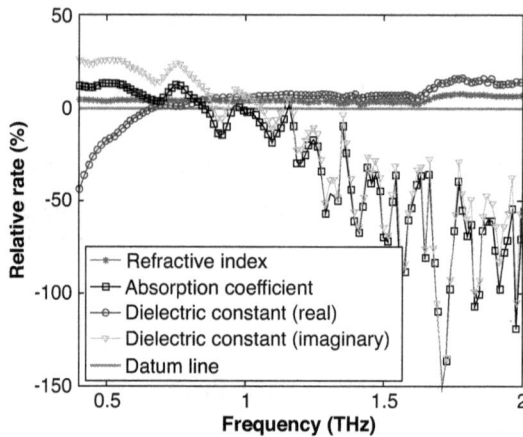

(a)

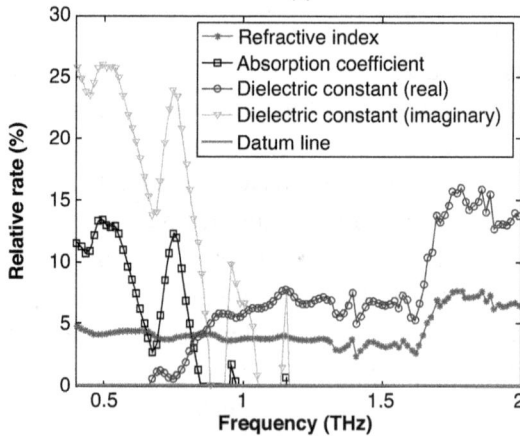

(b)

FIGURE 3.20 Relative rates of the refractive index, absorption coefficient, and dielectric constant. (a) The full curves and (b) the positive portions of the curves. ([152] © The Authors. Published by SPIE under a Creative Commons Attribution 3.0 Unported License.)

It is well regarded that brain glioma (and other cancer types viz. cervical, colorectal, etc.) has different water content as compared to normal tissues. The same has been argued for traumatic brain injury by Zhao et al. [154]. The authors in [154] imaged rat brain models with traumatic injury classified as sham, mild, moderate, and severe using THz CW imaging at 2.52 THz, magnetic resonance imaging (MRI), and white light. The *in-vivo* THz images of freshly excised brain samples correspond to the MRI images in distinguishing between three levels of injury and no injury (see Figure 3.21 [154]). It also highlights the contrast between white and gray matter of the brain samples in the sham group. This contrast is attributed to higher THz transmission from white matter areas which in turn is suggested to be due to the predominant lipid composition of myelin. A further investigation of absorption coefficient using THz-TDS of paraffin-embedded samples revealed that absorption coefficient increased with the severity of injury. However, clear distinction between mild and moderate injury cannot be made due to overlapping error bars. Nonetheless, this study highlighted that THz imaging is capable of producing meaningful

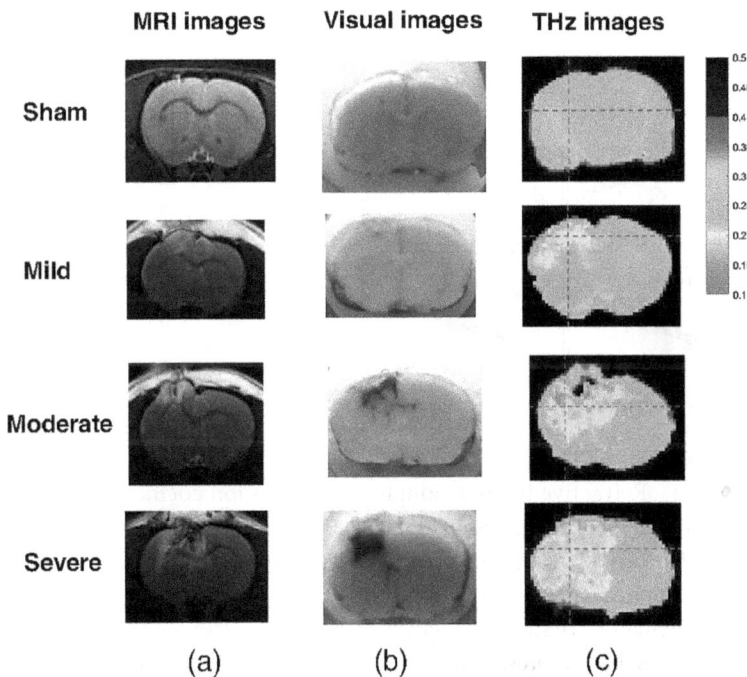

FIGURE 3.21 (a) MR (Magnetic Resonance), (b) visual, and (c) THz images of fresh brain tissues without and with different degrees of Traumatic brain injury (TBI). ([154] © 2018 Society of Photo Optical Instrumentation Engineers (SPIE).)

images and the absorption coefficient variation also shows that change in cell density most likely has nominal effect on THz absorption.

Another approach using gelatin for embedding the tissue has been used in [157]. The rationale is to prevent hydration changes of the tissue, and hence freshly excised tissues can be studied even after several hours without affecting its THz response. The authors in [157] used THz pulse system in reflection to extract n and α (in classical electrodynamics these two parameters can fully define wave–tissue interaction), *ex vivo*, from 26 human glioma samples. The glioma samples were graded I to IV as per WHO grading. The authors noted that while distinguishing between different grades of glioma as well as edematous and glioma tissues, the dispersion of n and α over the spectral range of 0.2 THz to 1.5 THz is evident in Figure 3.22 [157]. Dispersion of optical properties for grade IV (glioblastoma) were attributed to necrotic debris related inhomogeneity in the tissues. The authors also argue that instrument resolution could be a limiting factor for dispersion recorder for 0.3 THz or lower frequencies. Also, lack of resonant features for frequencies above 0.8 THz in tissues is argued to decouple the dispersion of n and α for these frequencies. Gavdush et al. in 2021 [160] in continuation

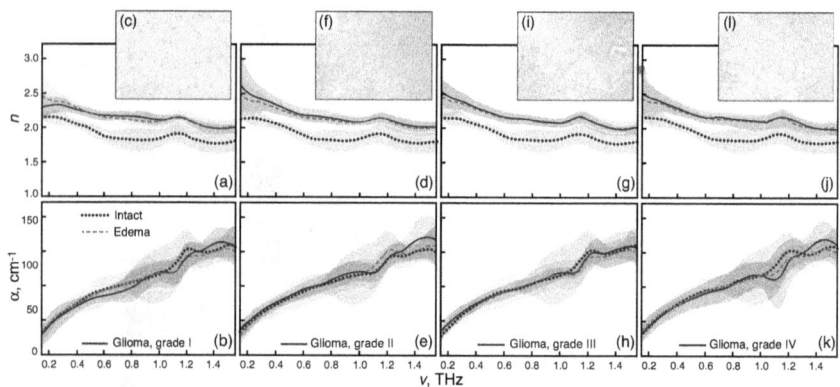

FIGURE 3.22 Refractive index n, amplitude absorption coefficient α, and H & E-stained histology of gelatin embedded human brain gliomas of different WHO grades *ex vivo*: (a)–(c) grade I; (d)–(f) grade II; (g)–(i) grade III; and (j)–(l) grade IV. The THz optical properties of gliomas are compared with equal data for the intact and edematous tissues, averages within the entire set of brain tissues specimens. The error bars represent a ±2.0σ confidential interval of measurements, assuming fluctuation of optical properties within each tissue sample and each tissue class. ([157] © The Authors. Published by SPIE under a Creative Commons Attribution 4.0 Unported License.)

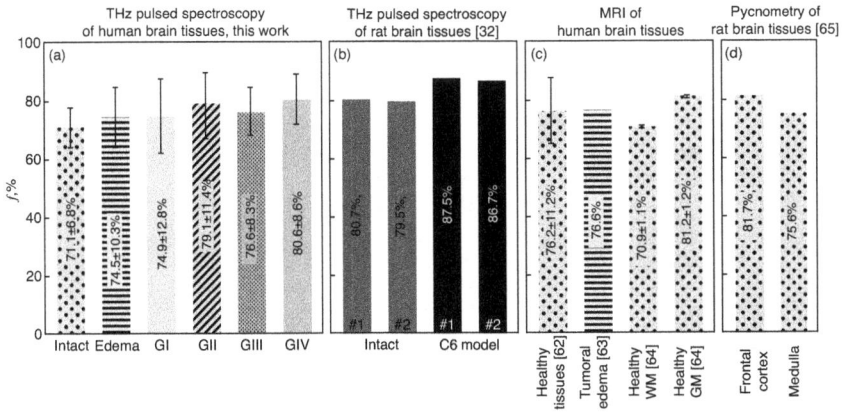

FIGURE 3.23 Water content in healthy and pathological tissues of the brain measured using different experimental techniques: (a) intact tissues, edema, and WHO Grade I–IV gliomas of the human brain *ex vivo* measured by the THz-pulsed spectroscopy in this work; (b) intact tissues and C6 glioma model from rat brain *ex vivo* measured by the THz-pulsed spectroscopy in Ref. [164]; (c) healthy human brain tissues and tumoral edema *in vivo* measured by MRI in Refs. [62–64], where WM and GM stand for white matter and gray matter, respectively; (d) healthy rat brain tissues *ex vivo* measured by a pycnometer in Ref. [65]. Here, error bars represent fluctuations of water content within the considered set of tissue specimens. ([160] © 2020 Optical Society of America under the terms of the OSA Open Access Publishing Agreement.)

to their previous work presented results showing the feasibility of using Double-Debye and double-overdamped-oscillator model to describe THz–brain tissue interactions. In particular, these models were used to estimate water content (see Figure 3.23 [160]) in intact and glioma tissues (WHO grade I-IV) of human brain by estimating the ratio of real and imaginary part of the complex dielectric permittivity (data measured using THz spectroscopy) [160].

CW THz reflection imaging (TRI) is used by Wu et al. [158] to distinguish orthotopic glioma and normal brain tissues in mouse. The imaging is done *in vivo* and *ex vivo* as shown in Figures 3.24 and 3.25 [158]. The THz images were compared with H&E, MRI, and white-light images and a good degree of correlation is observed between THz and other images regarding volume and location of glioma. The average reflectance values for normal and glioma regions in both *in vivo* and *ex vivo* settings differ by 5% or more. It is also noted that in THz images of *ex vivo* freshly excised samples glioma size is larger compared to MRI and H&E images.

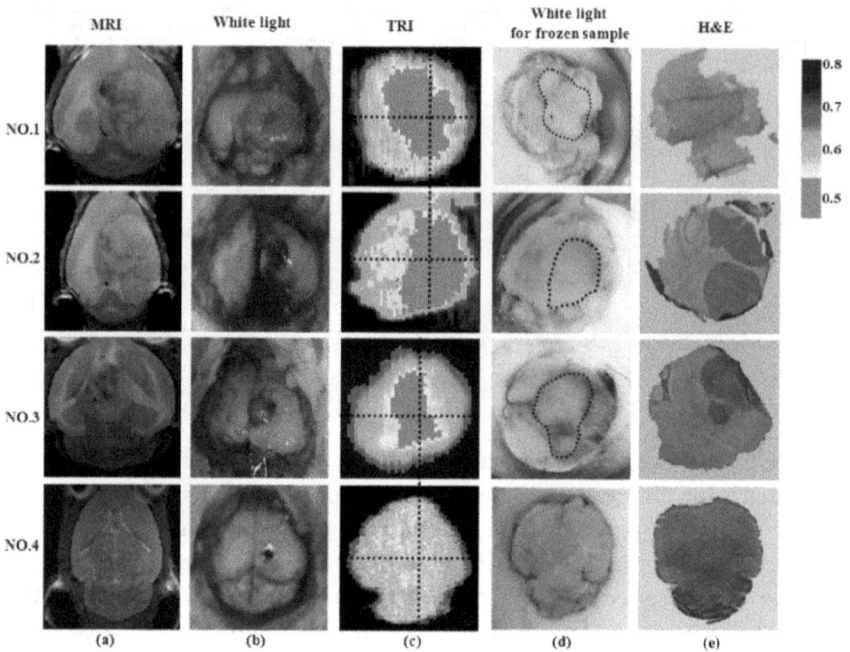

FIGURE 3.24   (a) MR, (b) visual of *in vivo*, (c) THz reflection, (d) visual of fresh excised and (e) H & E-stained images of whole brain images with (Nos. 1–3) and without (No. 4) tumors. ([158] © 2019 Optical Society of America under the terms of the OSA Open Access Publishing Agreement.)

Two probable reasons, namely lack of spatial resolution and non-discrimination of perifocal edema from normal tissue, are cited. They further used THz-TDS (0.6 THz - 2.8 THz) for studying spectral differences, namely n and α between two types of tissues and observed higher values for these parameters for glioma in comparison to normal tissues (see Figure 3.26) which is enhanced at higher THz frequencies [158].

THz reflection imaging is also used by Ji et al. to study *ex vivo* glioma. After establishing the feasibility of THz imaging with four *ex vivo* mouse samples in comparison with MRI, white light, OCT, fluorescence (ppIX and GFP), and H&E, it was used to study 14 human glioma samples [153]. In the mouse samples a good correlation between high-intensity areas of THz images and H&E and GFP fluorescence images is noted (see Figure 3.27) [153]. In human samples, a THz parameter (TP) "as a spectrum amplitude ratio at 0.5 THz from the region of interest (ROI)" [153] is defined for quantitative analysis. The difference in TP values of normal gray (0.8104) and normal white (0.7114) matter is observed and attributed to water and lipid contents. The authors

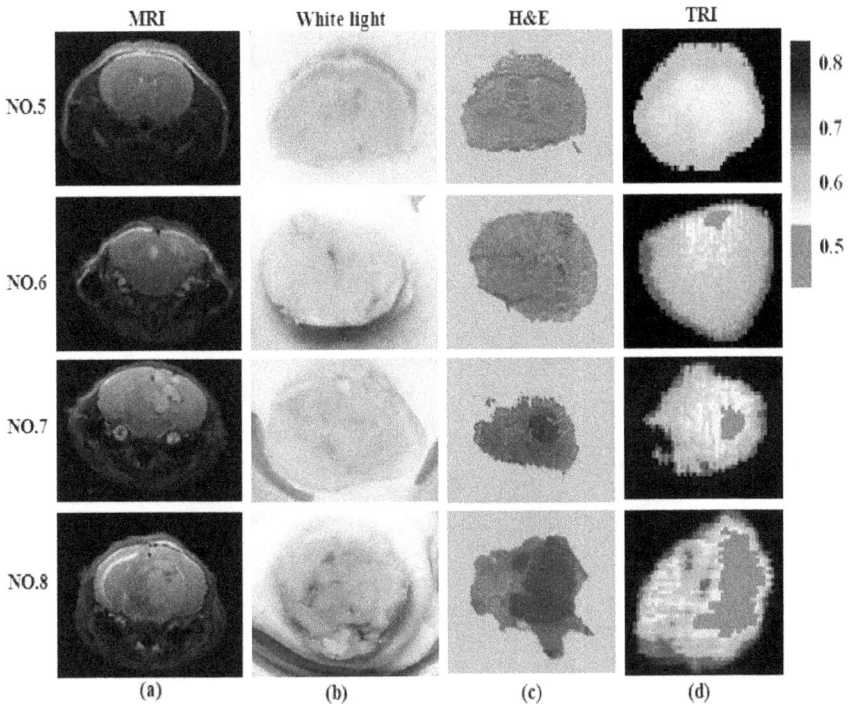

FIGURE 3.25 (a) MR, (b) Visual, (c) H & E-stained and (d) terahertz reflection images of fresh excised brain tissues without (No. 5) and with (Nos. 6–8) tumors. ([158] © 2019 Optical Society of America under the terms of the OSA Open Access Publishing Agreement.)

further define two TP values as threshold values TH1 and TH2 (corresponding to TP values+mean standard deviation+(a number)) to discriminate between tumor and normal cells (see Figure 3.28). In Figure 3.28c [153] the areas marked with a black square and the corresponding alphabet A-G along with the same gray scale area are tumors and they exceed TH1 values and are regarded as high-grade tumors (WHO grades III and IV). At the same time, areas immediately surrounding the above mentioned tumor areas can represent low-grade tumors (WHO grade II) or normal gray matter, and their TP values lie between TH1 and TH2. Nonetheless, the THz images reflect high sensitivity to variation of lipid and water content in different tissues. Thus, it can serve as a label-free tool for imaging glioma.

Wu et al. used CW THz reflectance imaging to differentiate and delineate orthotopic glioma and normal brain regions of mouse [162]. Toward this they first explored changes in THz optical parameters (i.e. n and α) of freshly excised brain tissues over a temperature range of −10°C to 20°C.

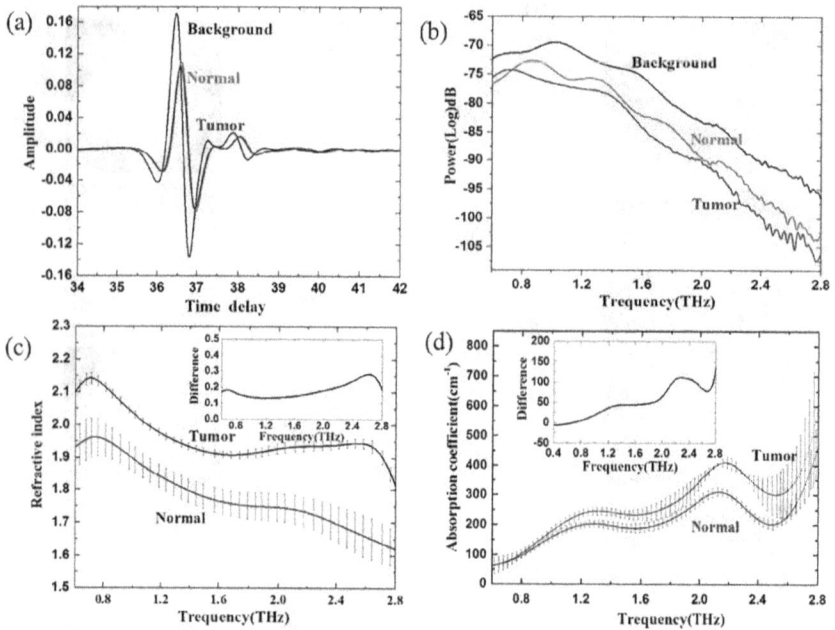

FIGURE 3.26 (a) The THz-TDS signal, (b) the power, (c) the refractive index, and (d) the absorption coefficient of the freshly excised brain tissue samples. The insets of (c) and (d) show the difference of the refractive index and the absorption coefficient between tumor and normal tissue, respectively. ([158] © 2019 Optical Society of America under the terms of the OSA Open Access Publishing Agreement.)

Using THz-TDS (0.4–2.53THz) the authors demonstrated greater variation of n at higher THz frequencies and temperatures as compared to α. Also, at all temperatures and frequencies, as expected, the refractive index and absorption coefficient of glioma regions is higher than the normal regions. Based on these observations the authors, using ATR imaging, imaged freshly excised brain tissues (see Figure 3.29c) and *in vivo* mice brain tissues (see Figure 3.30b) at 2.52 THz [162]. The highest contrast in freshly excised samples is observed for 35°C samples and the THz-ATR images were similar to the H&E images for glioma regions. The observed reduction in the size of tumor region for zero and sub-zero temperature is attributed to lower THz reflectance due to lower water content. Analysis of average reflectance revealed temperature dependence of average reflectivity in glioma, normal tissues, and water (see Figure 3.31 [162]). The *in vivo* THz-ATR images correlates well with white light/visual and H&E images thus providing a possibility of label-free technique for discriminating

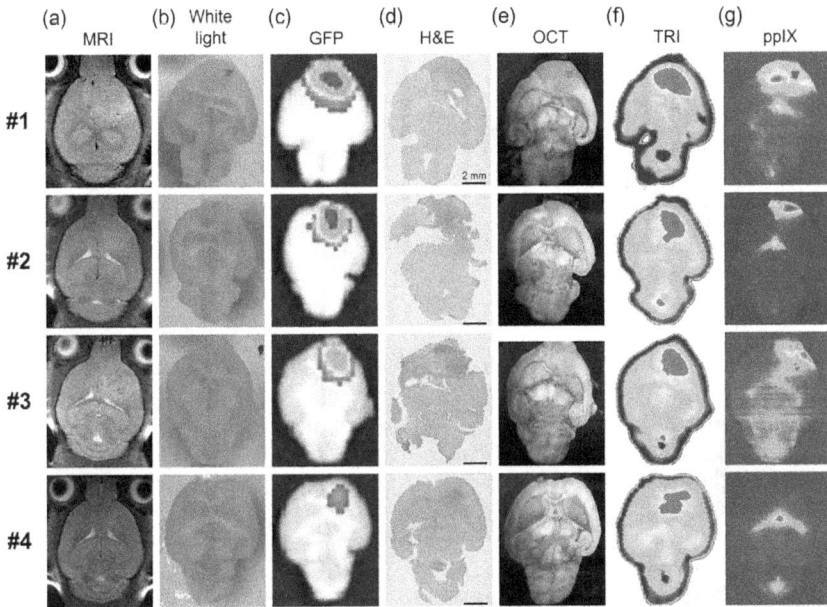

FIGURE 3.27 Tumor discrimination of enhanced green fluorescent protein (eGFP)-transfected human GBM tumorsphere (TS) (eGFP+ GSC-11) tumor-bearing mice ($n=4$) with TRI and multi-modality imaging. (a) Axial T2-weighted MRI images in living mouse for validation of tumor growth. (b) White light images of the excised brain samples. The tumors were invisible in the white light images as in human malignant gliomas. (c) GFP fluorescence images. (d) Hematoxylin and eosin (H & E)-stained image. Both modalities were used for visualization of tumor regions. (e) Optical coherence tomography (OCT) images. These images provide detailed information through the high-resolution anatomical structures. Although some regions with reduced scattering may correspond to the tumor region, it is not a common feature. (f) TRI images with peak-to-peak amplitude of time-domain signals. Relatively high-intensity regions (gray regions) in TRI images are well correlated with real tumor regions that are observed in GFP and H & E-stained images. We did not determine the precise threshold value in this preclinical experiment. (g) 5-ALA-induced ppIX fluorescence images. TRI images showed tumor regions more precisely than ppIX fluorescence images. Strong fluorescence in the center of the ppIX images of the mouse brains is emitted not from tumor but the ventricles. ([153] © The Author(s) 2016. This work is licensed under a Creative Commons Attribution 4.0 International License.)

normal and glioma tissues. At the same time, the authors note that THz-ATR imaging merits investigations for non-orthotopic models to establish its discrimination abilities for inherent complexities of glioma such as microvascularity, necrosis, etc.

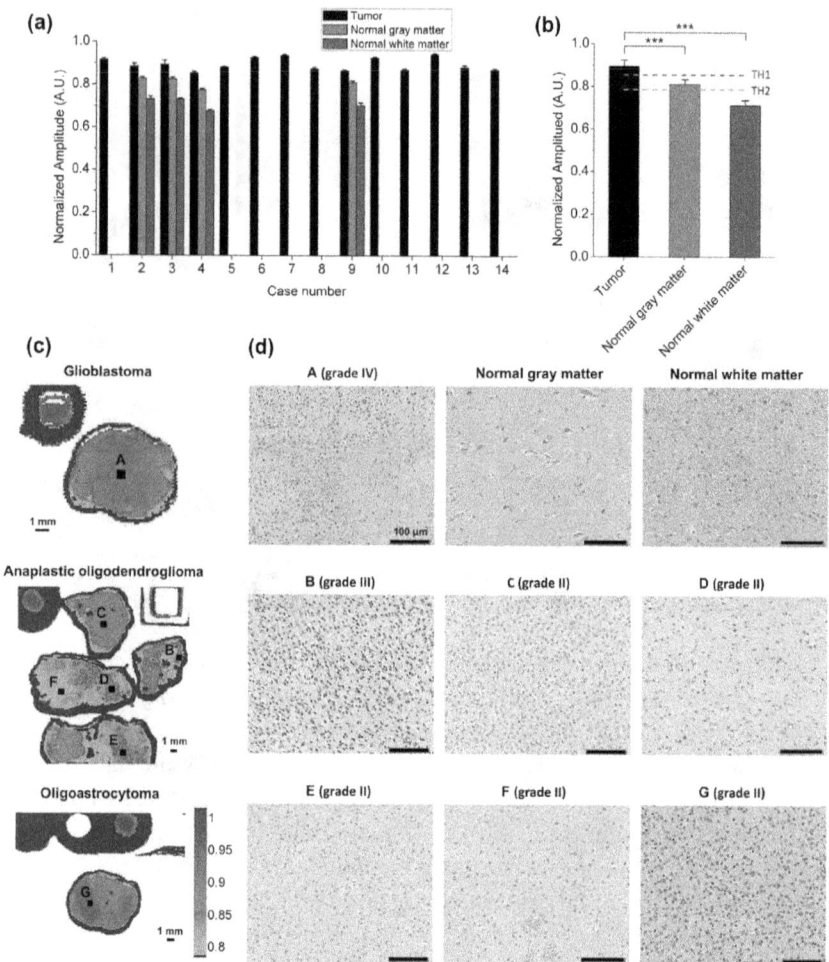

FIGURE 3.28 Discrimination of low and high grades of human gliomas with TRI. (a) Terahertz parameter (TP) values from regions of interest (ROIs) in tumors ($n = 14$), normal gray matters ($n = 4$), and normal white matters ($n = 4$). (b) Quantification of threshold value 1 (TH1) and TH2 (dashed lines,) for tumor discrimination using the data shown in (a). Data represent mean±SD. ***$P < 0.001$ (Kruskal–Wallis test.) Representative cases of grade IV, III, and II gliomas, characterized by (c) TRI images and (d) H & E-stained image. The capitals A–G shown in (d) correspond to the ROIs in (c). ([153] © The Author(s) 2016. This work is licensed under a Creative Commons Attribution 4.0 International License.)

Lastly, metamaterial-based biosensors in the THz range are an active topic of research toward discrimination of normal and glioma tissues [159]. The key change studied with these biosensors is the resonant

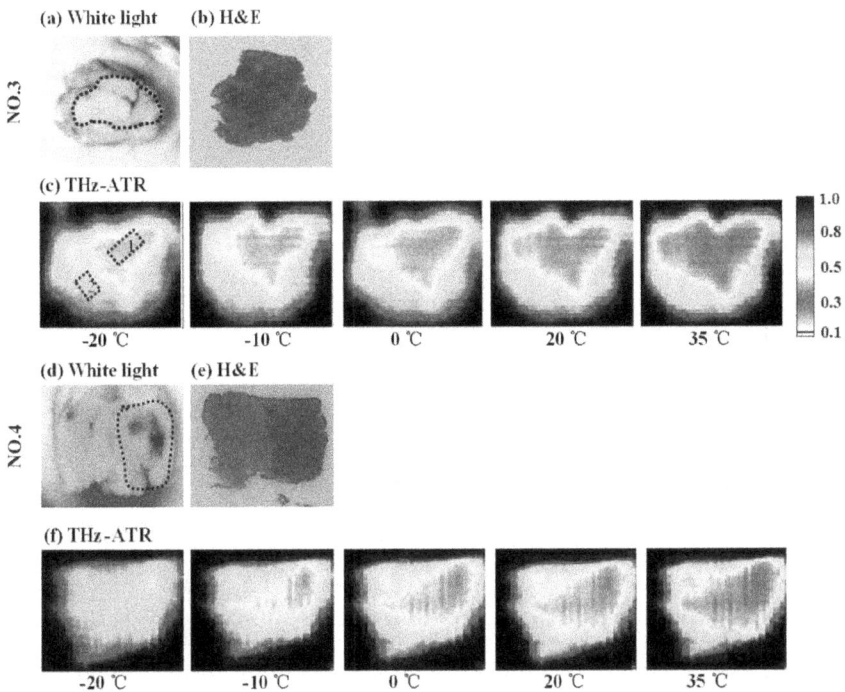

FIGURE 3.29 (a) Visual, (b) H & E-stained and (c) THz-ATR images of glioma samples at temperature of –20°C 35°C. The dark gray, light gray, and black areas of (c) and (f) were the tumor tissue, normal tissue, and background regions, respectively. The marked areas with dotted boxes 1 and 2 in (c) were the partial tumor and normal regions, respectively. ([162] © 2021 Optica Publishing Group under the terms of the Optica Open Access Publishing Agreement.)

frequency dip variation/shift in the THz spectrum of the sample/analyte. In the transmission mode, intracellular complexity, cell size, and other factors affect the resonant dip [159]. While red and blue shift of the resonant dip in transmission spectrum is being actively looked into as a characteristic feature to discriminate glioma, variation of magnitude of this dip has also been suggested to be considered simultaneously [161]. Zhang et al. proposed a combination of change of magnitude and shift of frequency dip for glioma classification and presented their findings on wild-type and mutant glioma cells [161]. Since the researchers are aware that isocitrate dehydrogenase (IDH) gene mutation for glioma patients is linked to better survival rates, such discrimination and detection techniques help customize the treatment [165]. Zhang et al. designed a polarization-independent biosensor for detection of glioma cells.

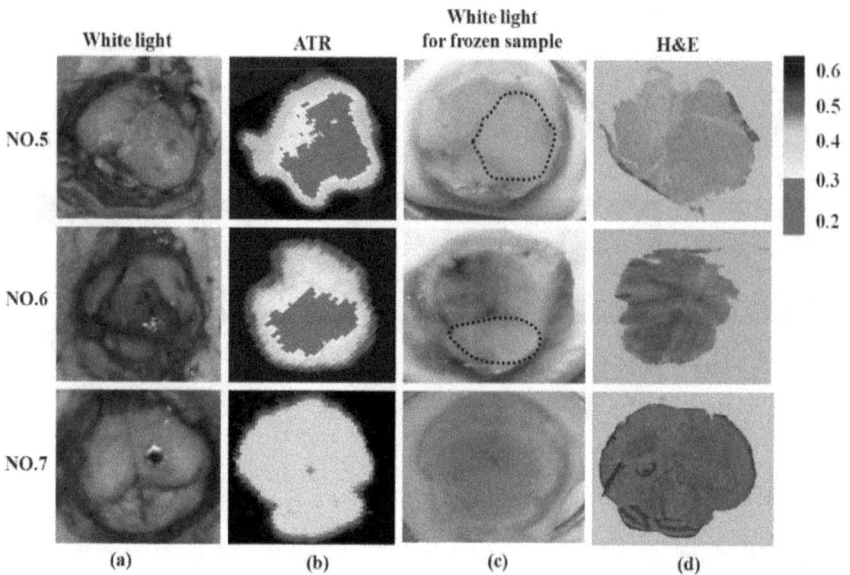

FIGURE 3.30 (a) *In vivo* visual image, (b) THz wave total reflection image, (c) freezing visual image, and (d) H & E-stained image for No. 5–7 samples. The dark gray, light gray, and black areas of (b) were the tumor tissue, normal tissue, and background regions, respectively. ([162] © 2021 Optica Publishing Group under the terms of the Optica Open Access Publishing Agreement.)

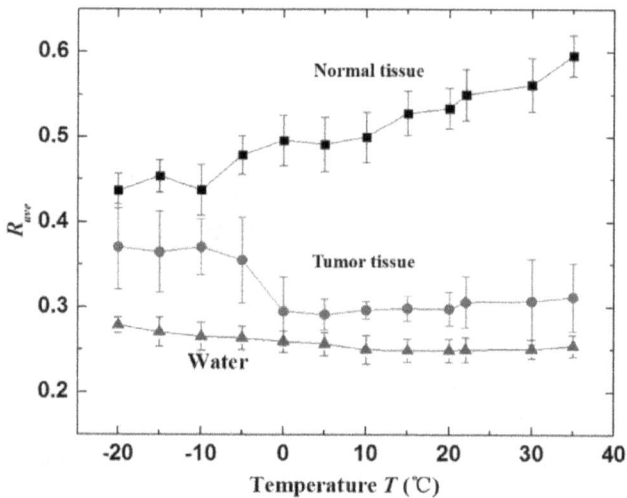

FIGURE 3.31 The averaged reflectivity in the tumor tissue, normal tissue, and distilled water at temperature interval of 5°C. ([162] © 2021 Optica Publishing Group under the terms of the Optica Open Access Publishing Agreement.)

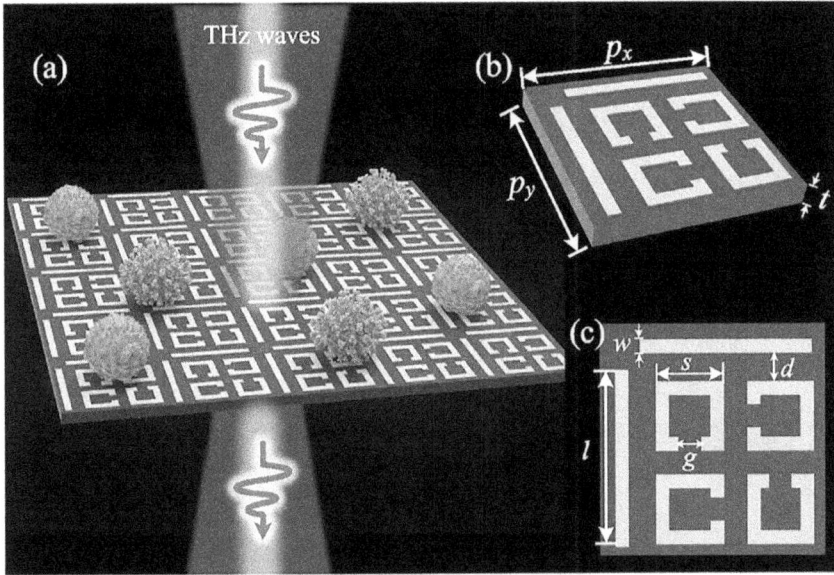

FIGURE 3.32 (a) Schematic illustration of the proposed metamaterial biosensor: THz beams normally penetrate through the devices on which different types of cells were cultured. (b) and (c) The structural configuration and the top view of unit cell consisting of metal patterns and substrate, respectively. The structure parameters are listed as: $p_x = p_y = 50\,\mu m$, $l = 38\,\mu m$, $w = 3\,\mu m$, $s = 15\,\mu m$, $g = 5\,\mu m$, $d = 6\,\mu m$, and $\varepsilon = 3.85$. ([161] ©2021 Elsevier B.V. All rights reserved.)

The metamaterial sensor, as shown in Figure 3.32, is made up of unit cells which consist of split ring resonators (SRRs) and metal cut wires to induce transparency at around 2.24 THz irrespective of polarization [161]. The frequency dip around 2.24 THz can be tuned by adjusting the dimensions of the SRR and/or the wires. The biosensor is then covered with the analyte and the transmission spectra is recorded for different cell concentration of glioma cells both mutant IDH and wild type. The shift in resonant frequency because of mutant IDH (0.12 THz) and wild type cells (0.2 THz) due to cell concentration is evident [161] in Figure 3.33. It can also be seen that unlike wild-type cells the variation in peak amplitude of the resonant dip for mutant IDH glioma cells is the distinguishing factor for cell concentration. It is also shown that for the same cell concentration the transmission spectrum for two cell types is different. A combination of variation in both frequency and peak amplitude allows for clear distinction between two cell types of glioma.

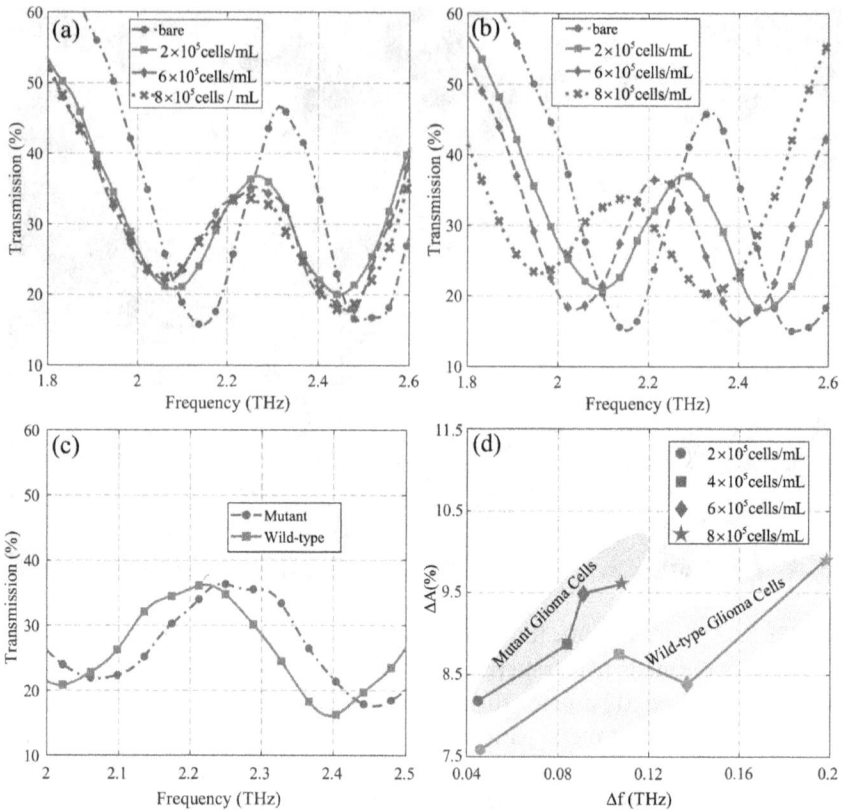

FIGURE 3.33 The measured transmission spectra of the proposed biosensor covered by (a) the mutant IDH glioma cells and (b) the wild-type IDH glioma cells. (c) The measured transmission spectra of two types of cells with same cells concentration of 4×10^5 cells/mL. (d) The resonate frequency shifts and the peak magnitude variations for mutant and wild-type glioma cells as the concentration changes. ([161] ©2021 Elsevier B.V. All rights reserved.)

3.4.4 Other Cancers

Earlier discussions in this chapter highlight that the THz radiation-based techniques for detection of diseased cancer tissue from healthy tissue study the change in absorption coefficient and refractive index between the two types of tissues to differentiate among them. The change in these properties of tissue samples is also studied for other types of cancers such as colorectal, cervical, liver, etc. In this section, we discuss progress made by THz-based techniques for such cancer types.

3.4.4.1 Colorectal Cancer

THz-TDS has been shown to discriminate between colon cancer and normal cells [166]. However, the comparatively simple and non-invasive liquid biopsy is gaining dominance over traditional pathological biopsy. In the case of human colon cancer, cell lines HT-29 and DLD-1 of colon adenocarcinoma are extensively studied for better understanding of its properties. It is expected that better discrimination between these cell lines and normal cell lines can improve the chances of colon cancer identification. Toward this, THz time-domain attenuated reflection (THz TD-ATR) spectroscopy has been used to study liquid-based samples namely HT-29 and DLD-1 cell lines. In such an experimental setup THz pulse from a conventional THz source is incident on an edge of a Si prism. The sample droplet is placed on the edge of the prism parallel to the ground. The THz pulse propagates within the prism and undergoes total internal reflection at the prism–sample boundary before emerging from the edge opposite to the incident edge. This reflected pulse contains the information, i.e. absorption coefficient, dielectric loss tangent (tan δ), and refractive index about the sample. Using THz TD-ATR and k-nearest neighbors (KNN) machine-learning method, Cao et al. [167] attempted to identify key parameters of reflected THz spectrum to distinguish between normal cells and cancer cells along with the classification/identification of cell lines mentioned earlier. They demonstrated a distinct non-linear dependence of absorption coefficient on cell concentration for HT-29 and DLD-1 cell lines. This distinction is attributed to different hydration states of the two cell lines. Further, after cleaning the measured data by removing the spectrum of culture medium and noise, the principal component analysis of the data performed and the output vector is fed to the KNN algorithm based cancer cell discrimination model. The model predicted absorption coefficient and tan δ as the sensitive parameters for cancer cell identification. Building upon the above-mentioned results and using THz TD-ATR, Cao et al. [168] in their current study showed a non-linear dependence between cell concentrations and refractive index especially in the frequency range of 08 to 1.4 THz. Furthermore, principal component analysis of absorption coefficient, tan δ, and refractive index is performed to identify strongly correlated components with cell types. Two principal components were identified and used with random forest algorithm to demonstrate distinction between the cancer cell line types.

3.4.4.2 Cervical Cancer

Cervical cancer is the most common gynecologic cancer worldwide. Early diagnosis of cervical cancer will greatly improve the treatment delivery. The most common method of diagnosis of such cancers to date is biopsy which is intrusive and invasive and analysis is dependent on the skill of the pathologist. THz-TDS is being investigated for diagnosis using micro-metastatic lump nodes [169] and cervical cell lines (SiHa and HeLa) [170,171] and has shown early promise and progress.

The first pilot study of micro-metastatic lump nodes for early-stage cervical cancer used the THz-TDS system for imaging [169]. The images for paraffin-embedded samples containing FIGO IB1 and squamous cell carcinoma (SCC) were produced using peak-to-peak amplitude and the changes in refractive index. The two set of images were more or less similar; however, regions of paraffin, non-metastatic, and metastatic portions were clearly delineated. The distinction between the two types of tissues are close to the level of methods used in histopathology. Prior to imaging, the difference between THz time-domain amplitude and Fourier-domain amplitude, revealed a contrast between paraffin, non-metastatic, and metastatic portions of the lymph nodes in reflection geometry THz-TDS [172].

The THz-TDs system in transmission mode has been used to extract refractive index and absorption coefficient of paraffin-embedded 52 dehydrated cervical samples (20 cancerous, rest normal) for classification using support vector machine (SVM and partial least squares-discriminant analysis (PLS-DA) [173]. This study focused on extending the THz-TDS system capabilities for diagnosis using machine learning for diagnosis based on classification metric. The key component of the study is to understand the effect of pre-processing methods, applied on refractive index and absorption coefficient data extracted from the THz-TDS of normal and diseased samples, on classification accuracy of SVM and PLS-DA. Four different pre-processing methods, separately and in combination, were used to treat experimental data before being fed to SVM and PLS-DA. It is then shown that both SVM and PLS-DA can predict classification between normal and diseased samples with 94±0.5% accuracy when TDS data (in this case absorption coefficient) is pre-processed with a Savitzky–Golay smoothing and first derivative and principal component orthogonal signal correction together [173].

THz-based metamaterial biosensors have also been investigated for identification of cervical cancer [174]. An array of SRR type (shown in Figure 3.34) is used to observe the frequency shift and amplitude

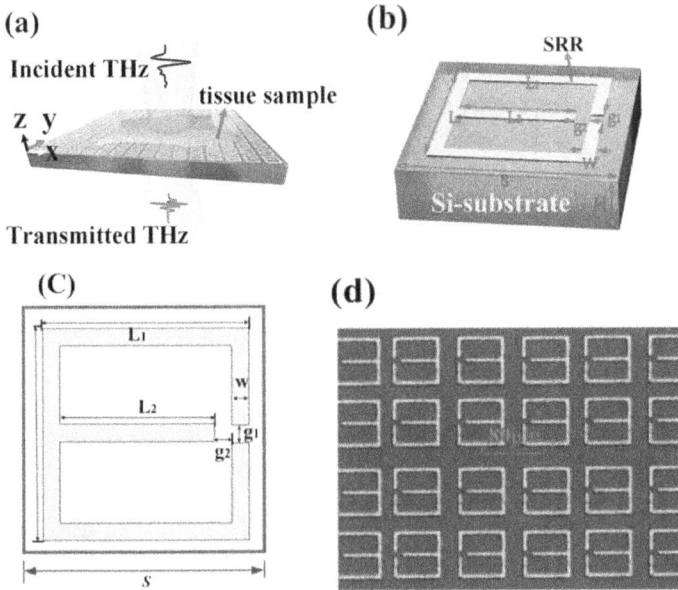

FIGURE 3.34   Structure and image of the MMs THz biosensor. (a) Schematic of MMs THz biosensor; (b) oblique view and (c) top view of a unit cell; (d) micrograph of sample. ([174] ©2021 IEEE.)

fluctuations in the two resonant dips (at lower and higher ends of the THz frequency spectrum between 0.2 and 1.0 THz) of the transmitted THz spectrum (see Figure 3.35a) [174]. It is observed that for such sensors a red shift of the resonant dips occurs when the sensor is loaded with diseased tissue or normal tissue. The amount of red shift for cancerous tissue is more than the normal tissue for both resonant dips with more contrast seen for higher frequency resonant dips. The amplitude of the transmitted signal also shows comparatively higher attenuation for cancer samples. Both the observations are linked to changes in complex permittivity of the system where the real part is affected by the frequency and the amplitude gets affected by the imaginary part [174].

While most of the studies on THz interaction with cervical (and other) cancer tissues are done with fixed tissues or imaging, an investigation on living HeLa cells has also been proposed [170]. A study of living cancer cell/tissue can shed light on macromolecules and kinematics within cells/tissue. Shi et al. [170] used a $LiNbO_3$ (for THz generation) and ZnTe (for detection) based transient THz-TDS system with tilted wave front for transient time-domain measurements. The data is recorded with a

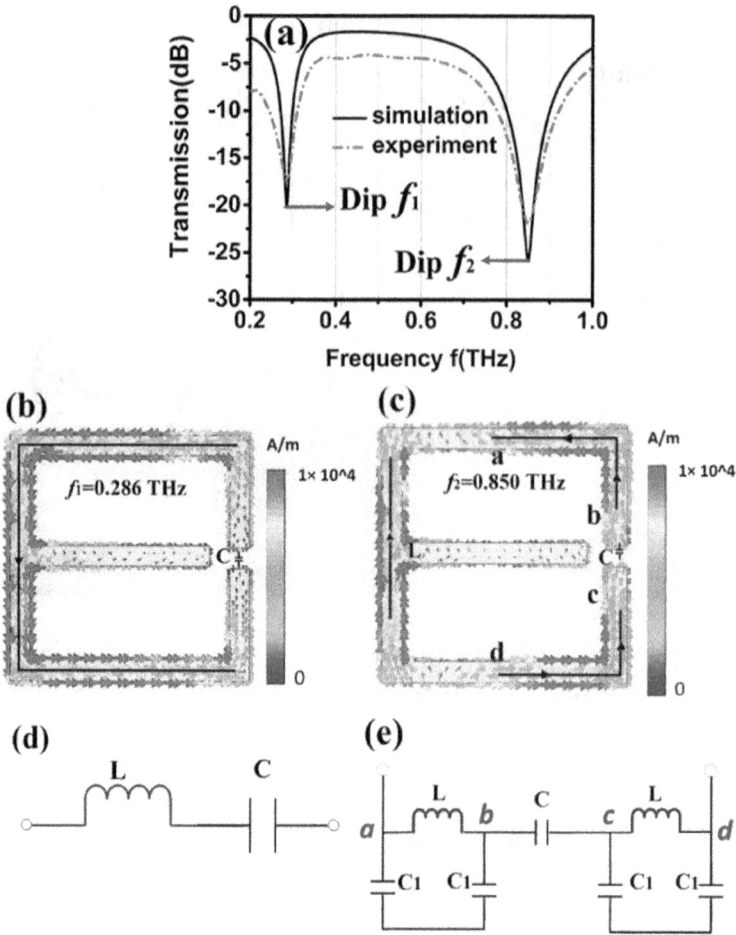

FIGURE 3.35 Transmission spectra, surface currents distribution, and equivalent circuit model. (a)Transmission spectra of the biosensor; surface current distribution at (b) 0.286 THz and (c) 0.850 THz; equivalent LC circuit models at (d) 0.286 THz and (e) 0.850 THz. ([174] ©2021 IEEE.)

CCD and is used to extract electric field in time domain and frequency domain. From the time-domain spectrum for three different concentration of HeLa cells as well as the empty glass side (reference signal), a variation in amplitude of the signal is expected but delay in THz pulse is not revealed. However, the expected high absorption (from 1.0 THz to 2.0 THz) for samples is confirmed. Further, calculation of characteristic absorption spectra for each concentration using Lambert–Beer law, after accounting for water absorption peaks [175], a variation in three characteristic THz frequencies (0.71, 1.04 and 1.07 [170]) is revealed for different HeLa cell concentrations. This technique has the potential to (a) reduce data collection time compared to conventional THz-TDS and (b) reveal characteristics of living cells/tissue at a picosecond scale.

3.4.4.3 Liver Cancer

TPI, i.e. THz-TDS in reflection geometry has been used to contrast between healthy and unhealthy (cirrhotic) liver tissue samples [176]. The increased water content in unhealthy (cirrhotic) liver tissue provides the basis for such a contrast in absorption coefficient. This contrast in absorption coefficient diminishes for formalin-treated samples [cite Sun et al. 2009 from [176]]. Since the contrast comparison is dependent on water content the hydration levels of samples during data collection can affect the results; thus, care is needed to keep dehydration minimal during data-acquisition time. Data-acquisition times for TPI and CW-THz imaging are of the order of minutes to hours depending on sample size, which is enough time for significant changes in the hydration levels of the samples.

THz in-line holography is another technique that can provide information on both the amplitude and the phase of the scattered signal. This information can be acquired in a single shot exposure of the sample, thus in principle rectifying time-dependent dehydration. However, current limitation on the area and pixel size of THz detectors prompts the need for sample-scanning methods to be employed. The acquired holographic data can be used to construct images by numerical reconstruction [cite 18 from [60]]. Rong et al. [60] studied hepatocellular carcinoma (HCC) tumor of liver by optics-free Gabor-type holography. In this study it is demonstrated that normalization and reconstruction-based in-line holography can be used to supplement liver cancer diagnosis. The technique produces images based on absorption and phase-shift distribution of the THz wave. The phase-shift information of the tissue samples is able to reproduce structural details, using error-reduction algorithm-based extrapolation and is more suited for diagnosis.

3.4.4.4 Tongue Cancer

Tongue cancer is an oral cancer type of very high incidence and patients will benefit from early diagnosis and clear demarcation of the affected area. THz-imaging technique based on reflection geometry for research on skin, breast, and other cancer types exploits the frequency-dependent refractive index change in cancer tissue samples due to high water content. Presence of higher water content is also true for tongue cancer samples. Increased content of water in diseased tissue indicates higher refractive index for THz frequencies. However, to some extent in the case of liver cirrhosis and predominantly in the case of tongue cancer tissue, the opposite of the expected behavior of refractive index change for THz radiation has been observed [177]. In a study conducted by Ji et al. [177] it is demonstrated that despite higher water content in the keratinizing SCC of tongue a lower reflection of THz signal compared to normal tongue tissue is indicative of factors other than water content dominating the refractive index change. It is deliberated that other tissue ingredients such as keratin, lipids, glycoproteins, and collagens can affect the depressed response of water on refractive index of the diseased tissue. Keratin has been shown to have lower refractive index and absorption coefficient at THz frequencies from 0.3 to 0.7 THz [177]. This is an important result for keratinized SCC of tongue as these tissues contain higher amount of keratin in comparison to normal tongue tissue. This also indicates that the effect of contents of the tissue other than water can play an important role in different types of cancer detection and imaging by TPI.

3.4.4.5 Lung Cancer

Lung cancer is one of the prevalent forms of cancer across the human population. Histologically it manifests in different forms of carcinomas (squamous, small cell, adeno-, large cell, large cell neuroendocrine and many more). An early, easy and cost effective diagnosis is of great benefit in administering treatment. THz based detection approaches with plasmonic metasurfaces [178] and electric potential [179] are being investigated for lung cancer detection.

Personalized treatment is of great interest from the perspective of the patient and its efficacy due to targeted approach. Toward this analysis of genomes for cancer gene is an area of increasing interest. To analyze genome in a sample, an important step is precise quantitative measurement of the number of cancer cells. The conventional method involves fixing the sample, waiting for >24 hours, slicing, staining, and then observing it under an optical microscope with a trained eye. An alternative technique, called TCM, based on change in THz-wave amplitude due to change in electric potential of a sensing plate is proposed by the researchers at Graduate School of Interdisciplinary Science and Engineering in Health Systems, Okayama University, Japan. Using the procedure detailed in [179], the effect of the concentration of PC9 (adenocarcinoma cells) lung cancer that reacted to cytokeratin (antibodies) upon THz amplitude is studied. In this approach a change in electric potential of the SiO_2-sensing plate is induced by the reaction between the cancer cells and the antibodies.

This electric potential change, i.e. sensitivity of sensing plate, is shown to be dependent on cancer cell concentration as the amplitude of the reflected THz wave increased with increasing concentration of PC9 cells. The optical setup used for these measurements is a standard THz-TDS system with a PCA. In this approach, the incoming THz signal is never in contact with the sample, an important distinction in comparison to other THz-based approaches for cancer detection. It also offers the potential benefit of simpler and time-saving sample preparation along with addressing the shortage of skilled pathologists required for accurate quantitative measurements in conventional method.

In another approach for lung cancer detection, plasmonic metasurfaces are used as biosensors by observing the transmitted THz signal. The idea driving this approach is spectral shift and amplitude change of the incoming signal due to different physical parameters of the diverse biomolecules. Such changes are a result of highly strengthened light–matter interactions between the metasurfaces and the biomolecules (but analytes in general). This enhancement in interaction allows for the detection of changes in the transmitted signal due to variation in observed molecules size, conductance, and refractive index. Recently, plasmonic toroidal metasurfaces with asymmetric SRRs have been used to show the variation in resonance dip of the transmitted THz signal [178]. The simulations predict a spectral redshift of the resonance dip with increasing refractive index and increasing height of the analyte. A significant decrease in the amplitude of resonance dip is also seen for increasing dielectric loss, measured by dielectric dissipation factor (tan δ), for $0 \leq \tan \delta \leq 0.3$. A less pronounced amplitude shift is reported for variation in the height of the analyte. Such a parameter-dependent behavior of resonant dip of the transmitted THz signal can be used as a fingerprint to identify different types of lung cancer. The observations made are used to study the transmission of THz signal with THz-TDS system for Calu-1, A427, and 95D lung cancer cells cultured on toroidal metasurfaces with cell concentrations of 200, 400, and 600 cells/mm^2 [178]. A combination of spectral shift and amplitude change for the resonant dip of the transmitted THz signal is reported. The degree of variation, though varies for cell-type concentrations, is still able to discriminate among the three lung cancer cell types with clearly marked regions for each cell type on the THz frequency vs transmittance (%) plot. Such a distinction when extrapolated for other cell types of lung cancer can push this technique as a THz-based fingerprinting tool for lung cancer type detection.

3.4.4.6 Gastric Cancer

With the understanding of elevated hydration levels and water content of cancer cells THz-TDS and THz imaging have been employed to extract absorption coefficient and refractive index values for gastric carcinoma. From works cited in a review by Danciu et al. [180] it can be seen that the absorption spectrum for gastric carcinoma revealed spectral features in the frequency range of 0.2–0.5 THz and 1.0–1.5 THz. A higher refractive index and absorption coefficient for diseased tissue as compared to normal tissue observed for 21 samples also finds mention in [180]. More recently in 2020, a study on histologically classified gastric adenocarcinoma pT3 and pT4 using THz-TDS and imaging was performed by Wahaia et al. [181]. The room temperature measurements were performed to extract refractive index and absorption coefficient. From the results presented, it can be seen that refractive index parameter for frequencies between 0.125 and 0.5 THz can discriminate between pT3, pT4, normal, and cancer cells. At the same time, absorption coefficient for frequencies in the range of 1.0–2.0 THz shows distinction between pT3 and pT4 cancer cells. These studies indicate that THz spectroscopy and imaging can prove to be an important non-invasive tool for early diagnosis of gastric cancer.

3.4.4.7 Ovarian Cancer

Ovarian cancer has been identified as one of the leading causes of gynecological tumor-related deaths in women. It has been argued that since ovarian cancer can be cured effectively when diagnosed early, techniques that can overcome the limitations of the conventional methods and can increase the diagnosis rate from 40% or less with consistency can have a high impact on the patients' well-being [182]. Toward this, THz-based techniques are being investigated for diagnosis. THz vibrational spectroscopy has been investigated to identify molecular biomarkers in human serum. This investigation is informed from the understanding that human body fluids such as serum contain cell-free RNA and such circulating nucleoids can be leveraged by understanding their expression levels. The microRNA-200 family is of high interest due to their increased expression in cancer cells compared to normal cells. The THz frequency range from 0.315 to 0.480 THz (sub-THz) is of interest for such studies due to the presence of weak hydrogen bonds. These bonds and other vibrational modes at lower end of THz frequencies are correlated to 3D molecular structure [183]. The experimental results in [182] indicate a characteristic peak at a frequency of 13 cm^{-1} (0.389 THz), which stands out for SK-OV-3 and ES-2 histotypes. Absorbance spectra generated from molecular dynamic simulations for a mix of miR-200c and miR-200a seems to correlate with experimental absorbance spectra for ES-2 cell line and miR-141 with SK-OV-3 cell types. The correlation in both cases is observed around the 13 cm^{-1} (0.389 THz) frequency band with more peaks in simulated absorbance mimicking experimental data. The authors of [182] present high mismatch at one end of the overexpressed micro RNA as the likely explanation for the 13 cm^{-1} (0.389 THz) frequency band and the features in it. At the same time, it is noted that the points of disagreement between simulations and experimental THz absorption data need further investigation primarily due to lack of information around the structure of micro RNA in 3D. The same technique is then utilized to study absorbance of normal urine and saliva samples [183]. While the spectra for the samples taken at close interval of time showed good consistency, considerable differences were found for the samples taken 2 years apart. It is argued that the patient may have suffered from breast cancer during this period that would have led to significant physiological changes. This observation is supported by the comparison between Figure 3.36a (green line) and Figure 3.36b [183]. Globus et al. [184] in continuation of their previous work [182] compared the simulated absorbance of all four micro RNAs (i.e. miR-220a, miR-200b, miR-200c, and miR-141) combined (25%, 10%, 40%, and 25% respectively) with experimental absorption spectra of normal tissue sample with reasonable correlation. However, further research is needed for identifying spectral signatures for other molecular components especially proteins.

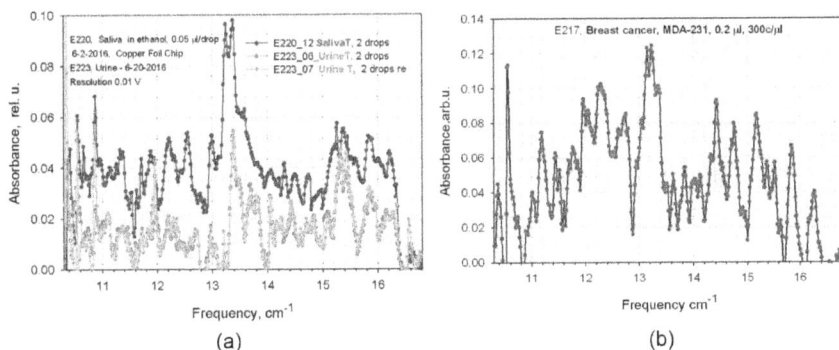

FIGURE 3.36 (a) Similarity of absorbance spectra of saliva and urine samples taken from the same patient at close time, June 2016; (b) absorption spectrum of Breast cancer sample MDA-MB-231. ([183] ©2018 Tatiana Globus (Open access).)

Moreover, a lack of reasonable correlation between experimental cancer spectra and simulated micro RNA spectra has been identified.

Limited resolution of peaks and contribution from other molecular components are cited as the probable causes for poor correlation [184].

CW THz spectroscopy is used in [185] to investigate difference between absorption spectra of high-grade serous ovarian cancer and normal tissue. The GaAs photomixer-based spectroscopy system produced a wide-band THz emission (0–1.8 THz) with 10 MHz resolution. The paraffin-fixed samples of increasing thickness (1.28, 1.54, 1.84 mm) were investigated in the frequency range of 0.4–1.5 THz. The transmission spectra for all three thicknesses demonstrated lower transmittance i.e. higher absorption compared to normal ovarian tissue. They also used area under the transmittance curve as a metric to highlight increased absorption by the cancer tissue which increases with thickness. For 1.28 mm thick sample the area under the transmittance curve for cancer sample is 50% smaller than the area for normal tissue curve.

3.4.4.8 Prostate Cancer

Prostate cancer is one of the malignant tumor types with an incidence of 1 in 8 men according to Prostate Cancer UK. Research with THz-based technologies has been employed to study their feasibility in identifying, imaging, and classifying prostate cancer [186,187]. A TPI system "TeraPulse4000" from Teraview with reflective module is used to study prostate tissue with both cancerous and normal regions in [186]. Here, the spectral and imaging data are obtained from the THz beam reflected from the sample surface as well as reflected beam passing twice from the tissue sample before and after reflection at the mirror–tissue interface. Absorption coefficient and refractive index of each point of the 15×5 mm tissue sample with a resolution of 0.2 mm is extracted from conventional THz-TDS data. The time-domain and frequency-domain spectra of normal (N), tumor (T), and muscle (M) sections for surface reflection and tissue–mirror interface reflection when compared showed that both data sets are capable of distinguishing three cell types. However, the interface reflection data showed distinct changes in time-domain spectra w.r.t intensity as well as shape. The latter indicates an impact on frequency components of the input signal. This is confirmed in the frequency domain picture with frequency components at frequencies >2THz were missing. This demonstrates a greater interaction of THz wave with the components of the tissue under investigation. A clear distinction in the extracted refractive index values 2.12, 2.0, and 1.9 for T, N and, M, respectively, at 1.0 THz and absorption coefficient spread over the range of 1.0–2.5 THz supplements the observations made from spectral data. The authors further used machine learning for classification by extracting two principal components with principal component analysis. These principal components were then used as input for the least squares support vector machine (LS-SVM) algorithm with good results [186]. A similar methodology of THz-TDS and machine learning is used for discrimination and classification of prostate cancer (Gleason scale 4 and 8) and normal tissue in [187]. Knyazkova et al. [187] also performed parameter i.e. refractive index and absorption coefficient from spectral data followed by principal component analysis and SVM algorithm. Knyazkova et al. [187] claim 100% accuracy for classification using SVM with "majority vote". Both these studies impress the usefulness of THz spectroscopy for prostate cancer analysis. Zhang et al. [186] also showed clear demarcation between regions of N, T, and M tissues using frequency domain slice imaging. It must also be noted that these studies were performed on paraffin-embedded tissue samples without any impact on data retrieval and analysis from paraffin or paraffin and plastic in the case of [187].

3.5 OTHER BIOMEDICAL APPLICATIONS OF THz SPECTROSCOPY AND IMAGING

3.5.1 Ophthalmologic Applications of THz Radiation

In THz-TDS and TPI, ophthalmology found a powerful diagnostic tool, as the ability to properly regulate water content is known to be a good indicator of corneal health, and deviations from normal hydration are significant indicators of many corneal diseases. Bennett et al. [188] studied THz reflectivity of the porcine cornea with different water content and found an approximately linear relationship between THz reflectivity and water concentration. For these experiments, they used THz-TDS setup for spectroscopy and replaced the detector PCA with an ultrafast Schottky diode for imaging. Liu et al. [189] characterized corneal samples with THz-TDS in transmission.

In vivo corneal sensing by THz radiation was reported by Ozheredov et al. [190] in normal incidence reflective THz-TDS setup (Figure 3.6d). One of the main results of the study is shown in Figure 3.37.

Real-time cornea hydration THz-TDS monitoring within a several-minute time window shows its gradual drop followed by full recovery

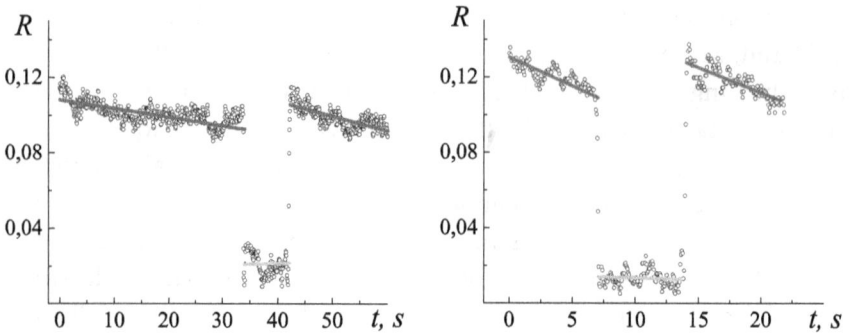

FIGURE 3.37 Results of the *in vivo* measurements of corneal THz reflectivity. Points, experimental data; lines, linear approximation. Left: 45-year-old man not wearing glasses. Right: 26-year-old man wearing glasses. ([190] ©IOP Publishing £125.)

of its initial state after blinking. Chen et al. [191] also focused on corneal phantom hydration dynamics monitoring with similar THz-TDS layout. To directly connect the THz reflectivity data with water content, a mass of the sample was monitored during the measurement. As the mass loss is associated with water evaporation only, the connection can be rather easily established. Moreover, authors look not only at the very first peak of the reflected signal, but also at the subsequent peaks of the THz pulse, and notice, then confirm by simulation, that while the amplitude of the first peak is decreasing with lowered water concentration, amplitudes of the following peaks grow as more radiation penetrates into the tissue and is reflected from inner layers. Further experimental THz-TDS studies of cornea include characterization of *ex vivo* human corneal stroma samples [192] with error correction method [193], *in vivo* long-term rabbit cornea monitoring [95,194], *ex vivo* rabbit cornea [195,196], and *ex vivo* rabbit and porcine eye studies confirming that THz-TDS is capable of intraocular pressure monitoring [197].

Iomdina et al. studied rabbit cornea and sclera hydration *in vitro* [53] in transmission and reflection and *in vivo* [53,198] in reflection layout with sub-THz CW setup (IMPATT source and different detectors were used). The results of the study give a bright perspective for CW sub-THz setups as a tool for remote cornea hydration monitoring providing much faster acquisition time and less complex alignment. Sung et al. [199] suggested CW system operating at 0.65 THz for *in vivo* imaging of human cornea, which was later updated [200], while Tamminen et al. [201] covered the 0.2–0.3 THz frequency range.

THz monitoring of minor changes of corneal hydration ability as well as its useful imaging depth promises a great potential of THz technology as a diagnostic tool in clinical ophthalmology.

3.5.2 Stomatologic Applications of THz Radiation

Teeth are made of probably the most ideal tissue for application of THz diagnostic tools as water content in the enamel is extremely low compared to other bodily tissues. Pilot study of the potential of TPI for dental imaging was published almost 20 years ago [202]. On the extracted tooth samples, the authors have demonstrated the ability of THz radiation to differentiate between caries and healthy enamel, between enamel and dentine, and even between hypomineralization and enamel caries, using both refractive index and absorption coefficient values. Later, bovine enamel-demineralized lesions were quantitatively studied *in vitro* [203,204]. Nazarov et al. [205], Smirnov et al. [206], and Kamburoglu et al. [207] confirmed these results for human teeth. Moreover, Kamburoglu et al. [208] compared THz properties of primary and permanent teeth, not finding a significant difference in THz properties, permanent being a little more transparent. Recently, Yadav et al. [209] showed that faster CW THz-imaging systems can help monitoring the dental health in real time. In the nearest future, we expect more results in this area of research with potentially achievable 3D dental images capable to replace significantly more dangerous X-ray used to date.

3.5.3 Hematologic Applications of THz Radiation

Some studies of blood were mentioned earlier in Section 3.2.3.1 in the context of glucose monitoring. Blood samples from the specimen rat with diabetes have lower absorption coefficient and higher refractive index than those of healthy ones [106,107]. Studies of rat blood serum have been demonstrated to differentiate between healthy and liver cancer-implanted specimen. The observed changes in the THz response are explained by a decrease in the number of protein molecules and bound water. Similar research has been reported for progressing Ehrlich carcinoma [210] and thyroid cancer [211].

3.5.4 Tissue Studies

Among biomedical studies, there have been more general measurements of tissues that either did not reveal any significant dependences or receive enough attention for the continuation of the studies. He et al. [212] studied skin, fat, and lean pork tissues in transmission THz-TDS (Figure 3.6a) and confirmed that all tissues have different frequency-dependent responses to terahertz radiation. Later, imaging was performed on dehydrated samples [213]. Nikoghosyan et al. [214] characterized THz spectral properties of human jawbone and cerabone–human bone substitute. Yang et al. [215] studied cultivated collagen samples. THz-TDS sensitivity to *ex vivo* liver injury severeness has been demonstrated in [216,217]. All studies were done in transmission.

Terahertz absorption and refractive index spectra of sugar, water, hemoglobin, lipids, human tooth enamel, and dentine were obtained by THz-TDS in transmission and reflection and reported in [205]. Spectroscopic differentiation between normal and Alzheimer's disease tissues by reflective THz-TDS is claimed in [218].

3.5.5 Remote Monitoring of Health Status

When talking about remote, we assume that this analysis is done from a reasonable distance of at least 10 cm in reflection layout. In addition to diabetes monitoring by the breath gases analysis mentioned in Section 3.2.3.1l, remote monitoring of heartbeat has been reported [219].

3.6 EFFECT OF THz RADIATION ONTO CELLS AND TISSUES

This section is relatively short as most focus of biomedical THz applications was aimed toward early cancer diagnostics, but with the appearance of numerous THz systems in the past couple of years, we expect a burst of discoveries in this field. So far, the sources were really low power for inducing a pronounced impact. Still, some results have been published.

3.6.1 Interaction of THz Radiation with DNA Molecules

As DNA are rather large molecules, they have strong absorption lines in THz spectrum associated with the vibration's degrees of freedom. Fischer et al. studied THz properties of the DNA nucleobases A, C, G, and T, recorded at room and cryogenic temperatures [220].

Each of the studied molecules: adenine, cytosine, guanine, and thymine demonstrated a distinct pattern of resonances (Figure 3.38), which authors identified as signatures of vibrational motion of hydrogen bonds responsible for the arrangement of the molecules in the microcrystalline structure. Later these results were argued by Tao et al. [221]. Sub-THz analysis of DNA molecules at frequencies between 0.1 and 0.3 THz is presented in [222].

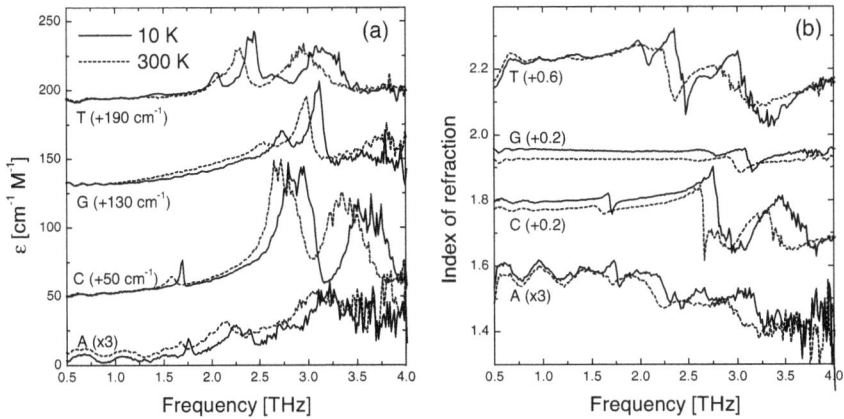

FIGURE 3.38 (a) Absorption coefficient and (b) index of refraction of the nucleo-bases A, C, G, and T, recorded at 10 K (solid curves) and 300 K (dashed curves). ([220] ©IOP Publishing £125.)

The research by Cheon et al. [223] highlights the ability of THz-TDS to spectroscopically differentiate DNA of cancerous and healthy tissues. Resonance signals can be quantified to identify the types of cancer cells, and some later studies confirm this finding [224]. The research by Tang et al. [225] reveals the potential of THz-TDS to monitor the DNA mutations.

Although no significant effect on the DNA molecules from THz radiation was reported in [226], later Wu et al. [227] discovered that the presence of THz radiation accelerates DNA unwinding.

This is a very new direction of THz research, and with the development of THz microscopic and nanoscopic techniques, we anticipate mapping of DNA molecular bonds with THz nanoscopic apparatus [228,229].

3.6.2 Interaction of THz Radiation with Living Cells and Tissues

As THz radiation is usually advertised as the safer alternative for X-ray in medical applications, it is essential to study the actual effects it has on cells, tissues, and living organisms. Since most available THz sources have very low power (in the orders of several μW), this type of research is accessible predominantly to the lucky users of THz-capable free-electron lasers (FEL) [230], or at least THz high-field amplified sources [4].

To date, the effect of THz radiation onto biological tissues was reported by several groups, and we will briefly overview these results. Most studies [26,59,231–236] are devoted to simulation and experimental verification of the heating effect of THz radiation on the samples. Despite different THz sources involved, all studies reported no noticeable thermal effect of THz radiation on tissues under study, even the ones where powerful radiation of FEL [237] and a gas laser [233] or a powerful amplified pulsed THz system [238–240] were used.

3.6.3 Therapeutic Action of THz Radiation

In [237–240] non-thermal effects of THz radiation were studied. Demidova et al. [237], using the radiation of an FEL on *E. coli* biosensor cells, discovered that different elements of *E. coli* stress response systems demonstrate different responses to THz radiation. Response was highest for genes involved in the oxidative stress response system. Hugh et al. [238] demonstrated that a high THz field from amplified ultrafast laser system pumped $LiNbO_3$ crystal induced a large genomic expression response in human skin tissue models (Figure 3.39).

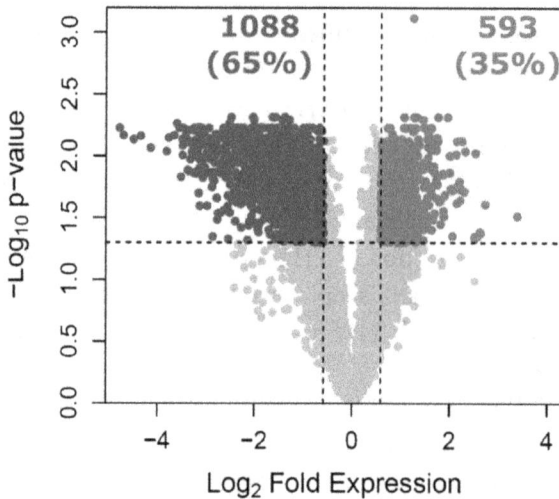

FIGURE 3.39 Volcano plot displaying the measured global differential gene expression profile induced by intense THz pulses in human skin tissue models. The statistical significance of each measurement is plotted as the adjusted p value (negative log10-transformed) against the magnitude of differential gene expression (log2-transformed fold-change of exposed vs. control tissues). Dotted black lines indicate conventional criteria for significance of gene expression. Of 9311 total genes detected in control probes, 1088 were downregulated and 593 were upregulated. ([238] © Springer Nature £85.)

Further research by the same team [240] unveiled the inhibition of Ras-signaling and calcium-signaling pathways by intense THz pulses, resulting in dysregulatory effects on cancer-related processes. Another research with similar $LiNbO_3$-based THz-pulsed system [241] also revealed the effect of THz radiation onto gene expression profiles in human eye cells.

These preliminary results are very promising as high-field THz radiation may potentially find novel clinical application with the goal of targeted inhibition of mitotic activity in cancerous cells [242–244].

3.7 CONCLUSION

In this chapter, we tried to cover the main outcomes of THz technology application to diagnostic, monitoring, and treatment of biomedical substances, cells, and tissues. As you could notice, THz radiation has found a plethora of applications in biomedical research. With the development and growth of the availability of THz setups, components, and methods in the past 3–4 years, a new avalanche of THz biomedical research has triggered, and we expect the number of research to grow even further – and move to the clinical research stage. With this review, we would like to encourage everyone involved in biomedical research to look into and give a chance to THz technology, and anyone from THz research to give some of their attention to the application possibilities opened by the biomedical avenues.

REFERENCES

1. P Uhd Jepsen, David G. Cooke, and Martin Koch. Terahertz spectroscopy and imaging - Modern techniques and applications. *Laser & Photonics Reviews*, 5(1): 124–166, 2011.
2. S S Dhillon, M S Vitiello, E H Linfield, A G Davies, Matthias C Hoffmann, John Booske, Claudio Paoloni, M Gensch, P Weightman, G P Williams, E Castro-Camus, D R S Cumming, F Simoens, I Escorcia-Carranza, J Grant, Stepan Lucyszyn, Makoto Kuwata-Gonokami, Kuniaki Konishi, Martin Koch, Charles A Schmuttenmaer, Tyler L Cocker, Rupert Huber, A G Markelz, Z D Taylor, Vincent P Wallace, J Axel Zeitler, Juraj Sibik, Timothy M Korter, B Ellison, S Rea, P Goldsmith, Ken B Cooper, Roger Appleby, D Pardo, P G Huggard, V Krozer, Haymen Shams, Martyn Fice, Cyril Renaud, Alwyn Seeds, Andreas Stöhr, Mira Naftaly, Nick Ridler, Roland Clarke, John E Cunningham, and Michael B Johnston. The 2017 terahertz science and technology roadmap. *Journal of Physics D: Applied Physics*, 50(4): 043001, 2017.
3. Aifeng Ren, Adnan Zahid, Dou Fan, Xiaodong Yang, Muhammad Ali Imran, Akram Alomainy, and Qammer H Abbasi. State-of-the-art in terahertz sens ing for food and water security – A comprehensive review. *Trends in Food Science & Technology*, 85: 241–251, 2019.

4. József András Fülöp, Stelios Tzortzakis, and Tobias Kampfrath. Laser-driven strong-field terahertz sources. *Advanced Optical Materials*, 8(3): 1900681, 2020.
5. David R Bacon, Julien Madéo, and Keshav M Dani. Photoconductive emitters for pulsed terahertz generation. *Journal of Optics*, 2021.
6. Enrique Castro-Camus, Martin Koch, and Daniel M Mittleman. Recent advances in terahertz imaging: 1999 to 2021. *Applied Physics B*, 128(1): 12, 2022.
7. E Pickwell and V P Wallace. Biomedical applications of terahertz technology. *Journal of Physics D: Applied Physics*, 39(17):R301–R310, 2006.
8. Edward Philip John Parrott, Yiwen Sun, and Emma Pickwell-MacPherson. Terahertz spectroscopy: Its future role in medical diagnoses. *Journal of Molecular Structure*, 1006(1–3): 66–76, 2011.
9. Shuting Fan, Yuezhi He, Benjamin S Ung, and Emma Pickwell-MacPherson. The growth of biomedical terahertz research. *Journal of Physics D: Applied Physics*, 47(37): 374009, 2014.
10. Calvin Yu, Shuting Fan, Yiwen Sun, and Emma Pickwell-Macpherson. The potential of terahertz imaging for cancer diagnosis: A review of investigations to date. *Quantitative Imaging in Medicine and Surgery*, 2(1): 33–45, 2012.
11. Hwayeong Cheon, Hee-jin Yang, and Joo-hiuk Son. Toward clinical cancer imaging using terahertz spectroscopy. *IEEE Journal of Selected Topics in Quantum Electronics*, 23(4): 1–9, 2017.
12. Ullrich R. Pfeiffer, Thomas Zimmer, Philipp Hillger, Ritesh Jain, Janusz Grzyb, Thomas Bucher, Quentin Cassar, Gaetan MacGrogan, Jean-Paul Guillet, and Patrick Mounaix. Ex vivo breast tumor identification: Advances toward a silicon-based terahertz near-field imaging sensor. *IEEE Microwave Magazine*, 20(9): 32–46, 2019.
13. Magda El-Shenawee, Nagma Vohra, Tyler Bowman, and Keith Bailey. Cancer detection in excised breast tumors using terahertz imaging and spectroscopy. *Biomedical Spectroscopy and Imaging*, 8(1–2): 1–9, 2019.
14. Zohreh Vafapour, Afsaneh Keshavarz, and Hossain Ghahraloud. The potential of terahertz sensing for cancer diagnosis. *Heliyon*, 6(12): e05623, 2020.
15. Yan Peng, Chenjun Shi, Xu Wu, Yiming Zhu, and Songlin Zhuang. Terahertz imaging and spectroscopy in cancer diagnostics: A technical review. *BME Frontiers*, 2020: 2547609, 2020.
16. Lulu Wang. Terahertz imaging for breast cancer detection. *Sensors*, 21(19): 6465, 2021.
17. Xiang Yang, Xiang Zhao, Ke Yang, Yueping Liu, Yu Liu, Weiling Fu, and Yang Luo. Biomedical applications of terahertz spectroscopy and imaging. *Trends in Biotechnology*, 34(10): 810–824, 2016.
18. Qiushuo Sun, Yuezhi He, Kai Liu, Shuting Fan, Edward P J Parrott, and Emma Pickwell-MacPherson. Recent advances in terahertz technology for biomedical applications. *Quantitative Imaging in Medicine and Surgery*, 7(3): 345–355, 2017.

19. O A Smolyanskaya, N V Chernomyrdin, A A Konovko, K I Zaytsev, I A Ozheredov, O P Cherkasova, M M Nazarov, J -P Guillet, S A Kozlov, Yu V Kistenev, J -L Coutaz, P Mounaix, V L Vaks, J -H Son, H Cheon, V P Wallace, Yu Feldman, I Popov, A N Yaroslavsky, A P Shkurinov, and V V Tuchin. Terahertz biophotonics as a tool for studies of dielectric and spectral properties of biological tissues and liquids. *Progress in Quantum Electronics*, 62(November): 1–77, 2018.

20. Michael S Shur. Subterahertz and terahertz sensing of biological objects and chemical agents. *Proc. SPIE*, 10531: 1053108, 2018.

21. Joo-Hiuk Son, Seung Jae Oh, and Hwayeong Cheon. Potential clinical appli cations of terahertz radiation. *Journal of Applied Physics*, 125(19): 190901, 2019.

22. Liu Yu, Liu Hao, Tang Meiqiong, Huang Jiaoqi, Liu Wei, Dong Jinying, Chen Xueping, Fu Weiling, and Zhang Yang. The medical application of terahertz technology in non-invasive detection of cells and tissues: Opportunities and challenges. *RSC Advances*, 9(17): 9354–9363, 2019.

23. Liu Wei, Liu Yu, Huang Jiaoqi, Huang Guorong, Zhang Yang, and Fu Weiling. Application of terahertz spectroscopy in biomolecule detection. *Frontiers in Laboratory Medicine*, 2(4): 127–133, 2018.

24. Liu Sun, Li Zhao, and Rui-Yun Peng. Research progress in the effects of tera-hertz waves on biomacromolecules. *Military Medical Research*, 8(1): 28, 2021.

25. I V Il'ina, D S. Sitnikov, and M B Agranat. State-of-the-art of studies of the effect of terahertz radiation on living biological systems. *High Temperature*, 56(5): 789–810, 2018.

26. Olga P Cherkasova, Danil S Serdyukov, Eugenia F Nemova, Alexander S Ratushnyak, Anna S Kucheryavenko, Irina N Dolganova, Guofu Xu, Maksim Skorobogatiy, Igor V Reshetov, Peter S Timashev, Igor E Spektor, Kirill I Zaytsev, and Valery V Tuchin. Cellular effects of terahertz waves. *Journal of Biomedical Optics*, 26(9): 090902, 2021.

27. Min Wan, John J Healy, and John T Sheridan. Terahertz phase imaging and biomedical applications. *Optics and Laser Technology*, 122: 105859, 2020.

28. Yaya Zhang, Chuting Wang, Bingxin Huai, Shiyu Wang, Yating Zhang, Dayong Wang, Lu Rong, and Yongchang Zheng. Continuous-wave THz imaging for biomedical samples. *Applied Sciences*, 11(1): 71, 2020.

29. Zhiyao Yan, Li-Guo Zhu, Kun Meng, Wanxia Huang, and Qiwu Shi. THz medical imaging: From in vitro to in vivo. *Trends in Biotechnology*, 40: 816–830, 2022.

30. Angelina I Nikitkina, Polina Y Bikmulina, Elvira R Gafarova, Nastasia V Kosheleva, Yuri M Efremov, Evgeny A Bezrukov, Denis V Butnaru, Irina N Dolganova, Nikita V Chernomyrdin, Olga P Cherkasova, Arsenii A Gavdush, and Peter S Timashev. Terahertz radiation and the skin: A review. *Journal of Biomedical Optics*, 26(4): 043005, 2021.

31. Kiarash Ahi, Nathan Jessurun, Mohammad-Parsa Hosseini, and Navid Asadizanjani. Survey of terahertz photonics and biophotonics. *Optical Engineering*, 59(6): 061629, 2020.

32. Aiping Gong, Yating Qiu, Xiaowan Chen, Zhenyu Zhao, Linzhong Xia, and Yongni Shao. Biomedical applications of terahertz technology. *Applied Spectroscopy Reviews*, 55(5): 418–438, 2020.

33. A Krotkus, R Viselga, K Bertulis, V Jasutis, S Marcinkevičius, and U Olin. Subpicosecond carrier lifetimes in GaAs grown by molecular beam epitaxy at low substrate temperature. *Applied Physics Letters*, 66(15): 1939, 1995.

34. Masahiko Tani, Shuji Matsuura, Kiyomi Sakai, and Shin-ichi Nakashima. Emission characteristics of photoconductive antennas based on low-temperature-grown GaAs and semi-insulating GaAs. *Applied Optics*, 36(30): 7853, 1997.

35. V G. Bespalov, A A. Gorodetskii, I Yu. Denisyuk, S A Kozlov, V N Krylov, G V Lukomski˘ı, N V Petrov, and S É Putilin. Methods of generating super-broadband terahertz pulses with femtosecond lasers. *Journal of Optical Technology*, 75(10): 636, 2008.

36. R B Kohlhaas, S Breuer, L Liebermeister, S Nellen, M Deumer, M Schell, M P Semtsiv, W T Masselink, and B Globisch. 637 μW emitted terahertz power from photoconductive antennas based on rhodium doped InGaAs. *Applied Physics Letters*, 117(13): 131105, 2020.

37. K Bertulis, A Krotkus, G Aleksejenko, V Pačebutas, R Adomavičius, G Molis, and S Marcinkevičius. GaBiAs: A material for optoelectronic terahertz devices. *Applied Physics Letters*, 88(20): 201112, 2006.

38. Moon Sik Kong, Ji Su Kim, Sang Pil Han, Namje Kim, Kiwon Moon, Kyung Hyun Park, and Min Yong Jeon. Terahertz radiation using log-spiral based low-temperature-grown InGaAs photoconductive antenna pumped by mode-locked Yb-doped fiber laser. *Optics Express*, 24(7): 7037, 2016.

39. Ross R Leyman, Andrei Gorodetsky, Natalia Bazieva, Gediminas Molis, Arunas Krotkus, Edmund Clarke, and Edik U Rafailov. Quantum dot materials for terahertz generation applications. *Laser & Photonics Reviews*, 10(5): 772–779, 2016.

40. Andrei Gorodetsky, Ivo T Leite, and Edik U Rafailov. Operation of quantum dot based terahertz photoconductive antennas under extreme pumping conditions. *Applied Physics Letters*, 119: 111102, 2021.

41. Sergey Lepeshov, Andrei Gorodetsky, Alexander Krasnok, Edik Rafailov, and Pavel Belov. Enhancement of terahertz photoconductive antenna operation by optical nanoantennas. *Laser & Photonics Reviews*, 11(1): 1600199, 2017.

42. Sergey Lepeshov, Andrei Gorodetsky, Alexander Krasnok, Nikita Toropov, Tigran A Vartanyan, Pavel Belov, Andrea Alú, and Edik U Rafailov. Boosting terahertz photoconductive antenna performance with optimised plasmonic nanostructures. *Scientific Reports*, 8(1): 6624, 2018.

43. Susan L Dexheimer. *Terahertz spectroscopy: principles and applications.* Boca Raton, FL: CRC Press, 2017.

44. C Vicario, M Jazbinsek, A V. Ovchinnikov, O V Chefonov, S I Ashitkov, M B Agranat, and C P Hauri. High efficiency THz generation in DSTMS, DAST and OH1 pumped by Cr:forsterite laser. *Optics Express*, 23(4): 4573, 2015.

45. Andrei Gorodetsky, Anastasios D. Koulouklidis, Maria Massaouti, and Stelios Tzortzakis. Physics of the conical broadband terahertz emission from two color laser-induced plasma filaments. *Physical Review A*, 89(3): 033838, 2014.

46. Anastasios D Koulouklidis, Claudia Gollner, Valentina Shumakova, Vladimir Yu Fedorov, Audrius Pugžlys, Andrius Baltuška, and Stelios Tzortzakis. Observation of extremely efficient terahertz generation from mid infrared two-color laser filaments. *Nature Communications*, 11(1): 292, 2020.

47. Jianming Dai, Jingle Liu, and Xi-Cheng Zhang. Terahertz wave air photonics: Terahertz wave generation and detection with laser-induced gas plasma. *IEEE Journal of Selected Topics in Quantum Electronics*, 17(1): 183–190, 2011.

48. T Seifert, S Jaiswal, U Martens, J Hannegan, L Braun, P Maldonado, F Freimuth, A Kronenberg, J Henrizi, I Radu, E Beaurepaire, Y Mokrousov, P M Oppeneer, M Jourdan, G Jakob, D Turchinovich, L M Hayden, M Wolf, M Münzenberg, M Kläui, and T Kampfrath. Efficient metallic spintronic emit ters of ultrabroadband terahertz radiation. *Nature Photonics*, 10(7): 483–488, 2016.

49. V G. Bespalov and A A Gorodetskiĭ. Modeling of referenceless holographic recording and reconstruction of images by means of pulsed terahertz radiation. *Journal of Optical Technology*, 74(11): 745, 2007.

50. Nikolay V Petrov, Maxim S Kulya, Anton N Tsypkin, Victor G Bespalov, and Andrei Gorodetsky. Application of terahertz pulse time-domain holography for phase imaging. *IEEE Transactions on Terahertz Science and Technology*, 6(3): 464–472, 2016.

51. Artëm T Turov, Maksim S Kulya, Nikolay V Petrov, and Andrei Gorodetsky. Resolution and contrast in terahertz pulse time-domain holographic reconstruction. *Applied Optics*, 58(34): G231, 2019.

52. Nikolay S Balbekin, Maksim S Kulya, Andrey V Belashov, Andrei Gorodetsky, and Nikolay V Petrov. Increasing the resolution of the reconstructed image in terahertz pulse time-domain holography. *Scientific Reports*, 9(1): 180, 2019.

53. E N Iomdina, S V. Seliverstov, A A Sianosyan, K O Teplyakova, A A Rusova, and G N Goltsman. Terahertz scanning for evaluation of corneal and scleral hydration. *Sovremennye Tehnologii v Medicine*, 10(4): 143, 2018.

54. Nikita V Chernomyrdin, Aleksander O Schadko, Sergey P Lebedev, Viktor L Tolstoguzov, Vladimir N Kurlov, Igor V Reshetov, Igor E Spektor, Maksim Skorobogatiy, Stanislav O Yurchenko, and Kirill I Zaytsev. Solid immersion terahertz imaging with sub-wavelength resolution. *Applied Physics Letters*, 110(22): 221109, 2017.

55. N V Chernomyrdin, A S Kucheryavenko, G S Kolontaeva, G M Katyba, I N Dolganova, P A Karalkin, D S Ponomarev, V N Kurlov, I V Reshetov, M Skorobogatiy, V V Tuchin, and K I Zaytsev. Reflection-mode continuous wave 0.15 λ -resolution terahertz solid immersion microscopy of soft biological tissues. *Applied Physics Letters*, 113(11): 111102, 2018.

56. Gombo Tzydynzhapov, Pavel Gusikhin, Viacheslav Muravev, Alexey Dremin, Yuri Nefyodov, and Igor Kukushkin. New real-time sub-terahertz security body scanner. *Journal of Infrared, Millimeter, and Terahertz Waves*, 41: 632–641, 2020.

57. Alfonso Alessandro Tanga, Valeria Giliberti, Francesco Vitucci, Domenico Vitulano, Vittoria Bruni, Andrea Rossetti, Gabriele Carmine Messina, Maddalena Daniele, Giancarlo Ruocco, and Michele Ortolani. Terahertz scattering microscopy for dermatology diagnostics. *Journal of Physics: Photonics*, 3(3): 034007, 2021.

58. Saikat Adhikari, Dinesh Bhatia, and Moumita Mukherjee. Super-lattice GaN/AlxGa1-xN nanoscale MITATT oscillator as terahertz radiation source: Novel application in breast cancer imaging. *Sensors International*, 1(June): 100014, 2020.

59. Torben T Kristensen, Withawat Withayachumnankul, Peter U Jepsen, and Derek Abbott. Modeling terahertz heating effects on water. *Optics Express*, 18(5): 4727, 2010.

60. Lu Rong, Tatiana Latychevskaia, Chunhai Chen, Dayong Wang, Zhengping Yu, Xun Zhou, Zeyu Li, Haochong Huang, Yunxin Wang, and Zhou Zhou. Terahertz in-line digital holography of human hepatocellular carcinoma tissue. *Scientific Reports*, 5(1): 8445, 2015.

61. Marcel J E Golay. Theoretical consideration in heat and infra-red detection, with particular reference to the pneumatic detector. *Review of Scientific Instruments*, 18(5): 347–356, 1947.

62. H D. Drew and A J Sievers. A^{3}He-cooled bolometer for the far infrared. *Applied Optics*, 8(10): 2067, 1969.

63. A Shurakov, Y Lobanov, and G Goltsman. Superconducting hot-electron bolometer: From the discovery of hot-electron phenomena to practical applications. *Superconductor Science and Technology*, 29(2): 023001, 2016.

64. Sheng-Hui Ding, Qi Li, Yun-Da Li, and Qi Wang. Continuous-wave terahertz digital holography by use of a pyroelectric array camera. *Optics Letters*, 36(11): 1993–1995, 2011.

65. Erwin Hack, Lorenzo Valzania, Gregory Gäumann, Mostafa Shalaby, Christoph Hauri, and Peter Zolliker. Comparison of thermal detector arrays for off-axis THz holography and real-time THz imaging. *Sensors*, 16(2): 221, 2016.

66. Andrei A Gorodetsky, Suzanna Freer, and Miguel Navarro-Cía. Assessment of cameras for continuous wave sub-terahertz imaging. *Proc SPIE*, 11499: 114990Y, 2020.

67. Suzanna Freer, Cong Sui, Pavel Penchev, Stefan Dimov, Andrei Gorodetsky, Stephen M Hanham, Liam M Grover, and Miguel Navarro-Cía. Hyperspectral terahertz imaging for human bone biometrics. *Proc SPIE*, 11827: 118270T, 2021.

68. Wai Lam Chan, Kriti Charan, Dharmpal Takhar, Kevin F Kelly, Richard G Baraniuk, and Daniel M Mittleman. A single-pixel terahertz imaging system based on compressed sensing. *Applied Physics Letters*, 93(12): 121105, 2008.

69. Rayko I Stantchev, David B Phillips, Peter Hobson, Samuel M Hornett, Miles J Padgett, and Euan Hendry. Compressed sensing with near-field THz radiation. *Optica*, 4(8): 989, 2017.

70. Lu Rong, Tatiana Latychevskaia, Dayong Wang, Xun Zhou, Haochong Huang, Zeyu Li, and Yunxin Wang. Terahertz in-line digital holography of dragon fly hindwing: Amplitude and phase reconstruction at enhanced resolution by extrapolation. *Optics Express*, 22(14): 17236, 2014.

71. Adrien Chopard, Elizaveta Tsiplakova, Nikolay Balbekin, Olga Smolyanskaya, Jean-Baptiste Perraud, Jean-Paul Guillet, Nikolay V Petrov, and Patrick Mounaix. Single-scan multiplane phase retrieval with a radiation of terahertz quantum cascade laser. *Applied Physics B*, 128(3): 63, 2022.

72. Erwin Hack and Peter Zolliker. Terahertz holography for imaging amplitude and phase objects. *Optics Express*, 22(13): 16079, 2014.

73. Lorenzo Valzania, Peter Zolliker, and Erwin Hack. Topography of hidden objects using THz digital holography with multi-beam interferences. *Optics Express*, 25(10): 11038, 2017.

74. Maryelle Bessou, Bruno Chassagne, Jean-Pascal Caumes, Christophe Pradère, Philippe Maire, Marc Tondusson, and Emmanuel Abraham. Three dimensional terahertz computed tomography of human bones. *Applied Optics*, 51(28): 6738, 2012.

75. Fasheng Zhong, Liting Niu, Weiwen Wu, and Fenglin Liu. Dictionary learning-based image reconstruction for terahertz computed tomography. *Journal of Infrared, Millimeter, and Terahertz Waves*, 42(8): 829–842, 2021.

76. Bryan E Cole, Ruth M Woodward, David A Crawley, Vincent P Wallace, Donald D Arnone, and Michael Pepper. Terahertz imaging and spectroscopy of human skin in vivo. *Proc. SPIE*, 4276: 1–10, 2001.

77. Priyamvada Tewari, Colin P Kealey, David B Bennett, Neha Bajwa, Kelli S Barnett, Rahul S Singh, Martin O Culjat, Alexander Stojadinovic, Warren S Grundfest, and Zachary D Taylor. In vivo terahertz imaging of rat skin burns. *Journal of Biomedical Optics*, 17(4): 040503, 2012.

78. Emma Pickwell, Bryan E Cole, Anthony J Fitzgerald, Michael Pepper, and Vincent Patrick Wallace. In vivo study of human skin using pulsed terahertz radiation. *Physics in Medicine and Biology*, 49(9): 1595–1607, 2004.

79. Z D Taylor, R S Singh, M O Culjat, J Y Suen, W S Grundfest, H Lee, and E R Brown. Reflective terahertz imaging of porcine skin burns. *Optics Letters*, 33(11): 1258, 2008.

80. Kyung Won Kim, Kwang-Sung Kim, Hyeongmun Kim, Sang Hun Lee, Jae Hak Park, Ju-Hee Han, Seung-Hyeok Seok, Jisuk Park, YoonSeok Choi, Young Il Kim, Joon Koo Han, and Joo-Hiuk Son. Terahertz dynamic imaging of skin drug absorption. *Optics Express*, 20(9): 9476, 2012.

81. Kirill I Zaytsev, Arseniy A Gavdush, Nikita V Chernomyrdin, and Stanislav O Yurchenko. Highly accurate in vivo terahertz spectroscopy of healthy skin: Variation of refractive index and absorption coefficient along the human body. *IEEE Transactions on Terahertz Science and Technology*, 5(5): 817–827, 2015.

82. Jiarui Wang, Rayko I Stantchev, Qiushuo Sun, Tor-Wo Chiu, Anil T Ahuja, and Emma Pickwell MacPherson. THz in vivo measurements: The effects of pressure on skin reflectivity. *Biomedical Optics Express*, 9(12): 6467, 2018.

83. Qiushuo Sun, Edward P J Parrott, Yuezhi He, and Emma Pickwell MacPherson. In vivo THz imaging of human skin: Accounting for occlusion effects. *Journal of Biophotonics*, 11(2): e201700111, 2018.

84. Hannah Lindley-Hatcher, A I Hernandez-Serrano, Qiushuo Sun, Jiarui Wang, Juan Cebrian, Laurent Blasco, and Emma Pickwell-MacPherson. A robust protocol for in vivo THz skin measurements. *Journal of Infrared, Millimeter, and Terahertz Waves*, 40(9): 980–989, 2019.

85. Lixia Wang, Sayon Guilavogui, Henghui Yin, Yiping Wu, Xiaofei Zang, Jingya Xie, Li Ding, and Lin Chen. Critical factors for in vivo measurements of human skin by terahertz attenuated total reflection spectroscopy. *Sensors*, 20(15): 4256, 2020.

86. Zoltan Vilagosh, Alireza Lajevardipour, and Andrew Wood. An empirical formula for temperature adjustment of complex permittivity of human skin in the terahertz frequencies. *Bioelectromagnetics*, 40(1): 74–79, 2019.

87. Xomalin G Peralta, Dawn Lipscomb, Gerald J Wilmink, and Ibtissam Echchgadda. Terahertz spectroscopy of human skin tissue models with different melanin content. *Biomedical Optics Express*, 10(6): 2942, 2019.

88. Shuting Fan, Benjamin S Y Ung, Edward P J Parrott, Vincent P Wallace, and Emma Pickwell-MacPherson. In vivo terahertz reflection imaging of human scars during and after the healing process. *Journal of Biophotonics*, 10(9): 1143–1151, 2017.

89. Priyamvada Tewari, James Garritano, Neha Bajwa, Shijun Sung, Haochong Huang, Dayong Wang, Warren Grundfest, Daniel B Ennis, Dan Ruan, Elliott Brown, Erik Dutson, Michael C Fishbein, and Zachary Taylor. Methods for registering and calibrating in vivo terahertz images of cutaneous burn wounds. *Biomedical Optics Express*, 10(1): 322, 2019.

90. Jiarui Wang, Qiushuo Sun, Rayko I Stantchev, Tor-Wo Chiu, Anil T Ahuja, and Emma Pickwell-MacPherson. In vivo terahertz imaging to evaluate scar treatment strategies: Silicone gel sheeting. *Biomedical Optics Express*, 10(7): 3584, 2019.

91. Omar B Osman, Timothy Jack Tan, Sam Henry, Adelaide Warsen, Navid Farr, Abbi M McClintic, Yak-Nam Wang, Saman Arbabi, and M Hassan Arbab. Differentiation of burn wounds in an in vivo porcine model using terahertz spectroscopy. *Biomedical Optics Express*, 11(11): 6528, 2020.

92. Jiarui Wang, Hannah Lindley-Hatcher, Kai Liu, and Emma Pickwell MacPherson. Evaluation of transdermal drug delivery using terahertz pulsed imaging. *Biomedical Optics Express*, 11(8): 4484, 2020.

93. Hannah Lindley-Hatcher, Jiarui Wang, Arturo I Hernandez-Serrano, Joseph Hardwicke, Gabit Nurumbetov, David M Haddleton, and Emma Pickwell MacPherson. Monitoring the effect of transdermal drug delivery patches on the skin using terahertz sensing. *Pharmaceutics*, 13(12): 2052, 2021.

94. Sota Sueda, Tomoya Niki, Kenji Sakai, and Toshihiko Kiwa. Evaluation of penetration speed of liquids into skin using a terahertz time-of-flight method. *Japanese Journal of Applied Physics*, 60(3): 032002, 2021.

95. Taihei Kuroda, Taiga Morimoto, Kenji Sakai, Toshihiko Kiwa, and Keiji Tsukada. Evaluation of penetration of cosmetic liquids using terahertz time of flight method. In *2018 43rd International Conference on Infrared, Millimeter, and Terahertz Waves (IRMMW-THz)*, pages 1–2. IEEE, 2018.

96. Tomoya Niki, Tomoki Kotani, Jin Wang, Kenji Sakai, and Toshihiko Kiwa. Evaluation of cosmetic liquid penetration using terahertz time-of-flight method. In *2021 46th International Conference on Infrared, Millimeter and Terahertz Waves (IRMMW-THz)*, pages 1–2. IEEE, 2021.

97. Gyuseok Lee, Ho Nmkung, Youngwoong Do, Soonsung Lee, Hyeona Kang, Jin-Woo Kim, and Haewook Han. Quantitative label-free terahertz sensing of transdermal nicotine delivered to human skin. *Current Optics and Photonics*, 4(4): 368–372, 2020.

98. Zachary D Taylor, Rahul S Singh, David B Bennett, Priyamvada Tewari, Colin P Kealey, Neha Bajwa, Martin O Culjat, Alexander Stojadinovic, Hua Lee, Jean-pierre Hubschman, Elliott R Brown, and Warren S Grundfest. THz medical imaging: In vivo hydration sensing. *IEEE Transactions on Terahertz Science and Technology*, 1(1): 201–219, 2011.

99. Qiushuo Sun, Rayko I Stantchev, Jiarui Wang, Edward P J Parrott, Alan Cottenden, Tor-Wo Chiu, Anil T Ahuja, and Emma Pickwell-MacPherson. In vivo estimation of water diffusivity in occluded human skin using terahertz reflection spectroscopy. *Journal of Biophotonics*, 12(2): e201800145, 2019.

100. Xuequan Chen, Qiushuo Sun, Jiarui Wang, Hannah Lindley-Hatcher, and Emma Pickwell-MacPherson. Exploiting complementary terahertz ellipsometry configurations to probe the hydration and cellular structure of skin in vivo. *Advanced Photonics Research*, 2(1): 2000024, 2021.

101. Hannah Lindley-Hatcher, A I Hernandez-Serrano, Jiarui Wang, Juan Cebrian, Joseph Hardwicke, and Emma Pickwell-MacPherson. Evaluation of in vivo THz sensing for assessing human skin hydration. *Journal of Physics: Photonics*, 3(1): 014001, 2021.

102. G G Hernandez-Cardoso, S C Rojas-Landeros, M Alfaro-Gomez, A I Hernandez-Serrano, I Salas-Gutierrez, E Lemus-Bedolla, A R Castillo Guzman, H L Lopez-Lemus, and E Castro-Camus. Terahertz imaging for early screening of diabetic foot syndrome: A proof of concept. *Scientific Reports*, 7(1): 42124, 2017.

103. G G Hernandez-Cardoso, M Alfaro-Gomez, S C Rojas-Landeros, I Salas Gutierrez, and E Castro-Camus. Pixel statistical analysis of diabetic vs. non-diabetic foot-sole spectral terahertz reflection images. *Journal of Infrared, Millimeter, and Terahertz Waves*, 39(9): 879–886, 2018.

104. O A Smolyanskaya, I J Schelkanova, M S Kulya, E L Odlyanitskiy, I S Goryachev, A N Tcypkin, Ya V Grachev, Ya G Toropova, and V V Tuchin. Glycerol dehydration of native and diabetic animal tissues studied by THz-TDS and NMR methods. *Biomedical Optics Express*, 9(3): 1198, 2018.

105. Olga Cherkasova, Maxim Nazarov, and Alexander Shkurinov. Noninvasive blood glucose monitoring in the terahertz frequency range. *Optical and Quantum Electronics*, 48(3): 217, 2016.

106. O P Cherkasova, M M Nazarov, I N Smirnova, A A Angeluts, and A P Shkurinov. Application of time-domain THz spectroscopy for studying blood plasma of rats with experimental diabetes. *Physics of Wave Phenomena*, 22(3): 185–188, 2014.

107. O P Cherkasova, M M Nazarov, A A Angeluts, and A P Shkurinov. Analysis of blood plasma at terahertz frequencies. *Optics and Spectroscopy*, 120(1): 50–57, 2016.

108. Anastasiya A Lykina, Maksim M Nazarov, Maria R Konnikova, Ilia A Mustafin, Vladimir L Vaks, Vladimir A Anfertev, Elena G Domracheva, Mariya B Chernyaeva, Yuri V Kistenev, Denis A Vrazhnov, Vladimir V Prischepa, Yulia A Kononova, Dmitry V Korolev, Olga P Cherkasova, Alexander P. Shkurinov, Alina Y Babenko, and Olga A Smolyanskaya. Terahertz spectroscopy of diabetic and non-diabetic human blood plasma pellets. *Journal of Biomedical Optics*, 26(4): 1–14, 2021.

109. Yu V Kistenev, A V Teteneva, T V Sorokina, A I Knyazkova, O A Zakharova, A Cuisset, V L Vaks, E G Domracheva, M B Chernyaeva, V A Anfert'ev, E S Sim, I Yu Yanina, V V Tuchin, and A V Borisov. Diagnosis of diabetes based on analysis of exhaled air by terahertz spectroscopy and machine learning. *Optics and Spectroscopy*, 128(6): 809–814, 2020.

110. Nick Rothbart, Olaf Holz, Rembert Koczulla, Klaus Schmalz, and Heinz Wilhelm Hübers. Analysis of human breath by millimeter-wave/terahertz spectroscopy. *Sensors*, 19(12): 2719, 2019.

111. Panagiotis C Theofanopoulos and Georgios C Trichopoulos. A novel finger print scanning method using terahertz imaging. In *2018 IEEE International Symposium on Antennas and Propagation and USNC/URSI National Radio Science Meeting*, pages 2463–2464. IEEE, 2018.

112. Norbert Pałka and Marcin Kowalski. Towards fingerprint spoofing detection in the terahertz range. *Sensors*, 20(12): 3379, 2020.

113. Aleksandr Bespalov, Anton Barchuk, Anssi Auvinen, and Jaakko Nevalainen. Cancer screening simulation models: A state of the art review. *BMC Medical Informatics and Decision Making*, 21(1): 359, 2021.

114. Ruth M Woodward, Bryan E Cole, Vincent P Wallace, Richard J Pye, Donald D Arnone, Edmund H Linfield, and Michael Pepper. Terahertz pulse imaging in reflection geometry of human skin cancer and skin tissue. *Physics in Medicine and Biology*, 47(21): 3853–3863, 2002.

115. R M Woodward, V P Wallace, D D Arnone, E H Linfield, and M Pepper. Terahertz pulsed imaging of skin cancer in the time and frequency domain. *Journal of Biological Physics*, 29(2–3): 257–259, 2003.

116. Ruth M Woodward, Vincent P Wallace, Richard J. Pye, Bryan E. Cole, Donald D. Arnone, Edmund H. Linfield, and Michael Pepper. Terahertz pulse imaging of ex vivo basal cell carcinoma. *Journal of Investigative Dermatology*, 120(1): 72–78, 2003.

117. Vincent P Wallace, Anthony J Fitzgerald, Emma Pickwell, Richard J Pye, Philip F. Taday, Niamh Flanagan, and Thomas Ha. Terahertz pulsed spectroscopy of human basal cell carcinoma. *Applied Spectroscopy*, 60(10): 1127–1133, 2006.

118. Cecil S Joseph, Anna N Yaroslavsky, Munir Al-Arashi, Thomas M Goyette, Jason C Dickinson, Andrew J Gatesman, Brian W Soper, Christopher M Forgione, Thomas M Horgan, Elizabeth J Ehasz, Robert H Giles, and William E Nixon. Terahertz spectroscopy of intrinsic biomarkers for non-melanoma skin cancer. *Proc. SPIE*, 7215: 72150I, 2009.

119. Cecil S Joseph, Rakesh Patel, Victor A Neel, Robert H Giles, and Anna N Yaroslavsky. Imaging of *ex vivo* nonmelanoma skin cancers in the optical and terahertz spectral regions optical and terahertz skin cancers imaging. *Journal of Biophotonics*, 7(5): 295–303, 2014.

120. K I Zaitsev, N V Chernomyrdin, K G Kudrin, I V Reshetov, and S O Yurchenko. Terahertz spectroscopy of pigmentary skin nevi in vivo. *Optics and Spectroscopy*, 119(3): 404–410, 2015.

121. Anis Rahman, Aunik K Rahman, and Babar Rao. Early detection of skin cancer via terahertz spectral profiling and 3D imaging. *Biosensors and Bioelectronics*, 82: 64–70, 2016.

122. Kirill I Zaytsev, Nikita V Chernomyrdin, Konstantin G Kudrin, Arseniy A Gavdush, Pavel A Nosov, Stanislav O Yurchenko, and Igor V Reshetov. In vivo terahertz pulsed spectroscopy of dysplastic and non-dysplastic skin nevi. *Journal of Physics: Conference Series*, 735: 012076, 2016.

123. Bo Fan, Victor A Neel, and Anna N Yaroslavsky. Multimodal imaging for nonmelanoma skin cancer margin delineation. *Lasers in Surgery and Medicine*, 49(3): 319–326, 2017.

124. Rui Zhang, Ke Yang, Qammer Abbasi, Najah Abed AbuAli, and Akram Alomainy. Experimental characterization of artificial human skin with melanomas for accurate modelling and detection in healthcare application. In *2018 43rd International Conference on Infrared, Millimeter, and Terahertz Waves (IRMMW-THz)*, pages 1–2. IEEE, 2018.

125. A V Postnikov, K A Moldosanov, N J Kairyev, and V M Lelevkin. A device to inspect a skin cancer tumour in the terahertz range, transferring the image into the infrared. *EPJ Web of Conferences*, 195: 10010, 2018.

126. S X Huang, X Y Guo, and M Y Xia. Terahertz wave scattering by skin cancer tissues. In *2018 IEEE International Conference on Computational Electromagnetics (ICCEM)*, pages 1–3. IEEE, 2018.

127. R Srivastava, J Cucalon, A K Rahman, B Rao, and A Rahman. Terahertz reconstructive imaging: A novel technique to differentiate healthy and diseased human skin. *British Journal of Cancer Research*, 2(1): 228–232, 2019.

128. Zoltan Vilagosh, Alireza Lajevardipour, and Andrew W Wood. Computational phantom study of frozen melanoma imaging at 0.45 terahertz. *Bioelectromagnetics*, 40(2): 118–127, 2019.

129. Dandan Li, Zhongbo Yang, Ailing Fu, Tunan Chen, Ligang Chen, Mingjie Tang, Hua Zhang, Ning Mu, Shi Wang, Guizhao Liang, and Huabin Wang. Detecting melanoma with a terahertz spectroscopy imaging technique. *Spectrochimica Acta Part A: Molecular and Biomolecular Spectroscopy*, 234: 118229, 2020.

130. Safa Isam Hakeem and Zainab Abdullah Hassoun. Skin cancer detection based on terahertz images by using Gabor filter and artificial neural network. *IOP Conference Series: Materials Science and Engineering*, 928(3): 032025, 2020.

131. Ruth M Woodward, Vincent P Wallace, Bryan E Cole, Richard J Pye, Donald D Arnone, Edmund H Linfield, and Michael Pepper. Terahertz pulse imaging in reflection geometry of skin tissue using time-domain analysis techniques. *Proc. SPIE* 4625: 160–169, 2002.

132. Anthony J Fitzgerald, Vincent P Wallace, Mercedes Jimenez-Linan, Lynda Bobrow, Richard J Pye, Anand D Purushotham, and Donald D. Arnone. Terahertz pulsed imaging of human breast tumors. *Radiology*, 239(2): 533–540, 2006.

133. Philip C Ashworth, Emma Pickwell-MacPherson, Elena Provenzano, Sarah E Pinder, Anand D Purushotham, Michael Pepper, and Vincent P Wallace. Terahertz pulsed spectroscopy of freshly excised human breast cancer. *Optics Express*, 17(15): 12444, 2009.

134. Hua Chen, Te-Hsuen Chen, Tzu-Fang Tseng, Jen-Tang Lu, Chung-Chiu Kuo, Shih-Chen Fu, Wen-Jeng Lee, Yuan-Fu Tsai, Yi-You Huang, Eric Y. Chuang, Yuh-Jing Hwang, and Chi-Kuang Sun. High-sensitivity in vivo THz transmission imaging of early human breast cancer in a subcutaneous xenograft mouse model. *Optics Express*, 19(22): 21552, 2011.

135. Hua Chen, Juan Han, Dan Wang, Yu Zhang, Xiao Li, and Xiaofeng Chen. In vivo estimation of breast cancer tissue volume in subcutaneous xenotrans plantation mouse models by using a high-sensitivity fiber-based terahertz scanning imaging system. *Frontiers in Genetics*, 12(September): 1–6, 2021.

136. Benjamin St Peter, Sigfrid Yngvesson, Paul Siqueira, Patrick Kelly, Ashraf Khan, Stephen Glick, and Andrew Karellas. Development and testing of a single frequency terahertz imaging system for breast cancer detection. *IEEE Transactions on Terahertz Science and Technology*, 3(4): 374–386, 2013.

137. Tyler Bowman, Yuhao Wu, John Gauch, Lucas K. Campbell, and Magda El-Shenawee. Terahertz imaging of three-dimensional dehydrated breast cancer tumors. *Journal of Infrared, Millimeter, and Terahertz Waves*, 2017.

138. Tyler Bowman, Tanny Chavez, Kamrul Khan, Jingxian Wu, Avishek Chakraborty, Narasimhan Rajaram, Keith Bailey, and Magda El-Shenawee. Pulsed terahertz imaging of breast cancer in freshly excised murine tumors. *Journal of Biomedical Optics*, 23(2): 026004, 2018.

139. Nagma Vohra, Tyler Bowman, Paola M Diaz, Narasimhan Rajaram, Keith Bailey, and Magda El-Shenawee. Pulsed terahertz reflection imaging of tumors in a spontaneous model of breast cancer. *Biomedical Physics and Engineering Express*, 4(6): 065025, 2018.

140. Tanny Chavez, Tyler Bowman, Jingxian Wu, Keith Bailey, and Magda El Shenawee. Assessment of terahertz imaging for excised breast cancer tumors with image morphing. *Journal of Infrared, Millimeter, and Terahertz Waves*, 39(12): 1283–1302, 2018.

141. Tyler Bowman, Keith Bailey, Magda El-Shenawee, Tyler Bowman, Nagma Vohra, Keith Bailey, and Magda El-shenawee. Terahertz tomographic imaging of freshly excised human breast tissues. *Journal of Medical Imaging*, 6(2): 023501, 2019.

142. Nagma Vohra, Tyler Bowman, Keith Bailey, and Magda El-Shenawee. Terahertz imaging and characterization protocol for freshly excised breast cancer tumors. *Journal of Visualized Experiments*, (158): e61007, 2020.

143. Tanny Chavez, Nagma Vohra, Jingxian Wu, Keith Bailey, and Magda El Shenawee. Breast cancer detection with low-dimensional ordered orthogonal projection in terahertz imaging. *IEEE Transactions on Terahertz Science and Technology*, 10(2): 176–189, 2020.

144. Tanny Chavez, Nagma Vohra, Keith Bailey, Magda El-Shenawee, and Jingxian Wu. Supervised Bayesian learning for breast cancer detection in terahertz imaging. *Biomedical Signal Processing and Control*, 70(June): 102949, 2021.

145. Nagma Vohra, Tanny Chavez, Joel R Troncoso, Narasimhan Rajaram, Jingxian Wu, Patricia N Coan, Todd A Jackson, Keith Bailey, and Magda El Shenawee. Mammary tumors in Sprague Dawley rats induced by N-ethyl N-nitrosourea for evaluating terahertz imaging of breast cancer. *Journal of Medical Imaging*, 8(2): 1–17, 2021.

146. Maarten R Grootendorst, Anthony J Fitzgerald, Susan G Brouwer de Koning, Aida Santaolalla, Alessia Portieri, Mieke Van Hemelrijck, Matthew R Young, Julie Owen, Massi Cariati, Michael Pepper, Vincent P Wallace, Sarah E Pinder, and Arnie Purushotham. Use of a handheld terahertz pulsed imaging device to differentiate benign and malignant breast tissue. *Biomedical Optics Express*, 8(6): 2932, 2017.

147. Wenquan Liu, Rui Zhang, Yu Ling, Hongping Tang, Rongbin She, Guanglu Wei, Xiaojing Gong, and Yuanfu Lu. Automatic recognition of breast invasive ductal carcinoma based on terahertz spectroscopy with wavelet packet transform and machine learning. *Biomedical Optics Express*, 11(2): 971, 2020.

148. Quentin Cassar, Samuel Caravera, Gaëtan MacGrogan, Thomas Bücher, Philipp Hillger, Ullrich Pfeiffer, Thomas Zimmer, Jean-Paul Guillet, and Patrick Mounaix. Terahertz refractive index-based morphological dilation for breast carcinoma delineation. *Scientific Reports*, 11(1): 6457, 2021.

149. Eman M. Hassan, Ahmed Mohamed, Maria C. DeRosa, William G. Willmore, Yuki Hanaoka, Toshihiko Kiwa, and Tsuneyuki Ozaki. High-sensitivity detection of metastatic breast cancer cells via terahertz chemical microscopy using aptamers. *Sensors and Actuators B: Chemical*, 287(February): 595–601, 2019.

150. Kosuke Okada, Quentin Cassar, Hironaru Murakami, Gaëtan MacGrogan, Jean-Paul Guillet, Patrick Mounaix, Masayoshi Tonouchi, and Kazunori Serita. Label-free observation of micrometric inhomogeneity of human breast cancer cell density using terahertz near-field microscopy. *Photonics*, 8(5): 151, 2021.

151. Seung Jae Oh, Yong-Min Huh, Sang-Hoon Kim, Jaemoon Yang, Kiyoung Jeong, Yeonji Park, Chul Kang, Joo-Hiuk Son, and Jin-Suck Suh. Terahertz pulse imaging of fresh brain tumor. In *2011 International Conference on Infrared, Millimeter, and Terahertz Waves*, pages 1–2. IEEE, 2011.

152. Kun Meng, Tu-nan Chen, Tao Chen, Li-guo Zhu, Qiao Liu, Zhao Li, Fei Li, Sen-cheng Zhong, Ze-ren Li, Hua Feng, and Jian-heng Zhao. Terahertz pulsed spectroscopy of paraffin-embedded brain glioma. *Journal of Biomedical Optics*, 19(7): 077001, 2014.

153. Young Bin Ji, Seung Jae Oh, Seok-gu Kang, Jung Heo, Sang-Hoon Kim, Yuna Choi, Seungri Song, Hye Young Son, Se Hoon Kim, Ji Hyun Lee, Seung Joo Haam, Yong Min Huh, Jong Hee Chang, Chulmin Joo, and Jin-Suck Suh. Terahertz reflectometry imaging for low and high grade gliomas. *Scientific Reports*, 6(1): 36040, 2016.

154. Hengli Zhao and Tunan Chen. High-sensitivity terahertz imaging of traumatic brain injury in a rat model. *Journal of Biomedical Optics*, 23(3): 036015, 2018.

155. Kirill I Zaytsev, Nikita V Chernomyrdin, Arseniy A Gavdush, Sheyh Islyam T Beshplav, Kirill M Malakhov, Anna S Kucheryavenko, Gleb M Katyba, Irina N Dolganova, Sergey A Goryaynov, Valeriy E Karassik, Igor E Spector, Vladimir N Kurlov, Stanislav O Yurchenko, Gennadiy A Komandin, Alexander A Potapov, and Valery V Tuchin. In vitro terahertz spectroscopy of gelatin-embedded human brain tumors: A pilot study, *Proc. SPIE* 10716: 107160S, 2018.

156. Yan Peng, Wanqing Chen, and Yiming Zhu. Identification of biomarker (L-2HG) in real human brain glioma by terahertz spectroscopy. In *2018 Conference on Lasers and Electro-Optics (CLEO)*, pages 3–4. OSA, 2018.

157. Arseniy A Gavdush, Nikita V Chernomyrdin, Kirill M Malakhov, Sheyh Islyam T Beshplav, Irina N Dolganova, Alexandra V Kosyrkova, Pavel V Nikitin, Guzel R Musina, Gleb M Katyba, Igor V Reshetov, Olga P Cherkasova, Gennady A Komandin, Valery E Karasik, Alexander A Potapov, Valery V Tuchin, and Kirill I Zaytsev. Terahertz spectroscopy of gelatin-embedded human brain gliomas of different grades: A road toward intraoperative THz diagnosis. *Journal of Biomedical Optics*, 24(2): 027001, 2019.

158. Limin Wu, Degang Xu, Yuye Wang, Bin Liao, Zhinan Jiang, Lu Zhao, Zhongcheng Sun, Nan Wu, Tunan Chen, Hua Feng, and Jianquan Yao. Study of in vivo brain glioma in a mouse model using continuous-wave terahertz reflection imaging. *Biomedical Optics Express*, 10(8): 3953, 2019.

159. Olga Cherkasova, Yan Peng, Maria Konnikova, Yuri Kistenev, Chenjun Shi, Denis Vrazhnov, Oleg Shevelev, Evgeny Zavjalov, Sergei Kuznetsov, and Alexander Shkurinov. Diagnosis of glioma molecular markers by terahertz technologies. *Photonics*, 8(1): 22, 2021.

160. A A Gavdush, N V Chernomyrdin, G A Komandin, I N Dolganova, P V Nikitin, G R Musina, G M Katyba, A S Kucheryavenko, I V Reshetov, A A Potapov, V V Tuchin, and K I Zaytsev. Terahertz dielectric spec tros-copy of human brain gliomas and intact tissues ex vivo: Double-Debye and double-overdamped-oscillator models of dielectric response. *Biomedical Optics Express*, 12(1): 69, 2021.

161. Jin Zhang, Ning Mu, Longhai Liu, Jianhua Xie, Hua Feng, Jianquan Yao, Tunan Chen, and Weiren Zhu. Highly sensitive detection of malignant glioma cells using metamaterial-inspired THz biosensor based on elec-tromagnetically induced transparency. *Biosensors and Bioelectronics*, 185(February): 113241, 2021.

162. Limin Wu, Yuye Wang, Bin Liao, Lu Zhao, Kai Chen, Meilan Ge, Haibin Li, Tunan Chen, Hua Feng, Degang Xu, and Jianquan Yao. Temperature dependent terahertz spectroscopy and imaging of orthotopic brain glio-mas in mouse models. *Biomedical Optics Express*, 13(1): 93, 2022.

163. Ning Mu, Chuanyan Yang, Degang Xu, Shi Wang, Kang Ma, Ying Lai, Peiwen Guo, Shuixian Zhang, Yuye Wang, Hua Feng, Tunan Chen, and Jianquan Yao. Molecular pathological recognition of freshly excised human glioma using terahertz ATR spectroscopy. *Biomedical Optics Express*, 13(1): 222, 2022.

164. Sayuri Yamaguchi, Yasuko Fukushi, Oichi Kubota, Takeaki Itsuji, Toshihiko Ouchi, and Seiji Yamamoto. Origin and quantification of differ-ences between normal and tumor tissues observed by terahertz spectros-copy. *Physics in Medicine and Biology*, 61(18): 6808–6820, 2016.

165. Hairui Sun, Lianhu Yin, Showwei Li, Song Han, Guangrong Song, Ning Liu, and Changxiang Yan. Prognostic significance of IDH mutation in adult low grade gliomas: A meta-analysis. *Journal of Neuro-Oncology*, 113(2): 277–284, 2013.

166. Irmantas Kašalynas, Rimvydas Venckevičius, Linas Minkevičius, Aleksander Sešek, Faustino Wahaia, Vincas Tamošiunas, Bogdan Voisiat, Dalius Seliuta, Gintaras Valušis, Andrej Švigelj, and Janez Trontelj. Spectroscopic terahertz imaging at room temperature employing microbo-lometer terahertz sensors and its application to the study of carcinoma tis-sues. *Sensors*, 16(4): 432, 2016.

167. Yuqi Cao, Jiani Chen, Pingjie Huang, Weiting Ge, Dibo Hou, and Guangxin Zhang. Inspecting human colon adenocarcinoma cell lines by using tera-hertz time-domain reflection spectroscopy. *Spectrochimica Acta Part A: Molecular and Biomolecular Spectroscopy*, 211: 356–362, 2019.

168. Yuqi Cao, Jiani Chen, Guangxin Zhang, Shuyu Fan, Weiting Ge, Wangxiong Hu, Pingjie Huang, Dibo Hou, and Shu Zheng. Characterization and discrimination of human colorectal cancer cells using terahertz spectroscopy. *Spectrochimica Acta Part A: Molecular and Biomolecular Spectroscopy*, 256: 119713, 2021.

169. Euna Jung, Meehyun Lim, Kiwon Moon, Youngwoong Do, Soonsung Lee, Haewook Han, Hyuck-Jae Choi, Kyoung-Sik Cho, and Kyu-Rae Kim. Terahertz pulse imaging of micro-metastatic lymph nodes in early-stage cervical cancer patients. *Journal of the Optical Society of Korea*, 15(2):155–160, 2011.

170. Wei Shi, Yuezheng Wang, Lei Hou, Cheng Ma, Lei Yang, Chengang Dong, Zhiquan Wang, Haiqing Wang, Juan Guo, Shenglong Xu, and Jing Li. Detection of living cervical cancer cells by transient terahertz spectroscopy. *Journal of Biophotonics*, 14(1): 1–7, 2021.

171. Xiaoyue Yang, Mei Li, Qi Peng, Jian Huang, Lifen Liu, Ping Li, Chenggan Shu, Xing Hu, Jie Fang, Fei Ye, and Weipei Zhu. Label-free detection of living cervical cells based on microfluidic device with terahertz spectroscopy. *Journal of Biophotonics*, 15(1): 1–11, 2022.

172. Jae Yeon Park, Hyuck Jae Choi, Hwayeong Cheon, Seong Whi Cho, Seungkoo Lee, and Joo-Hiuk Son. Terahertz imaging of metastatic lymph nodes using spectroscopic integration technique. *Biomedical Optics Express*, 8(2): 1122, 2017.

173. Na Qi, Zhuoyong Zhang, Yuhong Xiang, Yuping Yang, Xueai Liang, and Peter De B Harrington. Terahertz time-domain spectroscopy combined with support vector machines and partial least squares-discriminant analysis applied for the diagnosis of cervical carcinoma. *Analytical Methods*, 7(6): 2333–2338, 2015.

174. Dongxia Li, Fangrong Hu, Haipeng Zhang, Zhencheng Chen, Gaoxiang Huang, Fang Tang, Shangjun Lin, Yingchang Zou, and Yuan Zhou. Identification of early-stage cervical cancer tissue using metamaterial terahertz biosensor with two resonant absorption frequencies. *IEEE Journal of Selected Topics in Quantum Electronics*, 27(4): 1–7, 2021.

175. A Roggenbuck, H Schmitz, A Deninger, I Cámara Mayorga, J Hemberger, R Güsten, and M Grüninger. Coherent broadband continuous-wave terahertz spectroscopy on solid-state samples. *New Journal of Physics*, 12(4): 043017, 2010.

176. Stanley Sy, Shengyang Huang, Yi-Xiang J Wang, Jun Yu, Anil T Ahuja, Yuan Ting Zhang, and Emma Pickwell-MacPherson. Terahertz spectroscopy of liver cirrhosis: Investigating the origin of contrast. *Physics in Medicine and Biology*, 55(24): 7587–7596, 2010.

177. Young Bin Ji, Jung Min Kim, Young Han Lee, Yuna Choi, Da Hee Kim, Yong Min Huh, Seung Jae Oh, Yoon Woo Koh, and Jin-Suck Suh. Investigation of keratinizing squamous cell carcinoma of the tongue using terahertz reflection imaging. *Journal of Infrared, Millimeter, and Terahertz Waves*, 40(2): 247–256, 2019.

178. Chiben Zhang, Tingjia Xue, Jin Zhang, Longhai Liu, Jianhua Xie, Guangming Wang, Jianquan Yao, Weiren Zhu, and Xiaodan Ye. Terahertz toroidal meta surface biosensor for sensitive distinction of lung cancer cells. *Nanophotonics*, 11(1): 101–109, 2021.

179. Yuichi Yoshida, Xue Ding, Kohei Iwatsuki, Katsuya Taniizumi, Hirofumi Inoue, Jin Wang, Kenji Sakai, and Toshihiko Kiwa. Detection of lung cancer cells in solutions using a terahertz chemical microscope. *Sensors*, 21(22): 7631, 2021.

180. Mihai Danciu, Teodora Alexa-Stratulat, Cipriana Stefanescu, Gianina Dodi, Bogdan Ionel Tamba, Cosmin Teodor Mihai, Gabriela Dumitrita Stanciu, Andrei Luca, Irene Alexandra Spiridon, Loredana Beatrice

Ungureanu, Victor Ianole, Irina Ciortescu, Catalina Mihai, Gabriela Stefanescu, Ioan Chirilă, Romeo Ciobanu, and Vasile Liviu Drug. Terahertz spectroscopy and imag ing: A cutting-edge method for diagnosing digestive cancers. *Materials*, 12(9): 1519, 2019.

181. Faustino Wahaia, Irmantas Kašalynas, Linas Minkevičius, Catia Carvalho Silva, Andrzej Urbanowicz, and Gintaras Valušis. Terahertz spectroscopy and imaging for gastric cancer diagnosis. *Journal of Spectral Imaging*, 9: 1–8, 2020.

182. Tatiana Globus, Igor Sizov, Jerome Ferrance, Amir Jazaeri, Jennifer Bryant, Aaron Moyer, Boris Gelmont, Mark Kester, and Alexei Bykhovski. Sub terahertz vibrational spectroscopy for microRNA based diagnostic of ovarian cancer. *Convergent Science Physical Oncology*, 2(4): 045001, 2016.

183. Tatiana Globus, Jerome Ferrance, Christopher Moskaluk, Boris Gelmont, Alexei Bykhovski, Aaron Moyer, Igor Gelmanov, and Varvara Peskova. Sub terahertz spectroscopic signatures from micro-rna molecules in fluid samples for ovarian cancer analysis. *Case Reports and Literature Review*, 2(2): 1–13, 2018.

184. Tatiana Globus, Christopher Moskaluk, Patcharin Pramoonjago, Boris Gelmont, Aaron Moyer, Alexei Bykhovski, and Jerome Ferrance. Sub-terahertz vibrational spectroscopy of ovarian cancer and normal control tissue for molecular diagnostic technology. *Cancer Biomarkers*, 24(4): 405–419, 2019.

185. Jinhua Zhang, Zhanghua Han, Cunzhong Yuan, Shujie Liu, Shu Yao, Kun Song, and Xuantao Su. Label-free characterization of cancerous ovarian tissues with continuous wave terahertz spectroscopy. *Proc. SPIE* 11562: 115620V, 2020.

186. Ping Zhang, Shuncong Zhong, Junxi Zhang, Jian Ding, Zhenxiang Liu, Yi Huang, Ning Zhou, Walter Nsengiyumva, and Tianfu Zhang. Application of terahertz spectroscopy and imaging in the diagnosis of prostate cancer. *Current Optics and Photonics*, 4(1): 31–43, 2020.

187. Anastasia I Knyazkova, Alexey V Borisov, Lyudmila V Spirina, and Yury V Kistenev. Paraffin-embedded prostate cancer tissue grading using terahertz spectroscopy and machine learning. *Journal of Infrared, Millimeter, and Terahertz Waves*, 41(9): 1089–1104, 2020.

188. David B Bennett, Zachary D Taylor, Pria Tewari, Rahul S Singh, Martin O Culjat, Warren S Grundfest, Daniel J Sassoon, R Duncan Johnson, Jean Pierre Hubschman, and Elliott R Brown. Terahertz sensing in corneal tissues. *Journal of Biomedical Optics*, 16(5): 057003, 2011.

189. Wen-Quan Liu, Yuan-Fu Lu, Guo-Hua Jiao, Xian-Feng Chen, Jin-Ying Li, Si-Hai Chen, Yu-Ming Dong, and Jian-Cheng Lv. Terahertz optical properties of the cornea. *Optics Communications*, 359: 344–348, 2016.

190. Ilya Ozheredov, Mikhail Prokopchuk, Mikhail Mischenko, Tatiana Safonova, Petr Solyankin, Andrey Larichev, Andrey Angeluts, Alexei Balakin, and Alexander Shkurinov. In vivo THz sensing of the cornea of the eye. *Laser Physics Letters*, 15(5): 055601, 2018.

191. Andrew Chen, Omar B Osman, Zachery B Harris, Azin Abazri, Robert Honkanen, and M Hassan Arbab. Investigation of water diffusion dynamics in corneal phantoms using terahertz time-domain spectroscopy. *Biomedical Optics Express*, 11(3): 1284, 2020.

192. Lin Ke, Qing Yang, Steve Wu, Nan Zhang, Zaifeng Yang, Erica Pei Wen Teo, Jodhbir S Mehta, and Yu-Chi Liu. Terahertz spectroscopy analysis of human corneal sublayers. *Journal of Biomedical Optics*, 26(4): 1–11, 2021.

193. Jiali Yao, Jiaonan Ma, Jiehui Zhao, Pengfei Qi, Mengdi Li, Lie Lin, Lu Sun, Xiaolei Wang, Weiwei Liu, and Yan Wang. Corneal hydration assessment indicator based on terahertz time domain spectroscopy. *Biomedical Optics Express*, 11(4): 2073, 2020.

194. Lin Ke, Nan Zhang, Qing Yang Steve Wu, Sergey Gorelik, Ali Abdelaziem, Zheng Liu, Erica Pei Wen Teo, Jodhbir S. Mehta, and Yu-Chi Liu. In vivo sensing of rabbit cornea by terahertz technology. *Journal of Biophotonics*, 14(9): 1–9, 2021.

195. Maya Mizuno, Hideaki Kitahara, Kensuke Sasaki, Masahiko Tani, Masami Kojima, Yukihisa Suzuki, Takafumi Tasaki, Yoshinori Tatematsu, Masafumi Fukunari, and Kanako Wake. Dielectric property measurements of corneal tissues for computational dosimetry of the eye in terahertz band in vivo and in vitro. *Biomedical Optics Express*, 12(3): 1295, 2021.

196. Lin Ke, Qing Yang, Steve Wu, Nan Zhang, Hong Wei Liu, Erica Pei Wen Teo, Jodhbir S Mehta, and Yu-Chi Liu. Ex vivo sensing and imaging of corneal scar tissues using terahertz time domain spectroscopy. *Spectrochimica Acta Part A: Molecular and Biomolecular Spectroscopy*, 255: 119667, 2021.

197. Andrew Chen, Arjun Virk, Zachery Harris, Azin Abazari, Robert Honkanen, and M Hassan Arbab. Non-contact terahertz spectroscopic measurement of the intraocular pressure through corneal hydration mapping. *Biomedical Optics Express*, 12(6): 3438, 2021.

198. Elena N Iomdina, Sergey V Seliverstov, Kseniya O Teplyakova, Elena V Jani, Viktorya V Pozdniakova, Olga N Polyakova, and Gregory N Goltsman. Terahertz scanning of the rabbit cornea with experimental UVB-induced damage: In vivo assessment of hydration and its verification. *Journal of Biomedical Optics*, 26(4): 1–10, 2021.

199. Shijun Sung, Elliott R Brown, Warren S. Grundfest, Zachary D Taylor, Skyler Selvin, Neha Bajwa, Somporn Chantra, Bryan Nowroozi, James Garritano, Jacob Goell, Alexander D Li, and Sophie X Deng. THz imaging system for in vivo human cornea. *IEEE Transactions on Terahertz Science and Technology*, 8(1): 27–37, 2018.

200. Yong Hu, Mariangela Baggio, Shahab Dabironezare, Aleksi Tamminen, Brandon Toy, Juha Ala-laurinaho, Elliot Brown, Nuria Llombart, Sophie Deng, Vincent Wallace, and Zachary Taylor. 650 GHz imaging as alignment verification for millimeter wave corneal reflectometry. *IEEE Transactions on Terahertz Science and Technology*, 12(2): 151–164, 2022.

201. Aleksi Tamminen, Samu-Ville Palli, Juha Ala-Laurinaho, Mika Salkola, Antti V Raisanen, and Zachary D Taylor. Quasioptical system for corneal sensing at 220–330 GHz: Design, evaluation, and ex vivo cornea parameter extraction. *IEEE Transactions on Terahertz Science and Technology*, 11(2): 135–149, 2021.
202. David A Crawley, Christopher Longbottom, Bryan E Cole, Craig M Ciesla, Don Arnone, Vincent P. Wallace, and Michael Pepper. Terahertz pulse imaging: A pilot study of potential applications in dentistry. *Caries Research*, 37(5): 352–359, 2003.
203. Emma Pickwell, Vincent P Wallace, Bryan E Cole, Sophia Ali, Christopher Longbottom, Richard J M Lynch, and Michael Pepper. A comparison of terahertz pulsed imaging with transmission microradiography for depth measurement of enamel demineralisation in vitro. Caries Research, 41(1): 49–55, 2007.
204. David Churchley, Richard J M Lynch, Frank Lippert, Jennifer Susan O'Bryan Eder, Jesse Alton, and Carlos Gonzalez-Cabezas. Terahertz pulsed imaging study to assess remineralization of artificial caries lesions. *Journal of Biomedical Optics*, 16(2): 026001, 2011.
205. M M Nazarov, A P Shkurinov, E A Kuleshov, and V V Tuchin. Terahertz time domain spectroscopy of biological tissues. *Quantum Electronics*, 38(7):647–654, 2008.
206. S V Smirnov, Ya V Grachev, A N Tsypkin, and V G Bespalov. Experimental studies of the possibilities of diagnosing caries in the solid tissues of a tooth by means of terahertz radiation. *Journal of Optical Technology*, 81(8): 464, 2014.
207. Kıvanç Kamburoğlu, Burcu Karagöz, Hakan Altan, and Dogukan Özen. An ex vivo comparative study of occlusal and proximal caries using terahertz and X-ray imaging. *Dentomaxillofacial Radiology*, 48(2): 20180250, 2019.
208. K Kamburoğlu, N Ö Yetimoglu, and H Altan. Characterization of primary and permanent teeth using terahertz spectroscopy. *Dentomaxillofacial Radiology*, 43(6): 20130404, 2014.
209. Nagendra Paradad Yadav, Guo-Zhen Hu, Zheng-Peng Yao, and Ashish Kumar. Diagnosis of dental problem by using terahertz technology. *Journal of Electronic Science and Technology*, 19(3): 100082, 2021.
210. O A Smolyanskaya, O V Kravtsenyuk, A V Panchenko, E L Odlyanitskiy, J P Guillet, O P Cherkasova, and M K Khodzitsky. Study of blood plasma optical properties in mice grafted with Ehrlich carcinoma in the frequency range 0.1–1.0 THz. *Quantum Electronics*, 47(11): 1031–1040, 2017.
211. M. Konnikova, O. Cherkasova, M. Nazarov, D. Vrazhnov, Y. Kistenev, and A. Shkurinov. Terahertz spectroscopy of blood plasma as a promising method for diagnosing of thyroid cancer. In *2020 45th International Conference on Infrared, Millimeter, and Terahertz Waves (IRMMW-THz)*, pages 1–2. IEEE, 2020.
212. Mingxia He, Abul K. Azad, Shenghua Ye, and Weili Zhang. Far-infrared sig nature of animal tissues characterized by terahertz time-domain spectroscopy. *Optics Communications*, 259(1): 389–392, 2006.

213. Yuezhi He, Kai Liu, Corinna Au, Qiushuo Sun, Edward P J Parrott, and Emma PickWell-MacPherson. Determination of terahertz permittivity of dehydrated biological samples. *Physics in Medicine and Biology*, 62(23): 8882–8893, 2017.

214. A S Nikoghosyan, H Ting, J Shen, R M Martirosyan, M Yu Tunyan, A V Papikyan, and A A Papikyan. Optical properties of human jawbone and human bone substitute Cerabone® in the terahertz range. *Journal of Contemporary Physics (Armenian Academy of Sciences)*, 51(3): 256–264, 2016.

215. Ke Yang, Nishtha Chopra, Qammer H Abbasi, Khalid A Qaraqe, and Akram Alomainy. Collagen analysis at terahertz band using double-debye parameter extraction and particle swarm optimisation. *IEEE Access*, 5(8): 27850–27856, 2017.

216. Pingjie Huang, Yuqi Cao, Jiani Chen, Weiting Ge, Dibo Hou, and Guangxin Zhang. Analysis and inspection techniques for mouse liver injury based on terahertz spectroscopy. *Optics Express*, 27(18): 26014, 2019.

217. Yuqi Cao, Pingjie Huang, Jiani Chen, Weiting Ge, Dibo Hou, and Guangxin Zhang. Qualitative and quantitative detection of liver injury with terahertz time-domain spectroscopy. *Biomedical Optics Express*, 11(2): 982, 2020.

218. W -G. Yeo, O Gurel, N K Nahar, C L Hitchcock, N L Lehman, S Park, and K Sertel. THz imaging of Alzheimer's disease: Spectroscopic differentiation between normal and diseased tissues. In *2014 39th International Conference on Infrared, Millimeter, and Terahertz waves (IRMMW-THz)*, volume 1, pages 1–2. IEEE, 2014.

219. Yu Rong, Panagiotis C Theofanopoulos, Georgios C Trichopoulos, and Daniel W Bliss. Cardiac sensing exploiting an ultra-wideband terahertz sensing system. In *2020 IEEE International Radar Conference, RADAR 2020*, pages 1002–1006, 2020.

220. B M Fischer, M Walther, and P Uhd Jepsen. Far-infrared vibrational modes of DNA components studied by terahertz time-domain spectroscopy. *Physics in Medicine and Biology*, 47(21): 3807–3814, 2002.

221. Yu Heng Tao, Stuart I Hodgetts, Alan R Harvey, Stephen Moggach, and Vincent P Wallace. Is there a terahertz absorption peak in frozen aqueous solutions of DNA nucleosides? In *2021 46th International Conference on Infrared, Millimeter and Terahertz Waves (IRMMW-THz)*, pages 1–2. IEEE, 2021.

222. M V Tsurkan, N S Balbekin, E A Sobakinskaya, A N Panin, and V L Vaks. Terahertz spectroscopy of DNA. *Optics and Spectroscopy*, 114(6): 894–898, 2013.

223. Hwayeong Cheon, Hee Jin Yang, Sang Hun Lee, Young A Kim, and Joo Hiuk Son. Terahertz molecular resonance of cancer DNA. *Scientific Reports*, 6(1): 37103, 2016.

224. Pingjie Huang, Piaoyun Chen, Zhangwei Huang, Yuqi Cao, Dibo Hou, and Guangxin Zhang. Terahertz spectral analysis of DNA based molecule cytosine and its methylated structure 5-methylcytosine. *Proc. SPIE* 11196, 111961V, 2019.

225. Mingjie Tang, Mingkun Zhang, Liangping Xia, Zhongbo Yang, Shihan Yan, Huabin Wang, Dongshan Wei, Chunlei Du, and Hong-Liang Cui. Detection of single-base mutation of DNA oligonucleotides with different lengths by terahertz attenuated total reflection microfluidic cell. *Biomedical Optics Express*, 11(9): 5362, 2020.

226. A N Bogomazova, E M Vassina, T N Goryachkovskaya, V M Popik, A S Sokolov, N A Kolchanov, M A Lagarkova, S L Kiselev, and S E Peltek. No DNA damage response and negligible genome-wide transcriptional changes in human embryonic stem cells exposed to terahertz radiation. *Scientific Reports*, 5(1): 7749, 2015.

227. Kaijie Wu, Chonghai Qi, Zhi Zhu, Chunlei Wang, Bo Song, and Chao Chang. Terahertz wave accelerates DNA unwinding: A molecular dynamics simulation study. *The Journal of Physical Chemistry Letters*, 11(17): 7002–7008, 2020.

228. Tyler L. Cocker, Vedran Jelic, Manisha Gupta, Sean J. Molesky, Jacob A J Burgess, Glenda De Los Reyes, Lyubov V. Titova, Ying Y. Tsui, Mark R Freeman, and Frank A Hegmann. An ultrafast terahertz scanning tunnelling microscope. *Nature Photonics*, 7(8): 620–625, 2013.

229. Oleg Mitrofanov, Leonardo Viti, Enrico Dardanis, Maria Caterina Giordano, Daniele Ercolani, Antonio Politano, Lucia Sorba, and Miriam S Vitiello. Near-field terahertz probes with room-temperature nanodetectors for subwavelength resolution imaging. *Scientific Reports*, 7(March): 44240, 2017.

230. P J Neyman, W B Colson, S C Gottshalk, A M M Todd, J Blau, and K Cohn. Free electron lasers in 2017 list of fels in 2017. In *38th International Free Electron Laser Conference*, page 6, 2018.

231. M V Duka (Tsurkan), Yu S Nesgovorova, O A Smolyanskaya, V G Bespalov, I V Kudryavtsev, A V Polevshchikov, M K Serebryakova, I V Nazarova, and A S Trulev. Study of the action of broad-band terahertz radiation on the functional activity of cells. *Journal of Optical Technology*, 80(11): 655, 2013.

232. M V Duka Tsurkan, M K Serebriakova, and I V Kudryavtsev. Influence of terahertz radiation with a frequency $0.05 \div 1.7$ THz on mitochondrial membrane potential of tumor cells. In *PIERS Proceedings*, pages 1523–1526, 2014.

233. Ibtissam Echchgadda, Jessica E. Grundt, Cesario Z. Cerna, Caleb C. Roth, Jason A. Payne, Bennett L. Ibey, and Gerald J. Wilmink. Terahertz radiation: A non-contact tool for the selective stimulation of biological responses in human cells. *IEEE Transactions on Terahertz Science and Technology*, 6(1): 54–68, 2016.

234. O A Smolyanskaya, E L Odlyanitskiy, S A Chivilikhin, I J Schelkanova, and S A Kozlov. Theoretical and experimental investigations of the heat transfer of eye cornea in terahertz field. In *2017 42nd International Conference on Infrared, Millimeter, and Terahertz Waves (IRMMW-THz)*, pages 1–2. IEEE, 2017.

235. Wenquan Liu, Yuanfu Lu, Rongbin She, Guanglu Wei, Guohua Jiao, Jiancheng Lv, and Guangyuan Li. Thermal analysis of cornea heated with terahertz radiation. *Applied Sciences*, 9(5): 917, 2019.

236. Yu-Chi Liu, Lin Ke, Steve Wu Qing Yang, Zhang Nan, Ericia Pei Wen Teo, Nyein Chan Lwin, Molly Tzu-Yu Lin, Isabelle Xin Yu Lee, Anita Sook-Yee Chan, Leopold Schmetterer, and Jodhbir S Mehta. Safety profiles of terahertz scanning in ophthalmology. *Scientific Reports*, 11(1): 2448, 2021.

237. Elizaveta V Demidova, Tatiana N Goryachkovskaya, Irina A Mescheryakova, Tatiana K Malup, Artem I Semenov, Nikolay A Vinokurov, Nikolay A Kolchanov, Vasiliy M Popik, and Sergey E Peltek. Impact of terahertz radiation on stress-sensitive genes of *E.coli* cell. *IEEE Transactions on Terahertz Science and Technology*, 6(3): 435–441, 2016.

238. Cameron M Hough, David N Purschke, Chenxi Huang, Lyubov V Titova, Olga Kovalchuk, Brad J Warkentin, and Frank A Hegmann. Topology-based prediction of pathway dysregulation induced by intense terahertz pulses in human skin tissue models. *Journal of Infrared, Millimeter, and Terahertz Waves*, 39(9): 887–898, 2018.

239. Cameron M Hough, David N Purschke, Chenxi Huang, Lyubov V Titova, Olga Kovalchuk, and J Brad. Global gene expression in human skin tissue induced by intense terahertz pulses. *Terahertz Science and Technology*, 11(1): 28–33, 2018.

240. Cameron M. Hough, David N. Purschke, Chenxi Huang, Lyubov V Titova, Olga V Kovalchuk, Brad J Warkentin, and Frank A Hegmann. Intense terahertz pulses inhibit Ras signaling and other cancer-associated signaling pathways in human skin tissue models. *Journal of Physics: Photonics*, 3(3): 034004, 2021.

241. Jin-Wu Zhao, Ming-Xia He, Li-Jie Dong, Shao-Xian Li, Li-Yuan Liu, Shao Chong Bu, Chun-Mei Ouyang, Peng-Fei Wang, and Long-Ling Sun. Effect of terahertz pulse on gene expression in human eye cells. *Chinese Physics B*, 28(4): 048703, 2019.

242. Lyubov V Titova, Ayesheshim K Ayesheshim, Andrey Golubov, Rocio Rodriguez-Juarez, Rafal Woycicki, Frank A Hegmann, and Olga Kovalchuk. Intense THz pulses down-regulate genes associated with skin cancer and psoriasis: A new therapeutic avenue? *Scientific Reports*, 3(1): 2363, 2013.

243. Hwayeong Cheon, Jin Ho Paik, Moran Choi, Hee-Jin Yang, and Joo-Hiuk Son. Detection and manipulation of methylation in blood cancer DNA using terahertz radiation. *Scientific Reports*, 9(1): 6413, 2019.

244. Hwayeong Cheon, Hee-Jin Yang, Moran Choi, and Joo-Hiuk Son. Effective demethylation of melanoma cells using terahertz radiation. *Biomedical Optics Express*, 10(10): 4931, 2019.

CHAPTER 4

Polarimetric and Spectral Imaging Approach for Meat Quality Control and Characterization of Biological Tissues

M. Peyvasteh and A. Bykov

University of Oulu

I. Meglinski

Aston University

CONTENTS

DOI: 10.1201/9781003228950-4

4.1 INTRODUCTION

Over the past years, there has been a growing interest in applying light to probe the structure and organization of living biological tissues [1]. Optical techniques have been widely used in biomedical applications because of their non-contact and non-destructive nature. Practically, probing biological, optically thick, turbid tissues is challenging due to multiple scattering and this causes difficulties achieving accurate measurements and proper interpretation of polarization parameters. Studies have shown that spectral properties of the scattered light carry information on the microstructure of biological samples and can be used in the diagnosis of cancerous tissues [2]. Apart from that, using polarization optical methods, healthy and cancerous tissues can be distinguished by measuring variations of polarization parameters [3]. Therefore, a combination of polarization and spectral techniques can contribute to novel and effective approaches for biomedical diagnosis [4,5]. Meat as a postmortem tissue has a random inhomogeneous, anisotropic medium which is similar to biological tissues while there is no need to consider ethical issues. Hence, studying the optical and polarization feature of meat samples can model biological tissue interaction with light and can be developed to create powerful assessment tools in biomedical and food applications. Due to the aforementioned reasons, meat samples were chosen to be examined in this study.

While the most common origin of foodborne outbreaks in the EU are animal products including meat and poultry [6], animal-based protein demand has been increasing specifically for pork (as the most widely consumed type of meat) in recent years [7,8]. The increasing concerns about the associated health risks of consuming contaminated and adulterated meat have encouraged the food industry to seek fast and non-invasive methods for accurate meat quality assessment [9]. Moreover, annually there are considerable amounts of spoiled meat and meat products amounting to approximately 3.5 billion kg of poultry and meat [10]. Therefore, finding accurate and real-time approaches for meat assessment at different points in the food supply chain will considerably reduce the financial losses from the disposal of meat products [11–13].

4.1.1 Interaction of Light and Tissue

The light–material interaction in biological tissues can be quantitatively characterized by optical properties, particularly scattering and absorption coefficients and the refractive index. When a photon hits the surface of a biological sample, it may be scattered, reflected, absorbed or transmits its energy to the molecules causing excitation of the molecular electronic, vibrational, or rotational states [14] (see Figure 4.1).

Scattering of light by particles in biological tissues can be described by the differences between the size of the particles and the wavelength λ. If the particles have the same size order as λ, then it is described by Mie theory and called *Mie scattering*. *Rayleigh scattering* is the Rayleigh limit of Mie scattering by particles much smaller than the wavelength of photons. In Mie scattering, the wavelength dependence of the light scattering is dependent on the size, shape, and index of refraction of the scattering particle [16,17].

During the propagation of light through a scattering medium such as biological tissues, scattering, anisotropy of the refractive index (birefringence), and the anisotropy of attenuation (diattenuation) will lead to the alternation of the polarization state of light within the medium. The propagation of polarized light through such a randomly inhomogeneous medium will cause partial or full depolarization, which depends on the tissue microstructure and the wavelength of incident light [18].

Studies on the interaction of polarized light with biological tissues have shown promising results in biomedical diagnostics and food

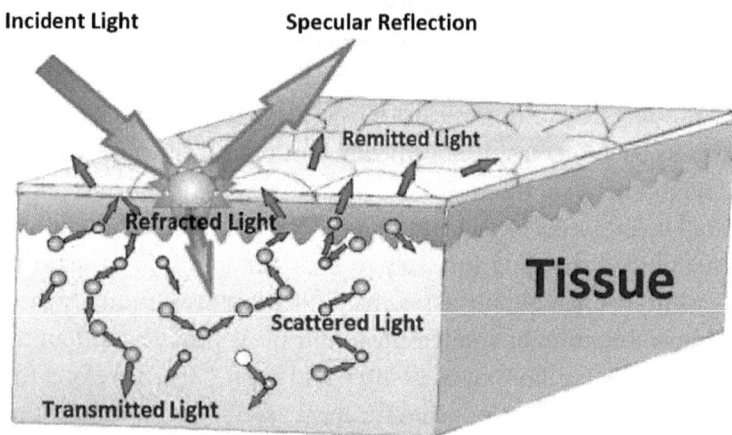

FIGURE 4.1 Schematic diagram of the interaction of light with matter. (Reprinted with permission, from [15] © 2013 SPIE.)

quality control applications. Biological tissues usually consist of a huge variety of microstructures and functional units. It is known that the cell dimensions are larger than the wavelength of the visible and near infrared (NIR) range for a postmortem tissue [19]. Therefore, tissue cells create inhomogeneities and optical anisotropy leading to dominant Mie scattering of transmitted or backscattered polarized light. The changes of the polarization state of the incident light due to the multiple scattering of light within biological optically thick tissue [20] may provide information about the level of food freshness [21–23]. The multiple scattering of polarized light within an optically thick tissue sample will be affected by the tissue state—either living or dead. As a postmortem tissue, dynamic temporal changes of meat are observed as a result of ongoing chemical processes and shape deformation due to water evaporation at both intracellular and extracellular levels. Polarization measurement techniques detect the changes in the polarization state of the reflected or transmitted light signal after its interaction with a sample. When probing meat with polarized light, the depolarization and rotation of the orientation of the polarization plane are dependent on the preferential orientation of the elongated muscle cells and meat aging [18,24]. The bulk of the meat constituents including fibrils and connective tissue fibers have a precise longitudinal arrangement of the proteins generating tissue birefringence [25].

4.1.2 Muscle Structure

The major components of meat muscle include 75% water, 20% protein, 3% fat, and 2% soluble non-protein substances [13,26]. The types of protein existed in the muscle are categorized as following [26]:

- *Myofibrillar* proteins (between 50% and 55%) including actin (thin filament) and myosin (thick filament);

- *Sarcoplasmic* proteins (approximately 30%–34%) are the soluble proteins of the sarcoplasm, to which belong myoglobin (Mb);

- *Connective tissue* proteins (10%–15%) including collagen, reticulin, and elastin are all fibrous proteins [26].

The muscle fibers constitute 75%–92% of the total muscle volume holding long, thread-like structures, the myofibrils, wherein the sarcomere, the smallest contractile unit, is aligned [26].

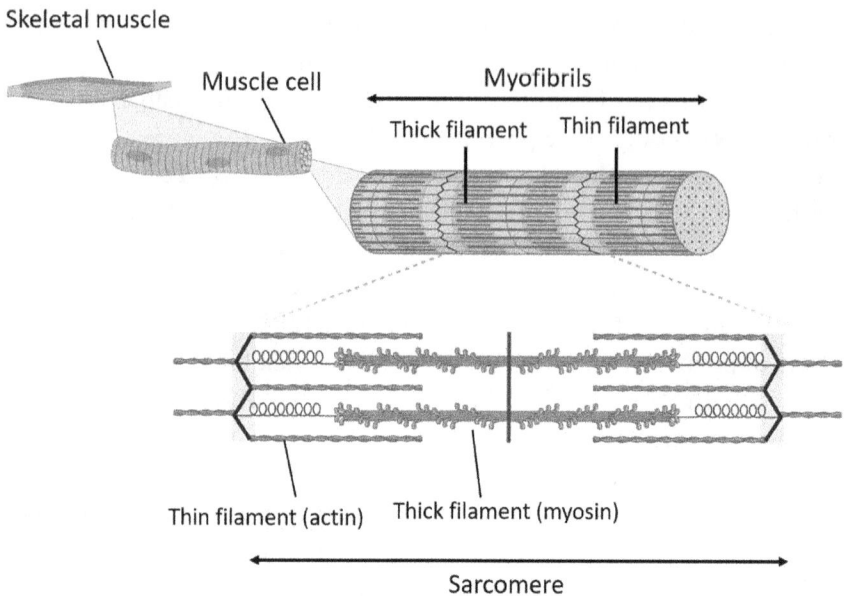

FIGURE 4.2 Schematic presentation of skeletal muscle structure.

Figure 4.2 illustrates the skeletal muscle structure including myofibrillar proteins (actin and myosin).

Specifically, there are several parameters affecting meat quality such as microstructural and appearance-related features as in the following:

- *Toughness* or the *degree of tenderness*, which mainly depends on the myofibrillar and conjunctive tissue [27];

- *Water content*, which is associated with juiciness and plays a crucial role in the freshness traits of a meat product. In the living muscles, water is preserved in the spaces between the thick (myosin) and thin (actin) filaments and changes in these spaces will lead to changes in the content and distribution of water within meat. Myofibrils shrink laterally postmortem, and the expelled fluid accumulates between the fiber bundles and fibers. Water can be evaporated from the raw meat surface or be exuded from the cut surfaces of drip. This concentrated solution of intracellular muscle proteins, including Mb, will lead to a red color of the muscle. In pale, soft, and exudative (PSE) pork, the amount of drip is expanded and by shrinkage of the myosin heads during denaturation, myofibrillar shrinkage increases [28].

- *pH content* changes associated with protein denaturation appear during the first 24 hours after slaughter and can be investigated through visible and NIR spectroscopy to study meat quality [29–33]. An overly low pH level can result in a poor water-holding capacity (WHC) [34]. The changes in pH content have been applied in, e.g., package labeling to differentiate the freshness level [33].

- *The fat content* is one of the chemical indicators of meat quality that can be determined using NIR techniques [8].

- *The collagen* content is the simplest way to assess the quality of protein in the product [35]. The collagen of meat has been studied using different approaches including ultrasound techniques, Raman scattering, visible spectroscopy and colorimetry [36], near infrared reflectance spectroscopy (NIRS) (for bovine meat) [37], and autofluorescence spectroscopy (for ground beef) [38].

- *Meat color,* which is dependent on the age of the animal and the color differences due to the various amount of Mb in the muscle [39]. Chromophores are responsible for absorbing a substantial amount of the electromagnetic spectrum in the visible range and include oxyhemoglobin (HbO_2), deoxyhemoglobin (Hb), etc. For these chromophores, light absorption in the ultraviolet and visible region is higher than the longer wavelength regions, and therefore they can be easily ignored in the NIR range as they contribute little to the overall attenuation. In the NIR region (900–2500 nm), there are other dominant chromophores including moisture, protein, and fat with distinctive absorption features at certain wavelengths [30].

Principally, the quality of meat products can be investigated by the nutritional content (fat, protein, vitamins, and minerals) and functional characteristics such as sensory properties of taste and appearance including color characteristics and surface texture which can be traditionally assessed by consumers and food experts [27,36].

4.1.3 Meat Chromophores

The color characteristics of meat and its major components (muscle, fat, and bone tissues) are crucial for its overall assessment, especially by consumers [8]. Meat color measurements including human visual evaluation and instrumental analysis are associated with the chemistry of Mb [40] which is the dominant chromophore in the visible spectra and is mainly responsible for the appearance of meat [41,42]. Meat color is primarily associated with the amount of different types of Mb as follows:

- *Carboxymyoglobin (COMb)* with a bright cherry-red color;

- *Oxymyoglobin (OxyMb)* due to Mb oxygenation after the exposure of fresh-cut meat to air within 30–60 minutes resulting in a cherry-red color typical for fresh meat found in shops.

This reaction is reversible through deoxygenation via oxygen partial pressure determining the partition between the two species [43]:

- *Deoxymyoglobin (DeoxyMb)* with a purplish-red color, a characteristic of recently sliced fresh meat;

- *Metmyoglobin (MetMb)* emerges brownish-red in color originating from the oxidation of the three other Mb forms in a ferric state and is responsible for meat discoloration [44,45].

Figure 4.3 represents the optical density of the major chromophores of muscle tissue including Mb, OxyMb, water, collagen, and fat [46–48]. In the visible region (400–700 nm), the dominant absorption of oxy- and deoxy-myoglobin is detected at different wavelengths, but with the same extinction coefficients (see Figure 4.3a). These common points on the graphs (isosbestic wavelengths) are typically chosen to quantify Mb pigment forms. According to Figure 4.3a, 525 nm is an isosbestic point for both pigment forms and it can be applied as a denominator of ratios of color calculations since it is referred to as the total Mb concentration regardless of the pigment form. The rest of isosbestic wavelengths are the extreme absorption points of one of the Mb forms [40].

Water has the greatest contribution compared to other chromophores in the shortwave near infrared (SW-NIR) range (700–1100 nm) (see Figure 4.3b), while in the NIR part of spectrum (1100–2400 nm, see Figure 4.3c) the spectra of water and collagen are comparable. Therefore, the structural and compositional variations within these components in these parts of the spectrum cause relative changes.

Meat color measurements can be determined using reflectance spectrophotometric techniques using mathematical manipulation of data including usage of the partial least squares (PLS) method or principal component analysis (PCA) from the selected wavelengths [30,40,49,50].

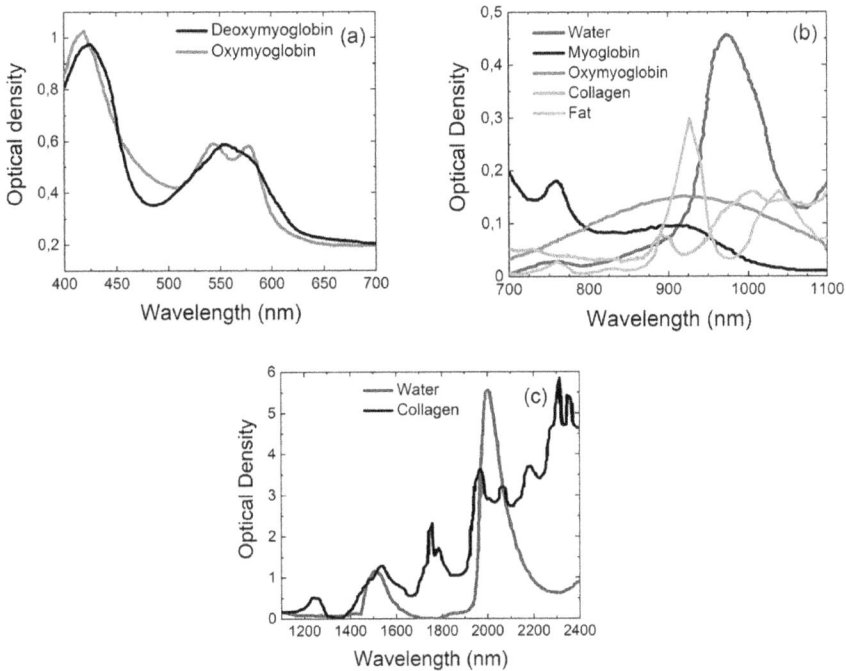

FIGURE 4.3 The optical density spectra of the main chromophores of muscle tissues, including: (a) myoglobin, oxymyoglobin (400–700 nm); (b) water, myoglobin, oxymyoglobin, collagen, fat (700–1100 nm); (c) water and collagen (1100–2400 nm). (Modified from [46–48].)

Specifically, for pork, the major part of the light is strongly scattered, absorbed (Mb will absorb most of the solid light), and reflected causing pork to appear pink to the observer [28]. The high degree of scattering originates from the denaturation of sarcoplasmic proteins which shortens the light path through the sample. Consequently, the chance for the selective absorbance by Mb is reduced and the meat looks less pink but more pale than normal due to scattering [28,51]. Therefore, the reflectance spectrum of the surface is because of the selective absorbance mainly by Mb imposed upon the spectrum from the scattered light that escapes from meat [51]. This may lead to the white appearance of PSE pork [52].

4.2 OPTICAL AND IMAGING TECHNIQUES

Since the absorption property of tissue varies with tissue components, especially water, fat, and collagen, the combination ratio of tissue constituents can be evaluated by decomposing the absorption spectrum to determine the light path length for each constituent [53]. Hence, spectroscopic-based approaches have been utilized in this study to examine absorption changes of meat chromophores associated with meat color and meat freshness.

The traditional methods of meat assessment (sensory evaluation, chemical and microbiological analysis) are still widely used although their contact and time- consuming nature is not appropriate for the online monitoring of meat production [54]. In recent years, a number of techniques have been developed to evaluate various quantities of meat quality, including chemical and microbiological analysis [8], ultrasound techniques, and microscopy approaches (optical and electron microscopy) [36]. However, the optical spectroscopy methods are highly promising compared to the aforementioned techniques because of their fast, non-contact, real-time ability to carry out online monitoring, as well as due to their economic and environment-friendly features [27]. Vis/NIR spectroscopy, Raman spectroscopy, hyperspectral imaging (HSI), and fluorescence spectroscopy are the most frequently applied optical techniques for meat quality assessment [29,36,55,56].

4.2.1 Optical Spectroscopy Techniques

4.2.1.1 Visible and Near Infrared Spectroscopy

NIR can penetrate relatively deeply into biological soft tissues [53] and unlike conventional methods, NIR spectroscopy shows promise due to its speed, adaptability, and relatively simple applicability in the examination of raw meat and meat products [8]. Most biological soft tissues have comparatively low light-absorption properties in the visible (400–800 nm) and NIR (750–1800 nm) spectral regions, especially between 600 and 1300 nm which is known as the "tissue optical window" or "therapeutic window" [57]. Outside of this region, light is absorbed by the tissue pigments (such as hemoglobin and melanin) in the visible spectral region and by the tissue water content in the long wavelength NIR spectral region [53]. Therefore, visible spectroscopy, with a scanning extension to the NIR region can be applied in the safety and quality control of meat products.

There have been several studies applying Vis/NIR spectroscopy to classify meat samples as either fresh or frozen-then-thawed [58], or to predict color, instrumental texture, and sensory attributes [31,59,60], and to predict the chemical composition [61]. NIR spectroscopy has shown promising results in the detection of chemical constituents such as fat [62], pH, and color values in pork samples [49]. In 2001, Liu and Chen examined visible spectra of chicken samples to investigate meat color variation under the conditions of cold storage and cooking process [41]. Knowing the absorbance bands for different pigments (485 nm; MetMb), 560 nm; OxyMb, and 635 nm; sulfmyoglobin), changes in the ratios of $R_1 = A_{485nm}/A_{560nm}$ and $R_2 = A_{635nm}/A_{560nm}$ were studied as a simple approach to monitoring the color changes where A is the light absorbance of the specific wavelength. In 2002, a Matlab-based 2D correlation was implemented utilizing Vis/NIR measurements by Chao et al. to analyze 2D visible spectra of irradiated chicken meat at various irradiation doses and storage times [44]. The results showed that the long-term discoloration of poultry meat was a consequence of the interaction between different forms of Mb. In 2005, García-Rey et al. studied Vis/NIR spectroscopy using fiber optics to predict the texture and color of dry-cured ham samples with promising results for NIRS [63]. The PCA and a K-nearest neighbors methods were applied to classify the samples into defective or no defective classes while the overall accuracy of the results for the pastiness and color were high. Another fiber optics application in Vis/NIR spectroscopy was examined by Hu et al. in the interactance mode to predict color values, chemical components, and other physical characteristics of fresh pork loin and had a high degree of accuracy with NIRS [50]. Lin et al. applied visible and SW-NIR diffuse reflectance spectroscopy (600–1100 nm) combined with PCA to assess the microbial loads in chicken meat and evaluate the onset of spoilage [64]. Ripoll et al. used NIR spectroscopy to predict sensory and texture characteristics of beef in which the tenderness was the best-predicted variable indicating the potential of NIR spectroscopy for the prediction of sensory variables [65]. In fact, accurate predictions of protein are still not achieved so far. In 2014, Girón et al. tested a non-destructive Vis-NIR spectroscopy (400–1000 nm) method to evaluate the degradation of freshness in commercially packaged cooked ham and turkey cold cuts by determining physico-chemical, biochemical, and microbiological properties such as the pH and total volatile basic nitrogen (TVB-N) [66]. A partial least squares discriminant analysis (PLS-DA) model was developed independently for packaged or unpackaged samples and using the second derivative of the spectra looked promising as a non-destructive tool for monitoring the freshness of commercial packages.

The potential of UV-visible (UV-vis), NIR, and mid-infrared (MIR) spectroscopy, coupled with chemometric techniques using PCA, linear discriminant analysis (LDA), and PLS were investigated by Alamprese et al. to detect minced beef adulteration with turkey meat [67]. The results showed that NIR and MIR spectroscopy were better compared to UV-vis, while SW-NIR spectroscopy (400–1000 nm) was reported to be suitable for moisture content and water activity examination. The PLS results showed that NIR and MIR, as non-selective analytical techniques, could provide fast and highly reliable support for traditional methods for species identification in minced meat products. Notably, NIR spectroscopy seems to be more suitable for quality control purpose, since instruments can be equipped with fiber-optic probes which are able to evaluate samples simply by surface contact [68]. Recently, there have been several machine-learning techniques combined with Vis and NIR spectroscopy to investigate meat samples [69].

4.2.1.2 Infrared Spectroscopy

Infrared (IR) spectroscopy is a spectroscopic method that deals with the IR region of the electromagnetic spectrum (from about 800–2500 nm). The principle of IR spectroscopy is that chemical bonds in organic molecules absorb or emit IR light when their vibrational state alters [36]. Pedersen et al. studied the potential of measuring fundamental vibrational information in IR absorption and Raman scattering in fresh porcine meat by using partial least squares regressions (PLSR) which indicated a high correlation between WHC and both IR and Raman spectra [70]. Fourier transform infrared (FTIR) spectroscopy is a rapid and non-invasive technique with considerable potential to apply in food industries. In 2002, Ellis et al. utilized FTIR spectroscopy directly on the surface of food to generate biochemically interpretable "fingerprints" by using PLS regression to detect early microbial spoilage [71]. The results indicated allowed the accurate estimation of bacterial loads directly measured from the meat surface in 60 seconds [71]. A machine-learning strategy and FTIR were applied by Argyri et al. to detect beef fillet spoilage in two storage conditions including chilled and abuse temperatures [72]. The artificial neural network algorithm correctly classified fresh samples with an accuracy of 91.7%, semi-fresh samples at 81.2% accuracy, and spoiled samples at 94.1% accuracy [72].

4.2.1.3 Fluorescence Spectroscopy

Fluorescence spectroscopy has been recognized as an efficient and promising tool to control food quality and authenticity due to its high selectivity and sensitivity [73]. It is a rapid and non-destructive method and is applicable to imaging techniques to determine the level of lipid oxidation in food such as fish and meat [74]. Wold et al. applied autofluorescence spectra for the rapid quantification of connective tissue and fat in ground beef showing promising results at 332 nm which could be an appropriate excitation wavelength to determine both fat and connective tissue [38]. In another study, the front face autofluorescence was measured from meat products including turkey meat to examine the capability of the approach to measure and predict lipid oxidation [75]. In 2003, Dufour et al. examined the intrinsic fluorescence of fish muscle to monitor fish freshness reporting that the method could be utilized as a fingerprinting technique to discriminate fresh and aged fish fillets [76].

4.2.1.4 Raman Spectroscopy

In the recent decades, Raman spectroscopy has appeared as a promising tool for biomedical diagnostics such as the detection and staging of cancer [77]. Raman spectroscopy can be also applied in food analysis due to multiple advantages because it is a fast and non-destructive method and it is simple to prepare the samples. This technique provides information about different food compounds including qualitative and quantitative analysis of components and their structural analysis [78]. Raman spectroscopy can be used as a practical tool for the detection of bacterial contamination in tissues or of foodborne microorganisms on food surfaces [79]. In 2003, a study by Pederson et al. was conducted on fresh porcine meat using IR absorption and Raman scattering to measure fundamental vibrational information and to investigate the feasibility of early WHC prediction of meat samples [70]. The main difficulties with the Raman method were the inherent poor signal-to-noise ratio and sample fluorescence, although time-resolved Raman scattering can serve as a technological solution. The IR region 1800–900 cm^{-1} involved the best predictive information for the WHC of the porcine meat.

In 2005, Ellis et al. developed an analytical approach based on Raman spectroscopy (using a NIR diode laser with excitation at 785 nm) and FT-IR combined with machine learning [80]. Raman spectroscopy combined with chemometrics was applied by Nache et al. to develop a fast and non-invasive method to check the early postmortem pH decrease in porcine muscle [81]. It showed that data pre-processing prior to modeling is necessary to eliminate irrelevant features in the Raman spectra that may reduce the modeling performance. Ebrahim et al. utilized a time-dependent Raman spectroscopic approach with a 671 nm microsystem diode laser for meat species identification and assessment of spoilage effects [82]. For data evaluation, PCA was applied showing an evident discrimination between beef and horse meat which can be associated with differences in the Mb content of both species [82].

4.2.1.5 Electrical Impedance Spectroscopy

Electrical impedance spectroscopy (EIS) is a method to analyze electrical properties of materials by inducing alternating electrical signals in them at different frequencies and measuring the responding signals [11]. EIS was first suggested as a skin characterization technique, but later further applications were found for it to characterize different materials [83]. Electrical impedance-based techniques are mainly applied for measuring tenderness and age-related shifts [84] in muscle fiber anisotropy [85].

4.2.2 Emerging Imaging Techniques

Emerging imaging techniques have been evolved based on different principles including mechanical and electromagnetic waves and can be utilized in biomedical applications [86], meat quality, and safety evaluation [87]. In the following section, the methods based on electromagnetic waves will be discussed and classified into optical, thermal, ultrasound, tomographic, and polarimetric imaging.

4.2.2.1 Hyperspectral Imaging

HSI techniques have been regarded as a smart and promising analytical tool for application in biomedical applications [86] and for food quality control [88]. HSI includes the integration of spectroscopy and imaging methods in one system to identify different sample components and their spatial distribution. In addition to its potential to characterize the quality of the visual attributes of meat such as the color, quality grade, and maturity, HSI can be applied to measure multiple chemical constituents simultaneously without sample preparation [88]. The water distribution within beef during dehydration was investigated using time series hyperspectral imaging (TS-HSI), which proved to be highly accurate (RMSECV of 1.280%) [89]. In 2018, Yang et al. [12] utilized HIS techniques and classified the freshness of cooked beef into three grades (freshness, medium freshness, and spoilage) according to measured total viable count (TVC).

4.2.2.2 Opto-Magnetic Imaging Spectroscopy

Opto-magnetic imaging spectroscopy (OMIS) is a novel method which utilizes diffuse and polarized light (wavelength range from 400 to 700 nm) as its key tool to extract information on tissues by converting digital images from reflectance properties into opto-magnetic spectra [83,90]. Using digital RGB images in this technique makes it faster and more cost-effective compared to HSI methods [83]. In 2017, Mileusnić et al. utilized OMIS and machine-learning algorithms to predict meat freshness degradation during refrigerated storage [83]. Detecting changes in the state of the water in tissues, the freshness decay period was evaluated according to the changes in meat hydration properties [83].

4.2.2.3 Raman Imaging

In recent years, Raman imaging has emerged as a novel technique in food quality and safety evaluation that combines the advantages of Raman spectroscopy and digital imaging. Compared to conventional techniques, Raman imaging provides more detail for the assessment of microbial contamination and the shelf life of food [91].

4.2.2.4 Fluorescence Imaging

Fluorescence imaging utilizes the fact that the objects absorbing light or other electromagnetic radiation emit fluorescence. Fluorescence imaging has been applied in several studies to detect contamination in pork [92], beef [93], lamb [93], and chicken meat [94], in addition to measuring lipid oxidation in pork [95] and chicken [96].

4.2.2.5 Thermal Imaging

Thermal imaging is a fast, non-invasive, and accurate technique to monitor meat safety and quality due to its ability to track moving targets in real time and generate a visual image by displaying temperature changes over a large area [87]. The basic principle of thermal imaging is to utilize the IR radiation emitted by a surface to create thermal images and represent the temperature distribution of the object [87]. IR thermography has been applied by Costa et al. to examine pork and ham quality on a slaughter line and showed better results for hams with less fat cover [97].

4.2.2.6 Ultrasound Imaging

Ultrasound imaging utilizes the acoustic features of the samples to provide internal images. It is a cost-effective and reliable technology that has been widely applied in meat quality and safety assessment [98,99]. There are two modes for ultrasound imaging: A-mode (amplitude modulation) and B-mode (brightness modulation), of which the B-mode is most common [87].

4.2.2.7 Tomographic Imaging

Tomographic imaging is another technique to evaluate meat quality and safety which can be divided into *X-ray imaging* and *magnetic resonance imaging* [87]. X-ray imaging utilizes X-rays to create tomographic images of scanned samples and has generally been applied to detect foreign objects in food samples [98]. However, it is an expensive and complicated approach which requires complex post-image processing procedures [87]. X-ray imaging techniques have been applied in the food industry to find foreign objects in food components although it is a complicated and costly approach requiring complex post-image processing. Compared to X-ray imaging, magnetic resonance imaging makes use of different characteristics in the electromagnetic spectrum to evaluate meat quality and safety because different biochemical properties in the tested objects can lead to different absorption and emission of energy in the electromagnetic spectrum [85,100,101].

4.2.2.8 Polarimetric Imaging

The multiple scattering at visible and NIR wavelengths cause difficulties for quantitative tissue spectroscopy and imaging due to their shallow penetration depth and the inhomogeneity of the tissue, which obscures the desired image information [102]. Therefore, there is a growing interest in applying polarimetric imaging techniques for the investigation of biological tissues due to the fact that diffusely scattered light is often partially polarized to an extent, which can be experimentally detected and provide additional information on tissue optical properties [4,103–108]. In the following section, two major polarimetric imaging techniques including *Stokes vector imaging* and *Mueller polarimetric imaging* that have been applied in this thesis will be presented.

4.2.2.8.1 Stokes Vector Imaging   The state of polarization and intensity of a light beam incident are defined by the 4×1 *Stokes vector S* in the following form:

$$I = \begin{bmatrix} I \\ Q \\ U \\ V \end{bmatrix} = \begin{bmatrix} S_0 \\ S_1 \\ S_2 \\ S_3 \end{bmatrix} \tag{4.1}$$

where $I \equiv S_0$ is the total intensity, $Q \equiv S_1$ is the polarization at 0° or 90° to the scattering plane, $U \equiv S_2$ is the polarization at ±45° to the scattering plane, $V \equiv S_3$ is the left or right circular polarization, and S_0, S_1, S_2, and S_3 represent four elements of the Stokes vector S [24].

Stokes vector-parametric formalism is usually applied to describe the interaction of polarized light with complex objects such as biological tissues. Stokes polarimetry is based on the principles of 'single-point' mapping, i.e. coordinate distributions of the azimuth and polarization ellipticity of microscopic images of histological sections from biological tissues [109]. The spatial distribution of the polarization for scattered radiation, especially the degree of depolarization, has a remarkable anisotropy. The existence of optical anisotropy can contribute to useful information on the structural characteristics of the biological sample. Stokes vector mapping on a Poincaré sphere has been applied as an approach to characterize malformations within biological tissues in several studies [110–112].

4.2.2.8.2 Mueller Polarimetric Imaging   Among novel emerging optical techniques, Mueller matrix (MM) polarimetry has demonstrated distinct advantages that are appropriate for diagnosis including the enhancement of the imaging contrast of superficial layers of tissues where more than 85% of cancers have their origins [113,114]. Furthermore, MM polarimetry can characterize the polarimetric properties (including diattenuation, dichroism, and depolarization) and provide abundant and comprehensive microstructural information on scattering media such as biological tissues [114–117], which means it can be used an effective label-free tool to study abnormal tissue areas [118,119]. Therefore, MM imaging polarimetry (MMIP) is becoming increasingly attractive for application in biomedical diagnostics and food quality control [107,116,120–128].

The principle of optical characterization of biological tissue within the framework of the Stokes–Mueller formalism is based on measuring the bulk tissue's polarimetric transfer function, known as its MM and contains the full polarization information reflecting the biophysical properties of the samples [118]. MM is a 4×4 matrix with real valued coefficients that transform a 4×1 Stokes vector representing a polarization state of the light impinging on the sample into another 4×1 Stokes vector representing a polarization state of the light emerging after the interaction with the sample [111,129]. This transformation is given by

$$S_{out} = M \cdot S_{in} = \begin{bmatrix} M_{11} & M_{12} & M_{13} & M_{14} \\ M_{21} & M_{22} & M_{23} & M_{24} \\ M_{31} & M_{32} & M_{33} & M_{34} \\ M_{41} & M_{42} & M_{43} & M_{44} \end{bmatrix} \cdot S_{in} \qquad (4.2)$$

where S_{in} and S_{out} are the Stokes vectors of incident and outgoing light beams, respectively, and M is the sample MM that contains all information about the optical properties [130,131]. The Stokes vector in this framework is given by

$$S = \begin{bmatrix} I \\ I_x - I_y \\ I_{+45} - I_{-45} \\ I_{LC} - I_{RC} \end{bmatrix} = \begin{bmatrix} S_0 \\ S_1 \\ S_2 \\ S_3 \end{bmatrix} \qquad (4.3)$$

where I is the total light intensity and I_x, I_y, I_{+45}, I_{-45}, I_{LC}, I_{RC} are the intensities measured through a linear polarizer with the transmission axis oriented along the x, y, $+45°$, and $-45°$ directions of the laboratory coordinate system, respectively, or through a left (LC) or right (RC) circular polarizer [132].

4.3 EXPERIMENT AND DATA ANALYSIS

4.3.1 Visible and Near Infrared Spectroscopy

Conventional Vis/NIR spectroscopy is used extensively for non-invasive *in vivo* characterization of human skin and other biological tissues [133]. Portable and cost-effective light sources (e.g. tungsten lamps) and detectors (e.g. silicon diode arrays) were used in the visible and NIR (750–1800 nm) spectral range [14,68]. The samples were chosen from porcine muscle meat purchased from local supermarkets on the first day after slaughter. Three samples for visible spectra, two samples for NIR spectra with the integrating sphere configuration, and 13 samples with an optical fiber configuration for each measurement were placed in a plastic Petri dish (5 cm in diameter, 1 cm high) with a hole (2×1 cm²) to provide direct penetration of light into the samples. To control moisture evaporation from the surface and to prevent drying, the samples were covered with a plastic film. Furthermore, the relative air humidity during the meat-aging process was controlled. Low air humidity would restrict bacterial growth, but increased water evaporation would cause dryness and the meat to be less juicy, while high humidity would facilitate spoilage bacteria growth leading to an unpleasant sticky surface. Therefore, the humidity in the laboratory was controlled (at 80%) and remained constant for all the measurements. The aim of this study was to detect early changes in the optical properties concerning the meat for a small area of the sample, and although water evaporation from the surface was restrained by covering the sample with plastic films, slight changes of humidity did not significantly affect the results [134].

The reflectance spectra of the samples were recorded every half an hour on average for 6 hours at room temperature (23°C). After calibration, reflectance spectra (R) were converted to absorbance spectra ($A=\log(1/R)$) [135] and a Savitzky–Golay fitting algorithm was run on the data to eliminate random variations in the measured spectra and clearly enhance the visual appearance of the spectra [136]. Finally, the isosbestic points within the absorption bands were detected which were responsible for the associated meat chromophores. By integrating the area between the isosbestic points, a new term 'integrated absorbance' was defined. Eventually, the dependence of the integrated absorbance values over time for each of the meat chromophores was named 'degradation kinetics' and these were studied to track the changes during the freshness decay [137].

Figure 4.4 presents the table-top configuration including the OL 400-LCS lamp source (Optronic Laboratories, USA), a monochromator (OL series 750-M), an integrating sphere attached to the monochromator to collect scattered light from the sample (see Figure 4.4; close-up view), two highly sensitive detectors (OL series 750), and a controller (OL 750-C) connected to a computer. The detectors operated within two wavelength ranges: 400–1100 nm (Si detector) and 1100–1800 nm (Ge detector). The probing spot of light on the surface of the sample was 10 mm in diameter for this setup [137].

In another configuration (see Figure 4.5), a standard portable spectrophotometer operated within the 400–1100 nm spectral range was utilized with an array of 11 fiber-optic probes (for illumination and light detection, see Figure 4.5; close-up view, left) with the maximal source-detector fiber separation of 5.3 mm, and minimal of 0.53 mm (see Figure 4.5; close-up view, right). This experimental setup included a light source Illuminator EK-1 Fiber Optic Light Source LE.5210-110 (EUROMEX, The Netherlands) with a halogen lamp and a compact CCS200 spectrometer (Thorlabs, USA), both connected to the fiber-optic probe [137].

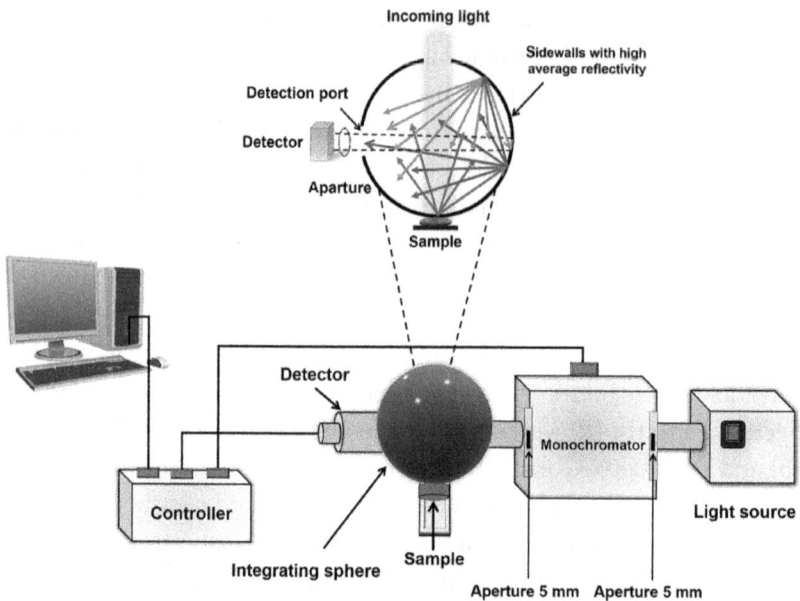

FIGURE 4.4 Schematic presentation of the experimental setup with an integrating sphere and a closer view of multiple reflections occurring in the integrating sphere [137].

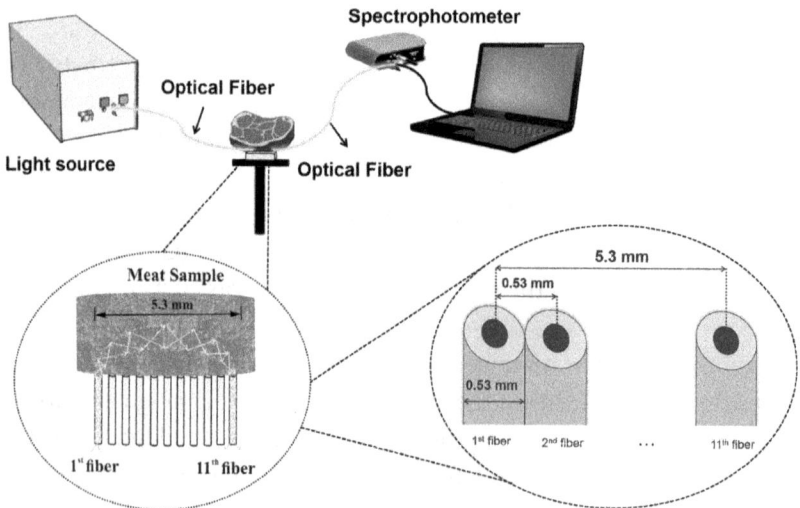

FIGURE 4.5 Schematic presentation of the experimental setup with a linear array of optical fibers. Left close-up view shows the contact with the meat sample and banana-shape trajectories of photons emitted by the first fiber and collected by the 11th fiber. Right close-up view shows the maximal and minimal source–detector fiber separation [137].

TABLE 4.1   Optical Properties of Meat (Muscle Tissue) [144]

λ, nm	μ_a, mm^{-1}	μ_s, mm^{-1}	g	n
632.8	0.059	17.9	0.858	1.381

4.3.1.1 Monte Carlo Simulation

A Monte Carlo (MC) simulation is a well-established and efficient method to model light propagation in turbid media such as biological tissues [138], which can track the photon transportation [139]. MC simulation comprises a sequential generation of trajectories of photon packets from the source (the entrance to the medium) to the detector (the area where the photon leaves the medium) [140]. Here, a free online simulation platform [141] implementing the MC method was applied to estimate a sampling volume [140,142] and a probing depth in each measurement configuration. The optical parameters used in the simulations corresponded to muscle tissue at 632.8 nm [139,143,144] and these are shown in Table 4.1.

The integrating sphere configuration composed of a collimated light beam (beam width of 10 mm) normally incident on a rectangular probing area ($20\times20\times5$ mm^3). Light reflected from the sample surface and deeper regions was collected from all directions within a 20 mm size area coincident with the incident beam. The fiber-optic configuration (see Figure 4.5, close-up views) with 300 μm source and detecting fibers for two separation distances was also simulated. In this configuration, the sample size was either $2.5\times2\times2$ mm^3 (source–detector distance of 0.53 mm) or $6\times2\times2$ mm^3 (source–detector distance of 5.3 mm) [137].

4.3.1.2 Principal Component Analysis

Multivariate statistical methods such as PCA can be applied to determine the main directions of variability in a multivariate data matrix and to present the results in a graphical plot [145]. PCA is a data analysis tool which is often applied to reduce the dimensionality (number of variables) of many interrelated variables, while retaining as much of the information (variation) as possible. The calculated factors or PCs as an uncorrelated set of variables are ordered in a way that the first few keep most of the variations present in all of the original variables [146]. There are a wide variety of PCA applications in different fields to classify large, scattered datasets. Specifically, it has been an effective and promising method utilized in meat quality assessment [67,146–150] such as beef characterization, as well as the classification of hairtail fish, beef, and pork [145,147,148]. In this study, the PCA method applied on the visible and NIR absorbance dataset was obtained from both experimental configurations to detect and discriminate sub- stages of freshness levels and was associated with chromophore changes over time, which might not be recognizable in spectroscopic analysis.

4.3.2 Mueller Matrix Imaging Polarimetry

A polarimetric imaging technique was used to evaluate the quality of meat samples to address the last research questions. MMIP was used to measure porcine muscle polarization properties over time. For this set of measurements, ten samples of fresh porcine muscle purchased from a local supermarket were used. The samples were about 1 cm in thickness and were cut into 3×3 cm² pieces, then placed in a glass container and covered with a glass slide to minimize the specular reflection from the uneven surface of the tissue. All samples were stored in air at room temperature (23°C) and measured several times a day, at average intervals of 2 hours, to observe the early changes in optical parameters due to the meat-aging process.

Basically, there must be at least 16 intensity measurements to build the MM of a sample [151]. The whole MM elements were normalized by M_{11} which generates dimensionless quantities varying from –1 to 1. There are several decomposition techniques to extract the information on polarization properties of the sample encoded in all 16 elements of the MM, e.g. the Mueller matrix polar decomposition (MMPD) [152] and the Mueller matrix transformation (MMT) [123,153]. A Lu–Chipman decomposition [152] was applied in this study, which shows that any physically detectable MM can be decomposed into a product of three MMs of the basic optical components including a diattenuator (D), a retarder (R), and a depolarizer (Δ) [152,154]. Biological tissues are considered highly scattering media comprised of cells, protein fibers, and optically active molecules. Therefore, they own such polarimetric properties as depolarization, linear birefringence, and optical activity [133]. Each of these properties can be achieved separately by using the MMPD (applied pixelwise in the case of MMIP) of

$$M = M_\Delta M_R M_D \qquad (4.4)$$

where M_Δ, M_R, and M_D are the matrices of a depolarizer, retarder, and diattenuator, respectively [127].

A custom-built multi-wavelength MM imaging polarimeter was used here which has been developed and installed in the Laboratory of Physics

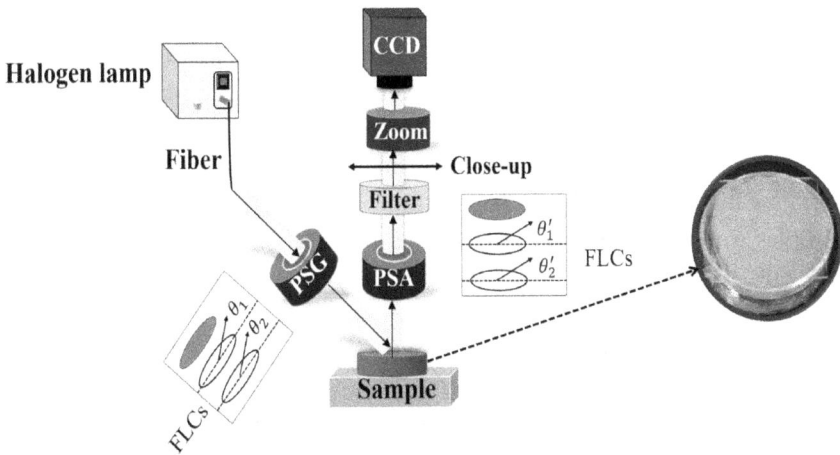

FIGURE 4.6 Schematic presentation of the imaging Mueller polarimeter used in the study. A photograph of a sample (porcine muscle). A glass slide was placed on top of the sample to flatten the surface.

of Interfaces and Thin Films, Ecole Polytechnique (LPICM), Palaiseau, France. A schematic presentation of the setup is shown in Figure 4.6 including a spectral filter zoom system, a charge-coupled device (CCD) camera, and a halogen lamp as the source of illumination.

To generate polarized light, a polarization state generator (PSG) consisting of a linear polarizer and two ferroelectric liquid crystals (FLCs) was utilized. Each liquid crystal (LC) originally operated as a wave plate with the fixed retardation whose fast axis orientation switched between θ and $\theta+45°$. The initial orientations of the fast axes of two LCs were fixed at the angles θ_1 and θ_2, respectively. In the detection arm, a polarization state analyzer (PSA) consisting of the same elements, but assembled in reverse order, was used to analyze the backscattered light [155]. A detailed description of the instrument can be found elsewhere [152,156].

The MMIP system operating in the visible wavelength range (450–700 nm) allowed the complete polarimetric characterization of the biological tissues by measuring the wide-field (up to 5×5 cm²) MM images of the sample. The PSG generated four different states of polarization of the incident light beam interacting with the sample and was projected sequentially on four polarization states of PSA, which were identical to those of the PSG. Therefore, 16 measurements were performed to obtain the complete MM images of the sample. The measurements were repeated typically 5–10 times for each state of polarization and averaged over the obtained images in order to achieve a satisfactory signal-to-noise ratio. The acquisition time for a complete set of 16 raw-intensity images was averaged over a few seconds for each measurement wavelength. Finally, a complete MM of the sample was acquired from the measured set of 16 raw-intensity images by using calibration data from measurements of the reference samples and applying a set of linear algebra operations. Polarimetric images of the meat samples were obtained over 26 hours at multiple wavelengths of 450, 500, 550, 600, 650, and 700 nm.

4.3.2.1 Analysis of MM Elements

To analyze the structural features of tissue samples in different states of freshness, a statistical analysis and frequency distribution histogram (FDH) were applied on the MM elements, as well as the total depolarization, and scalar retardance obtained by using the MMPD of the obtained MM [109,157].

For isotropic partially depolarizing samples, the MM had only non-zero elements on the diagonal and the absolute values of the M_{22} and M_{33} elements were equal, whereas for partially polarizing anisotropic samples, MM had both diagonal and non-diagonal non-zero elements due to the polarized light scattering and phase shift between its components related to sample anisotropic refractive index or birefringence [121,158]. The values of diagonal elements (M_{22}, $M_{33,}$ and M_{44}) were closely related to the depolarization and absorption properties of the samples [121,124].

4.3.2.2 Statistical Analysis

The MM data can be presented in the form of 2D ($m{\times}n$) distributions of matrix elements, known also as MM images and is indicated here as $M(m{\times}n)$.

For the quantitative evaluation of 2D distributions of $M(m{\times}n)$, a set of the central statistical moments of the first (Z_1; mean value), second (Z_2; variance), third (Z_3; skewness), and fourth (Z_4; kurtosis) orders are used [108,119,157,159]:

$$Z_1 = \frac{1}{N}\sum_{j=1}^{N} M_j;$$ (4.5)

$$Z_2 = \sqrt{\frac{1}{N-1}\sum_{j=1}^{N}(M_j - Z_1)^2};$$ (4.6)

$$Z_3 = \sqrt{\frac{1}{Z_2^3} \frac{1}{N} \sum_{j=1}^{N} (M_j - Z_1)^3} ; \qquad (4.7)$$

$$Z_4 = \sqrt{\frac{1}{Z_2^4} \frac{1}{N} \sum_{j=1}^{N} (M_j - Z_1)^4} . \qquad (4.8)$$

where $N = m \times n$ is the number of pixels of the CCD-camera register-ing inhomogeneously polarized field M_j of the jth element of MM, respectively.

A low value of the variance (Z_2) indicates that the distribution of the measured data would be close to the mean value (Z_1), while a high value of the variance shows that the data points are more spread out around Z_1 and from each other. The skewness (Z_3) indicates the asymmetry of the FDH and can be positive or negative. A negative (or positive) skewness value shows that the tail on the left side (or the right side) of the FDH is longer (or shorter) than that on the right side. The kurtosis (Z_4) charac-terizes the strength of the outliers of the distribution in FDH [119,160]. First, the 2D backscattering MM images of the samples were recorded, and then the pixelated images were transformed to FDHs. Finally, the statisti-cal analysis was applied to the FDHs of MM elements, total depolarization and retardance.

4.3.3 Two-Point Stokes Vector Diagnostic Approach

A two-point Stokes vector imaging approach was developed in this study to determine the diagnostic potential of Stokes correlometry of the pathological changes of biological tissues. The purpose of this work was to demonstrate a new method of Stokes-correlometric evaluation based on a correlation ("two-point") generalization of optically thin (attenua-tion coefficient $\tau < 0.01$) histological sections of optically anisotropic bio-logical tissues with different morphological structures. In this study, an experimental technique was developed to measure polarization–correla-tion maps, i.e., the coordinate distributions of the magnitude of the "two-point" Stokes vector parameters.

4.3.3.1 Theoretical Background

The complex amplitudes $E(r)$ of each point r of the object field of an optically anisotropic biological layer are described by the Jones vector [108,161,162] in the form

$$E_r = \begin{pmatrix} E_x \\ E_y \end{pmatrix}(r) = \begin{pmatrix} |E_x| \\ |E_y| exp(\delta y - \delta x) \end{pmatrix}(r) = \begin{pmatrix} 1 \\ tg\rho(\cos\delta + i\sin\delta) \end{pmatrix}(r)$$

(4.9)

Here, ρ is the orientation of the optical axis; $\tan \rho(r) = |E_y|(r)/|E_x|(r)$ and $\delta(r) = (\delta y - \delta x)(r)$ are the phase shifts between the orthogonal components $|E_x|(r)$ and $|E_y|(r)$ of the laser-wave amplitude. To describe the correlation structure of the stationary distributions of the fields of complex amplitudes of laser radiation converted by optically anisotropic layers, a biological matrix of mutual spectral density can be used in the form of [161,163]

$$W_{i,j}(r_1,r_2) = E^*(r_1)E_j(r_2),$$

(4.10)

where $(i, j) = (x, y)$ and r_1, r_2 are the coordinates of the neighboring points in the laser radiation field. This matrix operator can introduce the relations for the 'two-point' Stokes vector parameters

$$S_1 = W_{xx}(r_1,r_2) + W_{yy}(r_1,r_2),$$

(4.11)

$$S_2 = W_{xx}(r_1,r_2) - W_{yy}(r_1,r_2),$$

(4.12)

$$S_3 = W_{xy}(r_1,r_2) + W_{yx}(r_1,r_2),$$

(4.13)

$$S_4 = [W_{yx}(r_1,r_2) + W_{xy}(r_1,r_2)]$$

(4.14)

and

$$\begin{cases} W_{xx}(r_1,r_2) = E_x^*(r_1)E_x(r_2) \\ W_{yy}(r_1,r_2) = E_y^*(r_1)E_y(r_2) \\ W_{xy}(r_1,r_2) = E_x^*(r_1)E_y(r_2) \\ W_{yx}(r_1,r_2) = E_y^*(r_1)E_x(r_2) \end{cases}$$

(4.15)

The first Stokes vector parameter $S_1(r)$ in Eq. (4.11) characterizes the full intensity at the point r; $S_2(r)$ and $S_3(r)$ describe changes in the polarization azimuth and ellipticity, while $S_4(r)$ characterizes the value of polarization ellipticity. Further comprehensive analytical and experimental analyses were performed based on this to examine the potential of polarimetry of 'two-point' Stokes vector parameters using $S_3(r_1,r_2)$ and $S_4(r_1,r_2)$ as examples. For simplification, Eqs. (4.9)–(4.15) were considered in the approximation of a weak phase modulation [δ=0.12, $\cos(\delta_1-\delta_2) \to 1$; $\sin(\delta_1-\delta_2) \to (\delta_1-\delta_2)$]. Eventually, Eqs. (4.13) and (4.14) were reduced to

$$\begin{cases} |S_3| = 1 - ctg_{\rho2} tg_{\rho1} \\ |S_4| = 1 + ctg_{\rho2} tg_{\rho1} \end{cases} \tag{4.16}$$

where $|S_{i=3,4}|$ is the Stokes-correlometry parameter (SCP) modulus [164].

Figure 4.7 demonstrates a Stokes polarimeter used to measure the coordinate distribution values [162]. A low-intensity (5.0 mW) He-Ne laser radiation with a wavelength of 633 nm (Lasos HeNe Laser, Edmund Optics, USA) was applied as an optical probe. The collimator consisted of two microlenses with coincided foci which formed a parallel illuminating beam with a diameter of 2 mm. A circular polarization of the laser beam was created to recognize the conditions of azimuthally invariant SCP mapping. Consequently, a multifunctional polarizing filter was used including successively placed quarter-wave plates, a polarizer (B+W XS-Pro Polarizer MRC Nano, Kaesemann, Germany), and an achromatic true zero-order waveplate (APAW 15 mm, Astropribor, Ukraine). A histological section converted the circular polarization of the optical probe

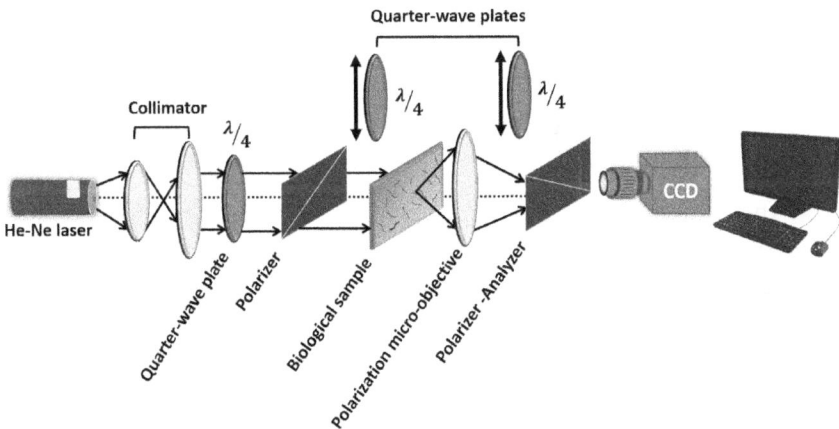

FIGURE 4.7 The optical scheme of the polarimeter consisted of a He-Ne laser; collimator; stationary quarter-wave plate; mechanically movable quarter-wave plates; polarizer and analyzer; biological sample (layer); polarization microobjective; CCD camera; computer [164].

according to the topographic structure of the optical anisotropic components of the biological tissue. Therefore, a polarization-inhomogeneous image of the biological sample was formed. A polarizing micro-objective (CFI Achromat P, focal length of 30 mm, numerical aperture of 0.1, magnification: 4x, Nikon, Japan) projected an image of a histological section of biological tissue into the matrix plane ($m{\times}n = 1280{\times}960$ pixels) of the photosensitive area of a digital CCD-camera (CFI Achromat P, focal length of 30 mm, numerical aperture: 0.1, magnification: 4x, Nikon, Japan) [164].

The achromatic true zero-order waveplate (APAW 15 mm, Astropribor, Ukraine) and an analyzer (B+W XS- Pro Polarizer MRC Nano, Kaesemann, Germany) were placed in front of the pixel matrix. The polarization filter passed several linear and circular polarization states of the image of the biological tissue sample. Accordingly, a set of digital (separated by the total number of pixels) polarization-filtered images of the histological section were formed. Eventually, an algorithmic calculation of the coordinate distributions of the SCP value was performed by computer. The measuring method of the absolute value $|(S_{i=3;4}(\Delta x, \Delta y))|$ of the SCP contains the following sequence of steps:

- The sample was illuminated by the circularly polarized laser beam providing a filter consisting of quarter-wave plates and a polarizer (see Figure 4.7);

- The axis of the polarizer–analyzer (in the absence of the quarter wavelength plate) was rotated by the angles $\theta=0°$, $\theta=90°$, $\theta=45°$, $\theta=135°$, and the intensities of the transmitted radiation $I_0^{\otimes}$, $I_{90}^{\otimes}$, $I_{45}^{\otimes}$, $I_{135}^{\otimes}$ were measured;

- The values of the 'one-point' first, second, and third Stokes vector parameters $S_1^{\otimes}=I_0^{\otimes}+I_{90}^{\otimes}$; $S_2^{\otimes}=I_0^{\otimes}-I_{90}^{\otimes}$; $S_3^{\otimes}=I_{45}^{\otimes}-I_{135}^{\otimes}$ were calculated within each pixel of CCD camera.

- A quarter-wave plate (8) was placed in front of the polarizer–analyzer, with the axis of the greatest speed oriented at the angles of $+45°$ and $-45°$ relative to the transmission plane of the polarizer;

- The 2D arrays of the values of the fourth Stokes parameter $S^{\otimes}=I^{\otimes}-I^{\otimes}$ were calculated.

- $|S_{i=3}(\Delta x;\Delta y)|$ and $|S_{i=4}(\Delta x;\Delta y)|$ were calculated by using the ratios of

$$\left\{ \begin{array}{l} |S_3| = \sqrt{\left[\sqrt{I_0(r_1)I_{90}(r_2)}\cos\delta_2 + \sqrt{I_0(r_2)I_{90}(r_1)}\cos\delta_1\right]^2} \\ + \left[\sqrt{I_0(r_1)I_{90}(r_2)}\sin\delta_2 - \sqrt{I_0(r_2)I_{90}(r_1)}\sin\delta_1\right]^2 \end{array} \right. \tag{4.17}$$

$$\left\{ \begin{array}{l} |S_4| = \sqrt{\left[\sqrt{I_0(r_2)I_{90}(r_1)}\sin\delta_2 + \sqrt{I_0(r_1)I_{90}(r_2)}\sin\delta_1\right]^2} \\ + \left[\sqrt{I_0(r_2)I_{90}(r_1)}\cos\delta_2 - \sqrt{I_0(r_1)I_{90}(r_2)}\cos\delta_1\right]^2 \end{array} \right. \tag{4.18}$$

and

$$(r) = arctan\left[\left(\frac{S_4(r)S_2(r)}{S_3(r)}\right)\left(\frac{1+\dfrac{I_{90}}{I_0}}{1-\dfrac{I_{90}}{I_0}}\right)\right] \tag{4.19}$$

Here I_0 and I_{90} are the intensities at the orientation of transmission plane of the polarizer at 0° and 90°; δ_i is the phase shift between the orthogonal components of the amplitude of the laser radiation at the points with coordinates r_1 and r_2 [164].

4.3.3.2 Biological Samples

The maps of the polarization parameters and the optical anisotropy of the fibrillary and parenchymal structures of biological tissues revealed correlations in the region of 'single-point' polarimetry [106,162–167]. These obtained results were oncologically efficient for the differential diagnosis of various stages of cancer [109,168–174], and therefore the technique of 'two-point' polarization–correlation mapping was tested in the present study. This method can provide a comparative analysis of the sensitivity of several polarimetric techniques and examine the diagnostic potential of Stokes correlometry of pathological changes in the orientation-phase structure of biological tissues.

Histological sections of biological tissues were prepared by a microtome from frozen samples. The following optically thin samples ($\tau < 0.01$) of histological sections were examined in this study:

- biological tissues with "ordered" birefringent fibrillary networks (atrium myocardium—see Figure 4.8, panels a, d);

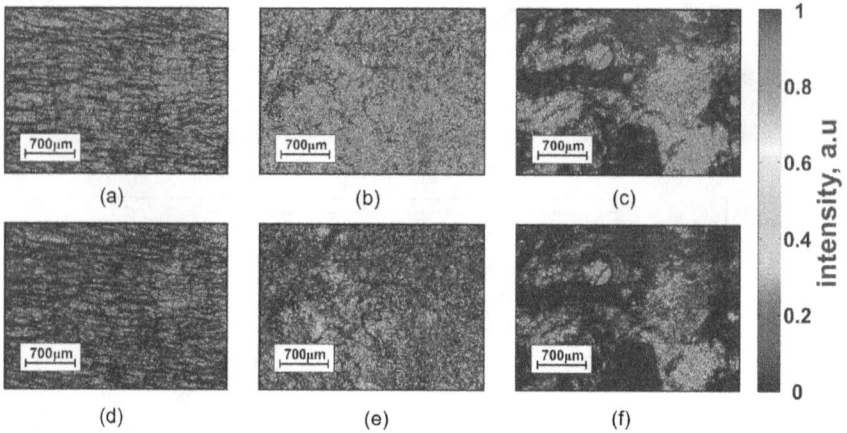

FIGURE 4.8 Polarization-inhomogeneous microscopic images of biological tissues with different morphological structures. Upper row (coaxial polarizer and polarizer–analyzer position): spatially ordered fibrillary (a), disordered (b) myosin myocardial networks and islet parenchymal structures of the colon wall (c). Bottom row (crossed polarizer and polarizer–analyzer position): optically anisotropic structures of myosin myocardial networks ((d), (e)) and colon wall parenchyma (f)).

- biological tissues with a "disordered" birefringent fibrillary network (ventricle myocardium—see Figure 4.8, panels b, e);

- biological tissues with "islet" structure (clusters of spatially non-oriented protein fibers) of optically anisotropic formations in the optically isotropic matrix (rectal wall—see Figure 4.8, panels c, f).

This selection of samples with different morphological structures (in terms of orientation and amorphous–anisotropic structure) provides comparative information about the patterns of changes in the polarization–correlation structure of microscopic images [164].

A comparative analysis of these microscopic images (see Figure 4.8) revealed their individual polarizationally inhomogeneous topographical structure—the coordinate distributions of different polarization states visualized as spots of varying intensity (see panels d–f in Figure 4.8). Such studies can determine objective statistical and correlation criteria that characterize the correlation coherence of optical anisotropy parameters and can form the basis for the differential diagnosis of birefringence changes in biological tissues [164].

4.3.3.3 Statistical Analysis

To determine the distributions of the module for the 'two-point' parameters of the Stokes vector for polarization-inhomogeneous microscopic images of biological tissues, a set of central statistical moments of the first to fourth orders (mean Z_1, variance Z_2, skewness Z_3 and kurtosis Z_4) was calculated according to the traditional method presented in [162].

4.4 RESULTS AND DISCUSSION

4.4.1 Spectroscopic Measurements

4.4.1.1 Analysis of Spectra

To track the changes of chemical component properties, the absorbance spectra in both configurations were analyzed over time. The major peaks associated with different meat chromophores (OxyMb, water, fat, and protein) were clearly detectable for the samples. Furthermore, there was a significant decrease in the absorbance values in both the visible and NIR spectral regions caused by changes in the chemical composition of the pork during the freshness decay.

Figure 4.9 shows absorbance spectra obtained from the configuration with the attached integrating sphere over different time measurements. The curves in Figure 4.9a are associated with the data obtained after 0 (solid), 3 (dash), and 6 (dot) hours of keeping the sample at room temperature, while in Figure 4.9b and c, they represent 0 (solid), 4 (dash), and 8 (dot) hours. The local absorbance peaks in the visible range (see Figure 4.9a) at around 540 and 575 nm wavelengths were attributed to the OxyMb content in the sample responsible for the meat color [175]. In the NIR region (see Figure 4.9b and c), the major peaks in the absorbance spectra emerged between 1100 and 1600 nm. The peak around 1200 nm in Figure 4.9b was correlated with the fat content in the samples, while the absorbance peak around 1450 nm (see Figure 4.9c), which had the largest amount of absorbance over the whole spectra, was related to water and water-bonded groups [14]. These results indicated that water was the dominant component in the NIR range of wavelengths which affected the mean spectrum of the pork samples. The local peak around 1525 nm (see Figure 4.9c) was attributed to the protein content [176].

For further analysis, the area between the isosbestic points under the absorbance spectra was integrated (termed 'integrated absorbance') within absorption bands attributed to the meat chromophores. The integrated area for each component was selected as follows: OxyMb (515–600 nm for the integrating sphere setup), fat (1175–1290 nm), water (1414–1490 nm), and

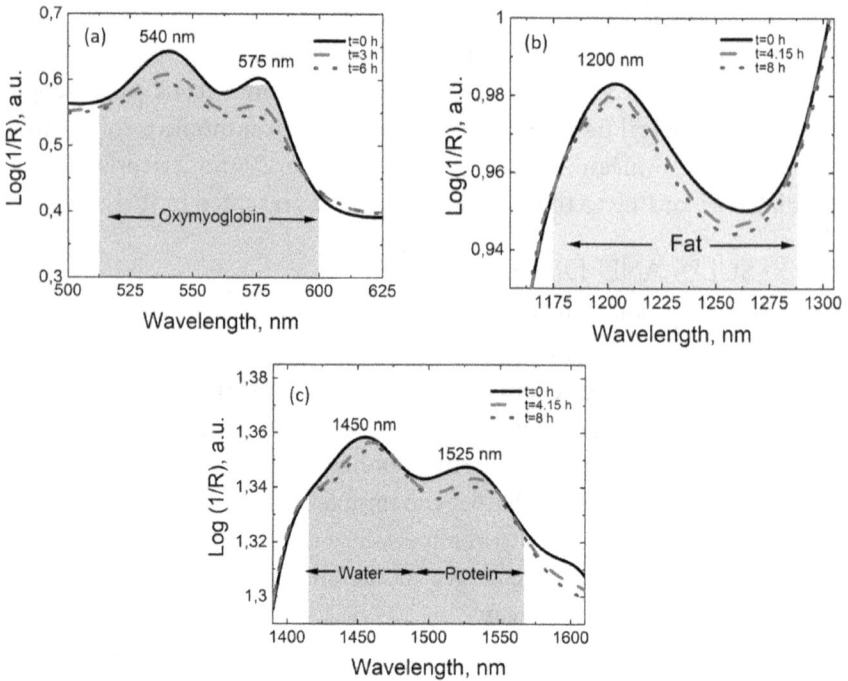

FIGURE 4.9   Absorbance spectra of the pork samples measured with the attached integrating sphere configuration at (a) 0 hours (solid), 3 (dash), and 6 (dot) hours; (b and c) 0 hours (solid), 4 (dash) hours, and 8 hours after keeping the sample at room temperature (23°C). The absorbance peaks indicate the presence of (a) oxymyoglobin (540 and 570 nm), (b) fat (1200 nm), (c) water (1450 nm), and proteins (1525 nm) [14,47,155].

proteins (1490–1567 nm); and these were plotted over time. Eventually, a new term called 'degradation kinetics' was introduced for each of the meat chromophores, defined by the dependence of the 'integrated absorbance' over time.

Figure 4.10 represents the changes in the integrated absorbance over time for the integrating sphere configuration in the visible (see Figure 4.10a) and NIR (see Figure 4.10b and c) spectral ranges for the selected areas referring to the meat chromophores. The integrated absorbance for different wavelengths decreased in the visible and NIR spectral regions indicating the degradation of the meat chromophores, which negatively affected freshness of the samples [14,27].

The degradation of OxyMb arising from color changes apparently started from the beginning (see Figure 4.10a), while in the NIR region

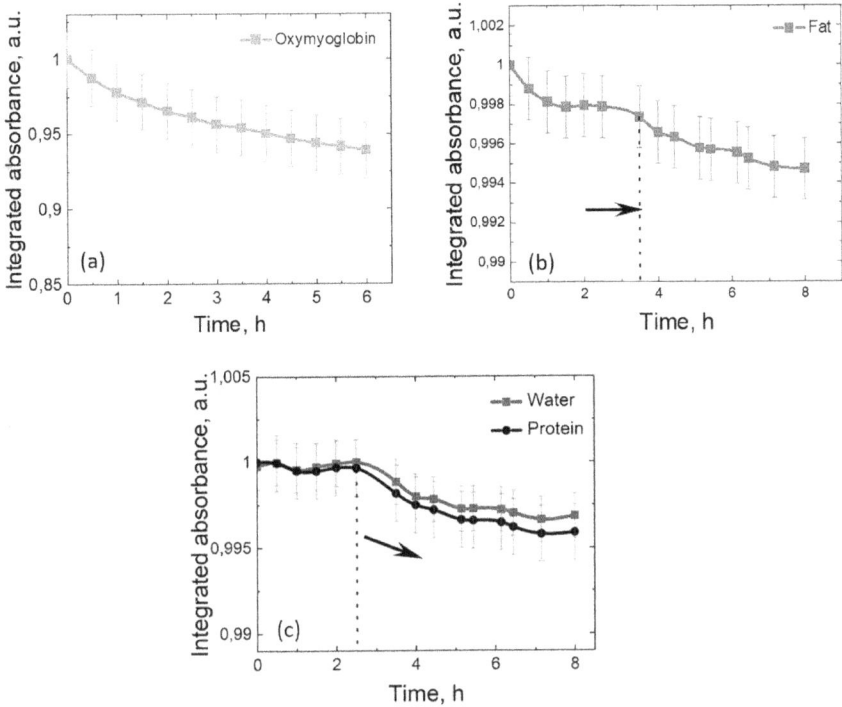

FIGURE 4.10 Integrated absorbance changes over time for (a) oxymyoglobin, (b) fat and (c) water (square), and proteins (circle) measured in the integrating sphere configuration. The dashed vertical lines in (b) and (c) indicate the transition time between the fresh and non-fresh pork samples [137].

(see Figure 4.10b and c) the integrated absorbance of water, fat, and protein reduced at a slower rate after approximately 2.5 hours, which could be interpreted as the beginning stage of the freshness deterioration process. The integrated absorbance for fat (see Figure 4.10b) did not experience a sharp reduction in contrast to the water and protein curves (see Figure 4.10c). This could be explained by the fat degradation occurring at a slower rate than the other considered components.

Similar experiments were performed with the fiber-optic configuration. Figure 4.11 shows the major peaks associated with the OxyMb absorbance measured at 0, 3, and 6 hours at room temperature (see Figure 4.11a) and the integrated absorbance changes with time over the selected region within 527–587 nm (see Figure 4.11b).

The integrated absorbance decreased over time in this case as well (see Figure 4.11b), although the drop in the integrated absorbance happened at

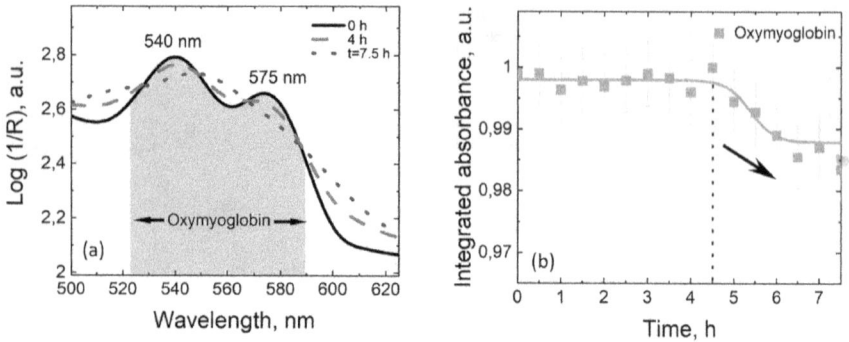

FIGURE 4.11 (a) Evolution of absorbance spectra in a pork sample measured with the fiber- optic configuration at 0 (solid), 4 (dash), and 7.5 (dot) hours after keeping the sample at room temperature (23°C). The 540 and 575 nm absorbance peaks indicate the presence of oxymyoglobin, and the shadowed area shows the integrated absorbance. (b) The changes of the integrated absorbance associated with oxymyoglobin over 7.5 hours. The dashed vertical line indicates the transition time between the fresh and non-fresh pork samples [137].

a slower rate after about 4.5 hours. Comparing the curves in Figures 4.10a and 4.11b (both referred to OxyMb absorbance changes over time measured with different configurations) revealed the difference between the decreasing trends. Since the pork samples were covered with a plastic film from all sides and were under stable and similar physiological conditions, we assumed that this difference stems from the difference in the probing depth of the configurations. With the configuration equipped with the optical fibers, the probing depth was shallower compared to the other configuration and therefore, it could principally detect superficial changes of the sample surface. Further discussion of the observed discrepancy will be elucidated through MC simulations in the following section.

4.4.1.2 Monte Carlo Simulations

Despite observing the same component (OxyMb), the integrated absorbance changes over time for the applied experimental configurations showed distinct trends: in the case of the integrating sphere (see Figure 4.10a) the degradation happened rapidly from the beginning, while for the fiber-optic setup (see Figure 4.11b) the degradation was noticeably delayed (after 4.5 hours). To elucidate this discrepancy in the degradation kinetics of OxyMb, MC simulations were applied for both configurations, and this revealed that the distinction from the optical point of view originated from the sensing depth. For the setup with an attached integrating sphere, the sensing depth was shallower due to higher contribution of the surface and subsurface reflected photons. In the configurations with the array of optical fibers, the probing depth was adjustable by modifying the source–detector separation and choosing the nth fiber as the detecting fiber, while the illuminating fiber was kept the same. Thus, the delay was generated by larger depths achieved by detected photons in the latter case.

Figure 4.12 represents the spatial distributions of the optical detected signals in the pork sample assessed by MC simulations for both experimental configurations and clearly illustrates this aspect. Figure 4.12a shows the spatial distributions of the fiber-optic configuration when there are only two fibers to detect signals, while Figure 4.12b demonstrates the spatial distributions for an array of 11 optical fibers (the same as the applied experimental configuration of this study). The depth and length of the probing area increased with the number of optical fibers used. Figure 4.12c simulates the spatial distributions of the experimental configuration with the attached integrating sphere and proves that the probing area was larger than the fiber-optic configuration, while the probability density for deeper areas was considerably lower than the other configuration.

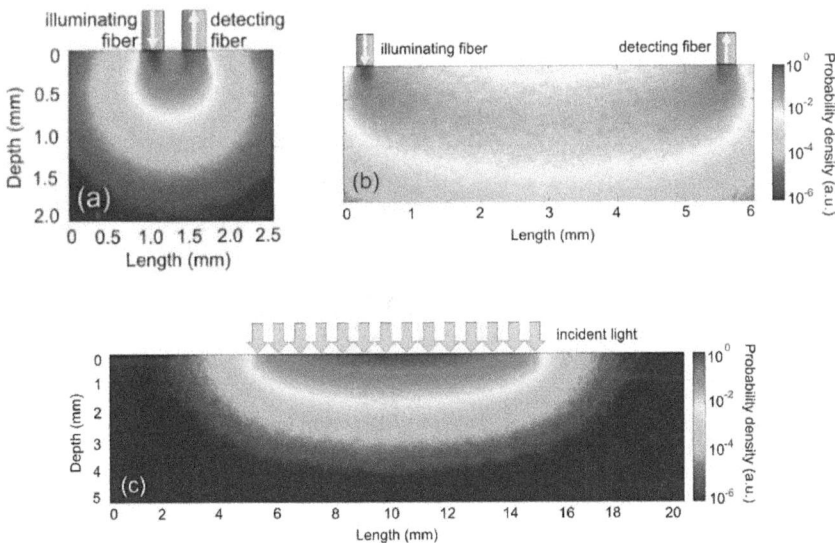

FIGURE 4.12 Spatial distributions of the detected optical signal in pork sample for the fiber optics with (a) two fiber optics, (b) 11 fiber optics and (c) integrating sphere configurations assessed by MC simulations. The distance between the illuminating and the detecting fibers is 0.53 mm (a) and 5.3 mm (b) [137].

4.4.1.3 Principal Component Analysis (PCA)

Figure 4.13 shows the corresponding scores plot of the pork samples and their spectra measured with two configurations in different spectral ranges (Vis/NIR) for the first and the second principal components. Figure 4.13a displays the scores plot of the visible spectra obtained from the configuration with the attached integrating sphere with 86.4% and 9.3% of the total variance in the dataset. Four distinct separations can be clearly detected to classify different levels of freshness according to PC 1 and PC 2. PC 1 indicated a clear division between the stages of freshness with negative values for the fresh sample and positive values for non-fresh sample. Moreover, PC 2 provided information about aging and spoilage, revealing the separation between the fresh sample (0 hour; solid cluster) and the non-fresh

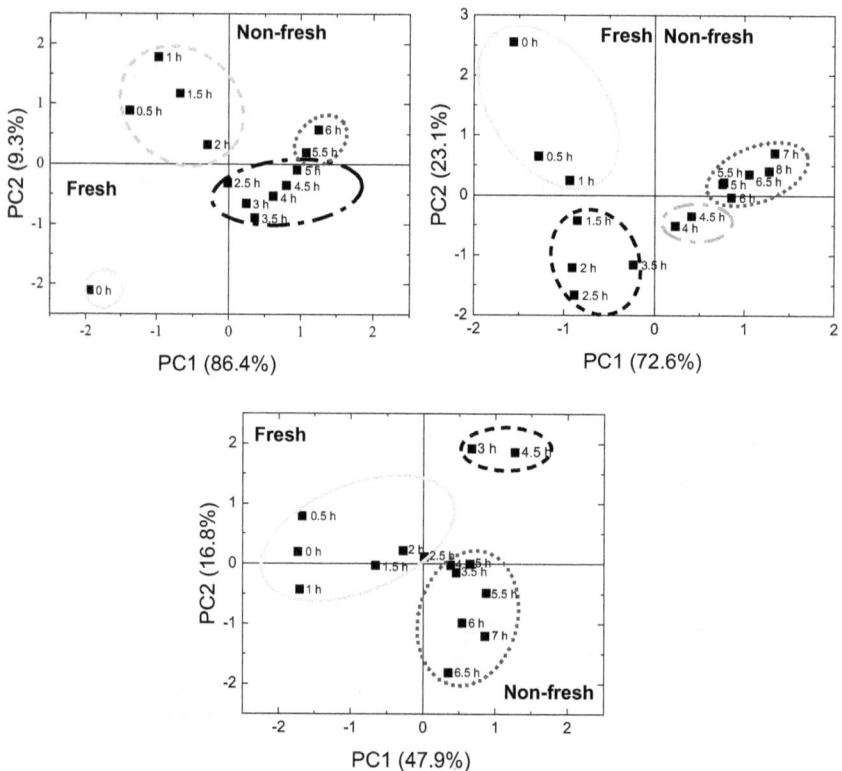

FIGURE 4.13   Representation of the score plots of the PCA performed on the absorbance spectra of a pork sample measured with the integrating sphere configuration in the visible (a) and NIR range (b), and with the fiber-optic configuration in the visible range (c). The clusters represent: fresh (solid cluster), less fresh (dash cluster), almost non-fresh (dash dot cluster), and non-fresh (dot cluster) [137].

sample (5.5 and 6 hours; dot cluster). Evidently, compared to the spectra analysis, the PCA method provided complementary information and distinguished the level of freshness between the totally fresh sample at the beginning of the measurement (0 hour; solid cluster) and the less fresh sample (0.5–2 hours; dash cluster) in addition to a mid-level classification between 2.5–5 hours (dash dot cluster) and 5.5–6 hours (dot cluster) for the non-fresh sample.

For the NIR spectra measured with the integrating sphere (see Figure 4.13b), the first three principal components were responsible for 98.7% of variability of the data; the first, second, and third principal components variability were 72.6%, 23.1%, and 3%, respectively. Similarly to visible spectra, PC 1 was the separator reference axis with negative values for the fresh sample and positive values for non-fresh sample. The transition to the non-fresh stage happened after 3.5 hours which was the same as the spectra analysis showed for the fat absorption (see Figure 4.13b), while for water and protein spectral changes were detected earlier after approximately 2.5 hours (see Figure 4.13c).

According to the PCA results, the stages of freshness could be divided into the following:

- 0–1 hour; fresh (solid cluster);
- 1.5–3.5 hours; less fresh (dash luster);
- 4–4.5 hours; almost non-fresh (dash dot cluster);
- 5–8 hours; totally non-fresh (dot cluster).

Figure 4.13c illustrates the scores plot for the visible spectra measured with the optical fibers configuration with 47.9% and 16.8% of the total variance in the dataset. Here, due to higher scattered data, it was difficult to categorize freshness sub-stages. The classification between the stages of freshness was defined using PC 1 with negative values referring to fresh sample (solid cluster) and positive values to less fresh and non-fresh samples (dash dot and dot clusters). Similar to the spectra analysis in Figure 13b, the freshness decay started after 4.5 hours although the data referring to 3.5 and 4 hours in the dash cluster were questionable.

4.4.2 Mueller Matrix Polarimetry Measurements

The possibilities of using MMIP to assess meat quality was explored by applying a custom-built wide-field MM imaging polarimeter. Fresh

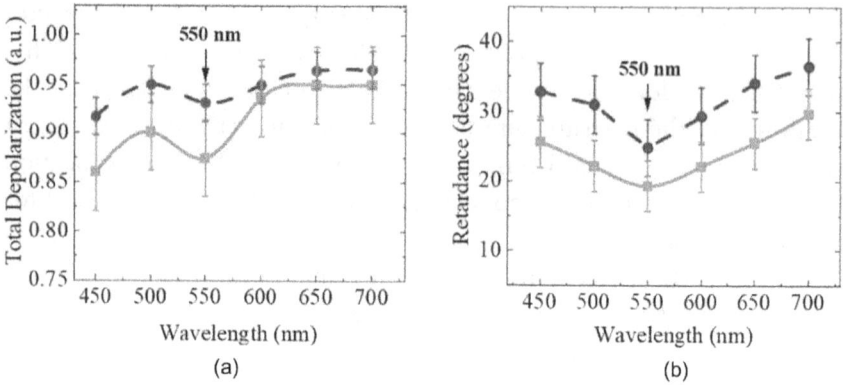

FIGURE 4.14 Wavelength dependence of total depolarization (left) and scalar retardance (right) for a fresh (0 hour; solid line) and an aged (26 hours; dash line) pork sample of 1 cm thickness stored at room temperature (23°C).

porcine muscles were imaged at room temperature over 26 hours to visualize the dynamics of the tissue polarization properties, including the total depolarization and scalar retardance.

The changes in total depolarization and scalar retardance spectra are shown in Figure 4.14a and b, respectively, for fresh (0 hour; solid line) and aged (26 hours; dash line) tissue samples, while the error bars represent the standard deviation of the parameters. The values of total depolarization and scalar retardance were averaged over 800×600 pixels of corresponding images measured at different wavelengths. For both parameters, an evident difference between the measured spectra for the fresh and aged sample could be easily observed. The total depolarization value increased with the wavelength for both freshness statements, except for the dip at the wavelength of 550 nm, which can be associated with Mb absorption (see Figure 4.14a). Similarly, for the scalar retardance spectra, the dip at 550 nm happened as well (see Figure 4.14b), which could be arguably interpreted by the higher concentration of Mb with a lower degree of scattering and birefringence.

Since the polarimetric parameters at 550 nm wavelength had a distinctive behavior compared to the rest of spectra (see Figure 4.14a and b), this wavelength was chosen for further analysis in this study.

4.4.2.1 MM Images and FDH Analysis

Figure 4.15 represents the backscattering 4×4 MM images of pork tissue (1 cm thick) measured at the 550 nm wavelength for a fresh (0 hour; see

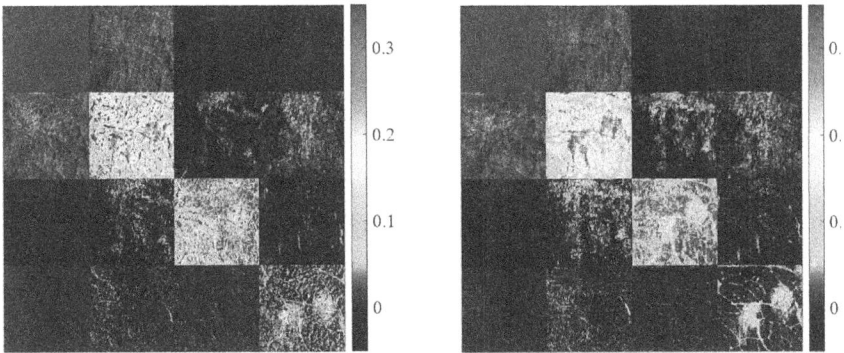

FIGURE 4.15   Experimental backscattering 4×4 MM images of a pork sample with a thickness of 1 cm measured at 550 nm wavelength: (Left) fresh (0 hour) and (Right) aged (26 hours) stored at room temperature (23°C). The field of view was 2×2 cm^2 and each element of polarimetric images was normalized by the corresponding pixel value of the M_{11} image [155].

Figure 4.15a) and aged (26 hours; see Figure 4.15b) sample stored in air at room temperature (23°C). According to Figure 4.15, the diagonal elements of MM changed significantly as the time of storing the sample at room temperature increased; the M_{22} value for the aged sample (see Figure 4.15b) was greater than the fresh sample (see Figure 4.15a) while the M_{33} and M_{44} values decreased after 26 hours which was attributed to a larger depolarization. The MM for both measurement times (0 hour and 26 hours) was non-diagonal, proving the anisotropic features of the tissue due to the well-aligned muscle fibers, although the values of the non-diagonal elements did not exceed 0.025. Although the 2D MM images include detailed spatial information of the sample, transforming the images into FDH curves can provide some intrinsic structural properties of tissue which might not be distinguishable with 2D images of MM.

Figure 4.16 shows the normalized FDH diagrams [121] of the MM elements of a glass-covered porcine muscle sample measured at a wavelength of 550 nm in fresh (0 hour; black line) and aged (26 hours; dash line) conditions stored in air at room temperature (23°C). The horizontal axis of each FDH illustrates the value of the pixel from the corresponding MM element, while the vertical axis shows the probability distribution. The FDHs of the diagonal elements (M_{33} and M_{44}) evolved noticeably with time.

To discover the origin of anisotropy, analyzing different groups of elements can help [108]. The FDHs of the non-diagonal elements including

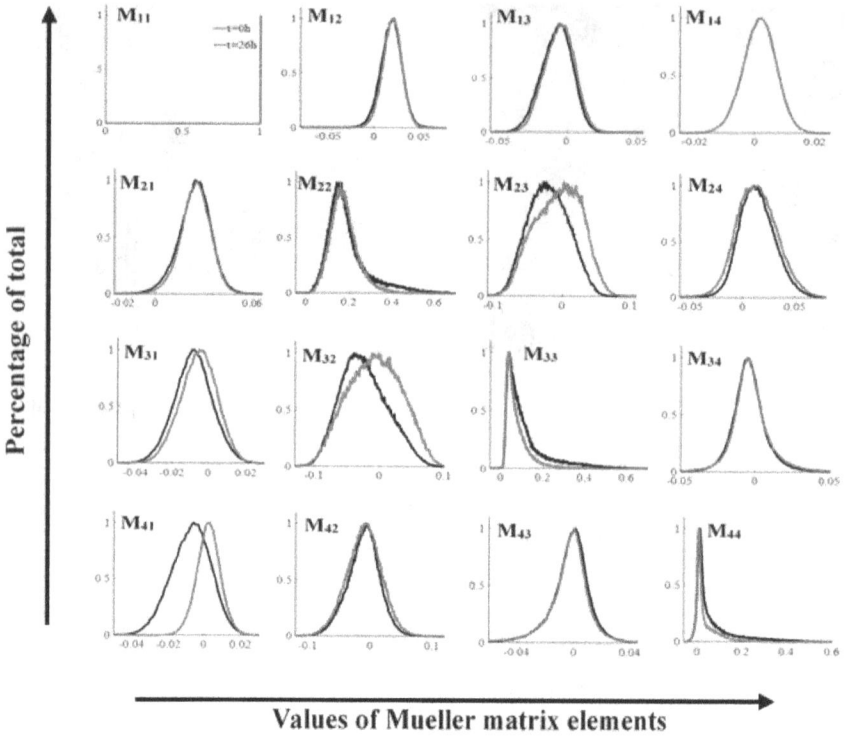

FIGURE 4.16 Normalized frequency distribution histograms (FDHs) of MM elements of a 1 cm thick pork sample in a fresh (0 hour) and aged (26 hours) state measured at a 550 nm light wavelength and stored at room temperature (23°C). The areas under the FDH are normalized to 1 [155].

M_{23}, M_{31}, M_{32}, M_{41}, and M_{42} measured after 26 hours shifted toward larger values confirming the increase in the sample anisotropy. However, this variation made it difficult to determine if the origin of anisotropy was due to the scattering properties of the tissue or its birefringence. In addition, the M_{23}, M_{32}, and M_{41} elements represented the most noticeable shift of FDHs toward larger values with time, which for M_{23} and M_{32} can be correlated with the direction of the aligned fibers or the birefringence.

4.4.2.2 Statistical Analysis

To provide further quantitative evaluation, 3D graphs of the statistical moments (Z_i) characterizing distributions of each MM element (normalized to M_{11}) of a glass-covered porcine muscle sample measured at 550 nm at fresh (0 hour; see Figure 4.17a, c, e, g) and aged (26 hours; see Figure 4.17b, d, f, h) state in air at room temperature are listed in Figure 4.17.

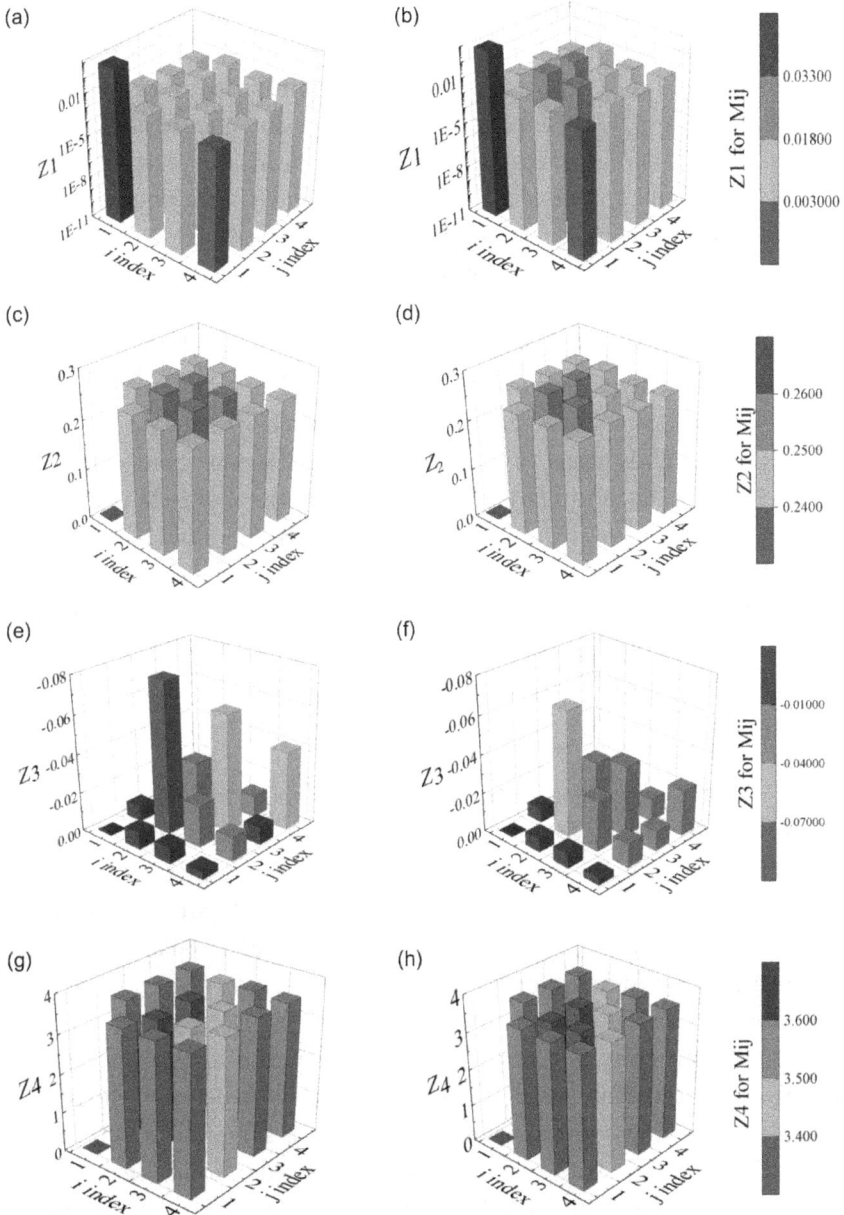

FIGURE 4.17 Statistical moments (Z_i) of the (a and b) first (Z_1; mean value), (c and d) second (Z_2; variance), (e and f) third (Z_3; skewness), and (g and h) fourth (Z_4; kurtosis) orders (normalized to M_{11}) characterizing the distributions of the MM elements of a glass-covered pork sample measured at 550 nm for fresh (0 hour; a, c, e, g) and aged (26 hours; b, d, f, h) in air at room temperature (23°C) [155].

According to Figure 4.17a, M_{22}, M_{23}, and M_{24} had the largest mean values for the fresh sample (0 hour), while for the aged sample (26 hours; see Figure 4.17b), M_{22}, M_{23}, M_{24}, M_{32}, and M_{33} had the largest mean values. In addition, M_{22} and M_{33} values of Z_1 increased over time, while Z_1 of M_{44} decreased considerably. Here, the differences in mean values of the M_{22} and M_{33} elements can be explained by the alignment of the fibers in almost the same direction [157]. The positive and low mean values of M_{34} and M_{43} elements can be contributed to the weak birefringence effect in this sample.

Meanwhile, the values of variance (see Figure 4.17c and d) for most of the elements hardly altered over time indicating that width distribution of the FDHs did not change noticeably with time. However, M_{22}, M_{23}, M_{32}, and M_{33} had slightly larger values for both freshness states compared to the other elements. According to Figure 4.17e and f, the skewness values considerably decreased over time. Moreover, the variance values of the central elements (M_{22}, M_{23}, M_{32}, M_{33}) and M_{41} were obviously higher than other elements for both states of freshness. The kurtosis values (see Figure 4.17g and h) of the central elements were smaller compared to the other elements for both measurement times, and the values of kurtosis slightly reduced over time.

4.4.2.3 Total Depolarization and Scalar Retardance Analysis

Figure 4.18 shows the total depolarization ($\Delta(x, y)$) (see Figure 4.18a–c) and scalar retardance ($R(x, y)$) (see Figure 4.18d–f) images obtained by MMPD applied pixel-wise to the measured MM. Figure 4.19 displays the corresponding histograms ($N(\Delta)$) of the total depolarization (see Figure 4.19a–c) and retardance (see Figure 4.19d–f) of a glass-covered porcine muscle sample of 1 cm thickness measured at 550 nm wavelength in air at room temperature (23°C). Obviously, the depolarization was strong (~0.9) and there were pronounced differences between the images over time showing some specific regions of the sample evolving differently over time. The strong depolarization observed in some regions of the measurement time points could be arguably elucidated by the presence of well-ordered myofibrils, most probably myosin, which has a thicker myofibrillar structure. Since for both parameters, there was no obvious shift in the histograms over time, the asymmetry of the distribution attributed to the skewness value (Z_3) should have been kept. Meanwhile, the tail heaviness of the histograms is due to the kurtosis (Z_4) of the total depolarization which was increasing over time and would need further studies.

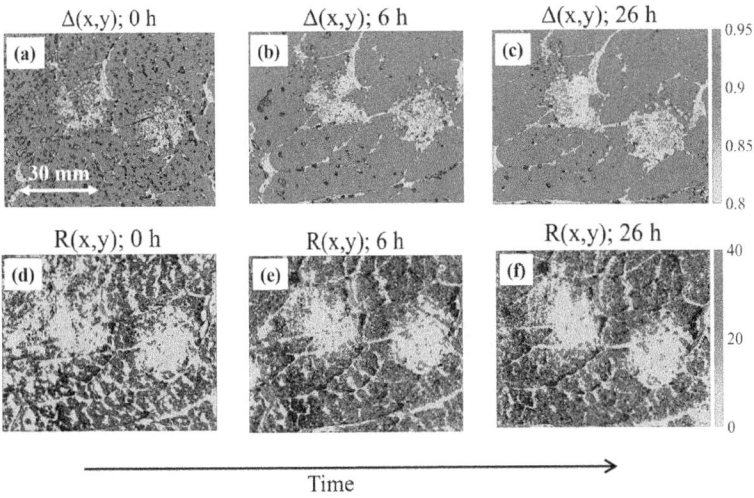

FIGURE 4.18   Images of the total depolarization ($\Delta(x, y)$; a–c) and scalar retardance ($R(x, y)$; (d–f) of a pork sample of 1 cm thickness measured at a 550 nm wavelength after 0 hours (a, d), 6 hours (b, e), and 26 hours (c, f) in air at room temperature (23°C) [155].

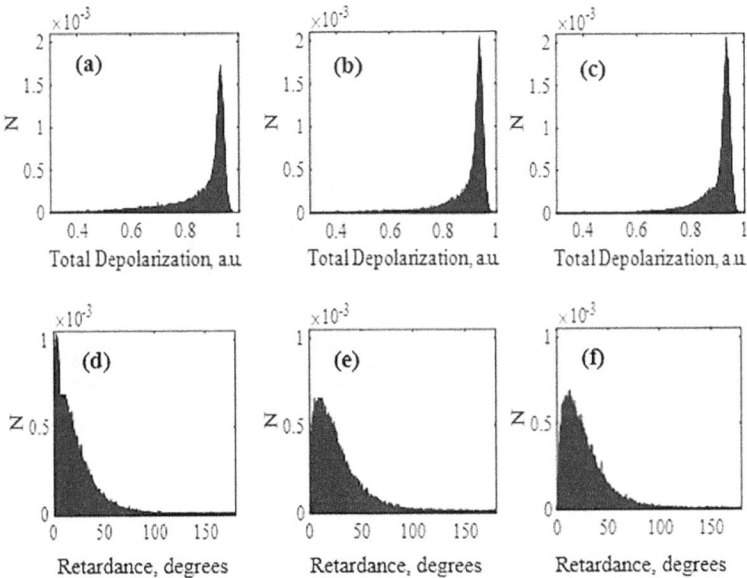

FIGURE 4.19   Histograms (N) of the total depolarization (a–c) and scalar retardance ($R(x, y)$; (d–f) of a pork sample of 1 cm thickness measured at a 550 nm wavelength after 0 hours (a, d), 6 hours (b, e) and 26 hours (c, f) in air at room temperature (23°C) [155].

The time dependency of the statistical moments of the polarization parameters was investigated to gain a deeper view of the changes occurring during the tissue storage at room temperature and as a quantitative description. The statistical moments of the total depolarization and scalar retardance histograms are shown after curve fitting in Figure 4.20 at a 550 nm wavelength.

The mean values of the total depolarization and scalar retardance (Z_1) increased smoothly with time, which can be elucidated by the increasing number of scattering events over time due to water evaporation and increasing spaces between muscle fiber bundles [177]. The variance values of the

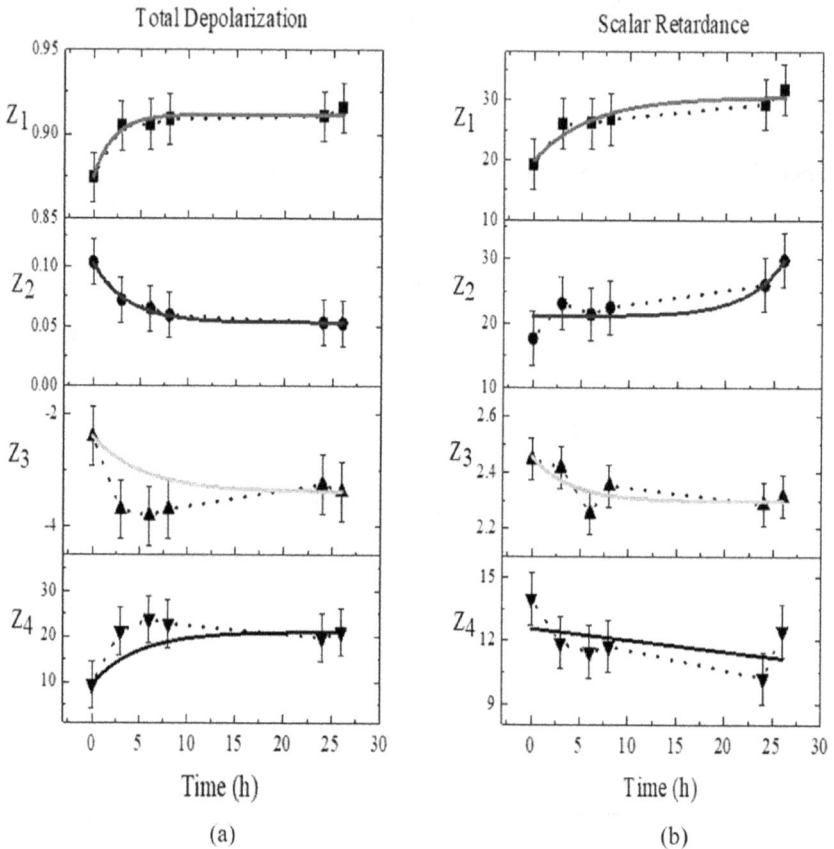

FIGURE 4.20 Images of statistical moments (Z_i) for (a) the total depolarization and (b) the scalar retardance of a pork sample of 1 cm thickness measured at a 550 nm wavelength over 26 hours at room temperature (23°C). The solid lines show the exponential fitting functions and the error bars represent the standard deviation of the statistical moments [155].

total depolarization (see Figure 4.20a (Z_2)) decreased over time indicating that the data points were distributed closer to the mean value, whereas for the scalar retardance (see Figure 4.20b (Z_2)) the data were distributed so that they were more spread around the mean value (Z_1). The skewness values showed that the distribution of the total depolarization values (see Figure 4.20a (Z_3)) was negatively skewed (wider left FDH tail toward lower values), while for the scalar retardance (see Figure 4.20b (Z_3)) they were positive indicating that the right FDH tail was wider and extended toward higher values. For both the total depolarization and scalar retardance values, the skewness noticeably reduced after 26 hours. Kurtosis values for total depolarization (see Figure 4.20a (Z_4)) increased with time, while for the scalar retardance (see Fig.4.20b (Z_4)) the kurtosis declined over time and contributed to the tail heaviness direction of the distribution.

4.4.3 Two-point Stokes Vector Diagnosis Approach

4.4.3.1 Tissue with Ordered (Rectilinear) Birefringent Fibrillar Networks – Myocardium Atrium

Figure 4.21 shows the 2D distributions of values $S_{i=3;4}(\Delta x; \Delta y)$ (see Figure 4.21a and c) and histograms N (see Figure 4.21b and d) of the SCP modulus distributions calculated for a polarizationally inhomogeneous microscopic image of the myocardium atrium.

An analysis of the obtained polarization–correlation maps of the SCP module showed the following:

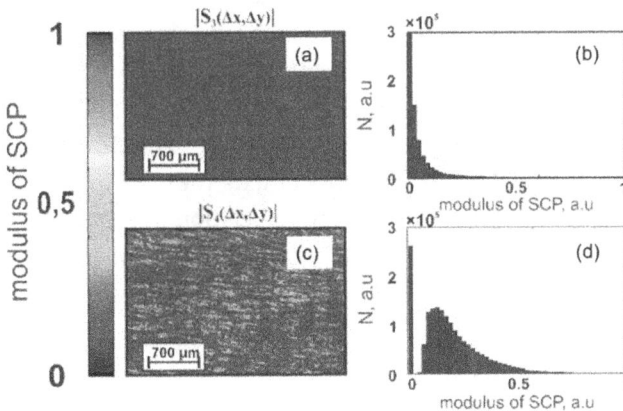

FIGURE 4.21   Stokes correlometry of spatially ordered birefringent fibrillary networks. Topographic (a and c) and statistical (b and d) SCP-map structure of the modulus of polarizationally inhomogeneous image of myocardium atrium [164].

- coordinate heterogeneity of the distributions of the third and fourth "two-point" parameters $S_{i=3;4}(\Delta x;\Delta y)$ of the Stokes vector for a spatially ordered network of myosin fibrils atrium myocardium (see Figure 4.21a and c);

- histograms of distributions of random variables $S_{i=3;4}(\Delta x;\Delta y)$ which were individual for the third and fourth "two-point" parameters (see Figure 4.21b and d);

- probabilistic distributions which were characterized by the presence of major extrema localized in the proximity of $S_{i=3;4}(\Delta x;\Delta y) =0$, as well as a significant scatter in the SCP asymmetry and peak acuity (see Figure 4.21b and d).

- From the physical perspective, in the 'one-point' approximation, the third parameter of the Stokes vector determined the magnitude of the polarization azimuth [162,167]. The magnitude of the polarization azimuth was proportional to the direction of the optical axis ρ (Eq. 4.6) of the biological tissue, which was defined by the spatial orientation of the birefringent fibrils [169,171,173]. Thus, the degree of correlation 'point-to-point' matching microscopic image of spatially ordered atrium myocardium ($|S_{i=3}(\Delta x;\Delta y)|$) of polarization azimuths at the points of the myosin fibrils practically did not change.

Correspondingly, the polarization–correlation map of this SCS parameter was quite homogeneous (see Figure 4.21a), and the distribution histogram was characterized by a pronounced extremum (see Figure 4.21b). The fourth 'one-point' parameter of the Stokes vector characterized the magnitude of the ellipticity of polarization [109,162,178]. This parameter was more noticeable in comparison to the azimuth which was associated with the direction of the optical axis ρ of the birefringent fibrils (Eq. 4.6). Accordingly, the degree of correlation 'point-to-point' matching ($S_{i=3;4}(\Delta x;\Delta y)$) of the ellipticity of polarization at the points in the microscopic image showing the myosin fibrils of the myocardium atrium was more sensitive to variations of ρ. As a result, the degree of correlation matching the ellipticity of polarization at different points declined. As a result, the coordinate heterogeneity of the polarization–correlation maps of this SCP parameter (see Figure 4.21c) increased and additional 'decorrelation' extremes (see Figure 4.21d) were formed in the distribution histogram.

4.4.3.2 Tissue with Disordered Birefringent Fibrillar
Networks— Myocardium Ventricle

Figure 4.22 represents the statistical and correlation characteristics of the values $S_{i=3;4}(\Delta x;\Delta y)$ distributions calculated for histological sections of the myocardium ventricle with the network of myosin fibers disordered by the packaging direction.

An analysis of the polarization–correlation mapping of the coordinate distributions of the amount of S_3 and S_4 (the third and fourth "two-point" parameters of the Stokes vector) of a histological section of the myocardium ventricle showed that:

- the coordinate heterogeneity of the distributions of $S_{i=3;4}(\Delta x;\Delta y)$ (see Figure 4.22a and c) increased compared to the Stokes correlometry data of the microscopic image of the histological section of the myocardium atrium (see Figure 4.21a and c);

- the magnitude of the main extrema characterizing the histograms of the distribution of $S_{i=3;4}(\Delta x;\Delta y)$ and the formation of additional local extrema (see Figure 4.22b and d) decreased.

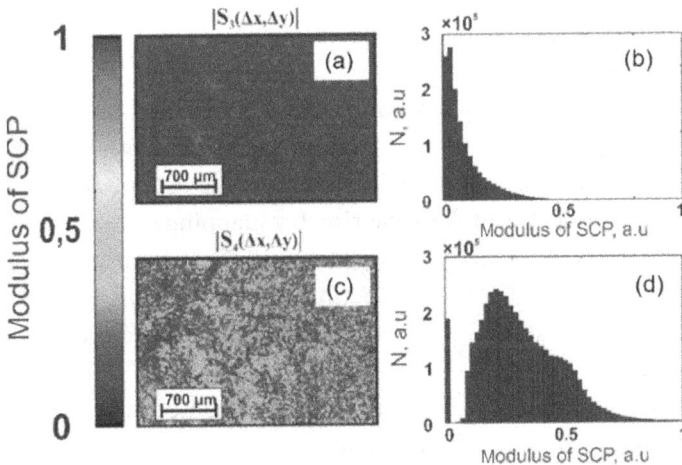

FIGURE 4.22 Stokes correlometry of spatially ordered birefringent fibrillary networks. Topographic (fragments (a),(c)) and statistical (fragments (b),(d)) distributions of the magnitude of the third and fourth 'two-point' parameters $\left|S_{i=3;4}\left(\Delta x,\Delta y\right)\right|$ of polarizationally inhomogeneous image of myocardium atrium [164].

The observed changes of the topographic and statistical structure of the distributions of the magnitude of S_3 and S_4 of the histological section of myocardium ventricle can be interpreted with a wider range of spatial orientations of the optical axes of myosin fibrils. Therefore, the degree of correlation between the azimuth and ellipticity of polarization would decrease for a polarizationally inhomogeneous image of a myocardial sample of this type.

According to the SCP-map structure (see Figure 4.22a and c), an increase in the decorrelation degree between the values of the Stokes vector parameters was observed at the points of the polarizationally inhomogeneous image of the myocardium ventricle. Quantitatively, it can be revealed in the reduction of the peak sharpness of the histograms $N\,(|S_{i=3}(\Delta x;\Delta y)|=0)$ and $N(|S_{i=4}(\Delta x;\Delta y)|=1)$, and in the increase in the value of the additional extremum $(|S_{i=4}(\Delta x;\Delta y)|\neq 0)$ of the distributions $N(|S_{i=4}(\Delta x;\Delta y)|$ (see Figure 4.22b and d).

These physically recognized features can be associated with an increase in the range of optical axes ρ orientations, which are determined by the packaging directions of birefringent myosin fibrils. Due to the increase in the differences between $\rho(r_1)$ and $\rho(r_2)$, an increase in the values of $|S_{i=3}(\Delta x;\Delta y)|$ and $|S_{i=4}(\Delta x;\Delta y)|$ would be detected (13).

4.4.3.3 Intergroup Statistical Analysis of the Modulus Distributions of SCP-Maps

The statistical $(Z_{i=1;2;3;4})$ analysis of coordinate distributions of the values of $S_{i=3;4}(\Delta x;\Delta y)$ of polarizationally inhomogeneous images of histological sections of the myocardium ventricle tissues (ordered and disordered) was performed in [164]. The Stokes-polarimetry mapping showed that the values of statistical moments of $Z_1(S_{i=3;4})$ (about 1.5–2 times), $Z_3(S_{i=3;4})$ (about 1.95 times), and $Z_4(S_{i=3;4})$ (about 2.5 times) were the most sensitive to the peculiarities of orientation-phase structure of the studied types of biological tissues [164].

The main objective of this work was to investigate scalar and polarized light interaction with a complex random inhomogeneous media including biological tissues by applying different methodologies and developing effective assessment tools in biomedical diagnostics in addition to food applications. The samples examined were chosen from porcine muscle meat due to the following reasons: meat as a postmortem tissue has a random inhomogeneous, anisotropic medium similar to biological tissues. Moreover, pork is the most widely consumed type of meat in the world, while concerns about contaminated and adulterated meat and the associated health risks are rising due to extensively spoiled meat products. The results of this work are applicable in biomedical diagnostics and food applications.

It was hypothesized that a polarization-based diagnostic approach could be highly sensitive to the structural changes within biological tissues caused by associated physiological and pathological malformations. Accordingly, utilizing a combination of optical spectroscopy and a polarization-based approach, healthy/fresh and cancerous/non-fresh tissues can be distinguished and characterized quantitatively.

In the first stage, spectroscopic techniques (Vis/NIR) were applied to detect the early stages of the loss of freshness in pork samples at room temperature with the aim of understanding the optical properties of ex vivo tissues over time. As presented in this chapter, it was possible to observe the decreasing light absorbance for different pork chromophores such as OxyMb, water, fat, and protein in the visible and NIR spectral ranges. Since a reduction of the absorbance caused by water loss and degradation of OxyMb can reduce the sample freshness, we considered this parameter to be a reference to address different freshness states of the samples.

An experimental configuration with an integrating sphere measured a larger probing area at a low depth and showed promise detecting superficial changes of the sample surface and could detect the early degradation stages of some chromophores including water, fat, and protein (after around 2.5 hours). The depth of probing was adjustable using another configuration with a compact linear array of optical fibers by changing the nth detecting fiber and keeping the illuminating fiber the same. According to the MC simulations, a higher n will provide a deeper probing depth according to the distance that light passes through.

The PCA method was applied to the absorbance database as a complementary analysis tool to label the different stages of freshness of the samples according to changes in the amount of chromophore absorbance of the meat. The approach was successful and detected stages which were not recognizable using the spectroscopic analysis method. The stages of freshness were called as fresh, less fresh, and non-fresh states.

The MMIP technique was applied to pork samples at room temperature to examine meat quality by investigating the polarization features of meat. Changes in the total depolarization ($\Delta(x, y)$) and scalar retardance ($R(x, y)$) images over time were considerable for fresh and non-fresh (26 hours) samples. An increase in the total depolarization with the wavelength could be explained by the decrease of light absorption by Mb in the red part of the visible light spectrum. The high depolarization value was associated with multiple scattering within a thick tissue. The least value of depolarization at the 550 nm wavelength could be arguably interpreted by the highest absorption of Mb, which is associated with meat color and freshness. Thus, the changes in the increasing slope of the total depolarization mean values over time at the 550 nm wavelength were explained by decreases in Mb absorption over time and the disordering of the fibrillary structure of the samples. These changes in the depolarization of fresh and non-fresh meat samples were clearly detected in polarimetric images and time-dependent graphs and could provide quantitative metrics for a non-invasive assessment of meat freshness.

The increase of scalar retardance over time was attributed to water evaporation, causing the densification and alignment of myosin bundles which increased the anisotropy of the refractive index, including the sample birefringence. Furthermore, compared to the long-path photons that were absorbed, the detected photons traveled a shorter distance within the sample. Consequently, short-path photons were less depolarized because they experienced fewer scattering events and accumulated less phase shift, which is proportional to the length of photon trajectory within the birefringent sample [117].

The analysis of FDHs showed that the non-diagonal elements including M_{23}, M_{31}, M_{32}, M_{41}, and M_{42} measured after 26 hours shifted toward larger values showing the increase in the sample anisotropy. Moreover, M_{23}, M_{32}, and M_{41} elements represented the most pronounced shift of FDHs toward higher values over time which for M_{23} and M_{32} is probably due to the direction of the aligned fibers or the birefringence.

Although further studies are still required to discover the relationships between tissue morphology and the statistical moments of MM elements, an analysis of statistical changes in moment elements over time revealed that the values of Z_2, Z_3, and Z_4 of the MM elements were partially sensitive to time and, as a consequence, to the meat freshness level. Therefore, they were quite good quantitative indicators of the microstructural changes over time.

A two-point Stokes vector approach was developed to determine the diagnostic potential of Stokes correlometry to evaluate pathological changes of biological tissues. The method reveals coordinate distributions of the modulus of 'two-point' Stokes vector parameters of polarizationally inhomogeneous images for optically thin (optical thickness smaller than

0.01) histological sections of biological tissues with different morphological structures.

The results from the Vis/NIR spectroscopic approach could be utilized as primary studies which could then be further developed for meat freshness investigations in the food industry and could help to reduce the costs and accelerate meat quality monitoring. The configuration with an integrating sphere can be utilized to detect superficial contamination on the sample surface while the fiber-optic configuration can be applied as a basis for further studies to design a portable low-cost sensor of meat freshness which could become available for use in markets.

The polarimetric approach with MMIP can be applied as guidelines to study ex vivo tissues in different conditions (healthy/cancerous or fresh/non-fresh) in biomedical diagnosis in addition to food investigations.

The results from the two-point Stokes vector diagnostic approach can be applied in differential diagnoses of changes in optical anisotropy of human biological tissues with different morphological and physiological states.

Here we describe the spectroscopic and polarimetric imaging techniques that showed promising results in probing biological tissues through non-invasive approaches, which could be applied in the biomedical and food industry.

4.5 SUMMARY AND CONCLUSIONS

Rising concerns about adulterated meat have encouraged the food industry to seek novel non-invasive methods for rapid and accurate meat quality assessment. Dominant meat chromophores (Mb, oxy-myoglobin, fat, water, collagen) are characterized by close comparable absorbance values in the visible and NIR spectral regions. Thus, structural and compositional variations in meat can cause relative differences in light absorption. Here, we found specific times of transition to lower stages of freshness for pork samples kept at room temperature according to the absorbance changes of the meat chromophores by utilizing a fiber-optic probe and integrating sphere. The absorbance spectra were analyzed using PCA and freshness levels discriminated by different clusters could be related to 3–4 stages of freshness. The transition times from a fresh to non-fresh condition nearly matched the results from a spectroscopic analysis, although the PCA method revealed more details of the sub-stages of freshness which were not evident in a spectroscopic analysis. The results showed promise for the use of visible-to-NIR spectroscopy to assess changes in meat quality by monitoring the relative absorbance alternation of OxyMb and Mb in visible spectral ranges, and fat, water, and collagen in NIR spectral ranges combined with a PCA method as a complementary analysis tool.

Along with meat assessment studies, the possibilities of using MMIP were explored to investigate meat quality by analyzing the polarization properties. In this case fresh glass-covered porcine muscles were imaged with a custom-built wide-field MM imaging polarimeter at room temperature over 26 hours to visualize the dynamics of the optical properties of the tissue by applying a Lu–Chipman decomposition. The FDHs and statistical analysis of the MM elements showed prominent shifts over time. The wavelength spectra of both the total depolarization and scalar retardance values continuously increased over time while they experienced a dip at 550 nm. The increasing values of the total depolarization over time was linked to the increasing number of scattering events and decrease of Mb absorption in the red part of visible spectra related to the meat color and freshness, while for the scalar retardance it was associated with the increase in birefringence and meat tenderness. The obtained results are promising for the development of a novel, fast, non-contact optical technique for the monitoring of meat quality.

A two-point Stokes vector method was applied to examine the diagnostic potential of Stokes correlometry concerning pathological changes of biological tissues. This approach could provide a comparative analysis of the sensitivity of different polarimetric techniques and indicate the diagnostic potential of Stokes correlometry to examine pathological changes in the orientation-phase structure of biological tissues. The results showed that direct Stokes polarimetry mapping can be a basis for the differential diagnosis of changes in optical anisotropy of human biological tissues with different morphological and physiological states.

REFERENCES

1. I. Meglinski, C. Macdonald, A. Doronin, and M. Eccles, "Screening cancer aggressiveness by using circularly polarized light," in *Bio-Optics: Design and Application, BODA 2013*, 2013, p. 2013, doi: 10.1364/boda.2013. bm2a.4.
2. V. Backman et al., "Detection of preinvasive cancer cells," *Nature*, vol. 406, no. 6791, pp. 35–36, 2000, doi: 10.1038/35017638.
3. I. A. Vitkin and R. C. N. Studinski, "Polarization preservation in diffusive scattering from in vivo turbid biological media: Effects of tissue optical absorption in the exact backscattering direction," *Opt. Commun.*, vol. 190, no. 1–6, pp. 37–43, 2001, doi: 10.1016/S0030-4018(01)01080-X.

4. A. Pierangelo et al., "Multispectral Mueller polarimetric imaging detecting residual cancer and cancer regression after neoadjuvant treatment for colorectal carcinomas," *J. Biomed. Opt.*, vol. 18, no. 4, p. 046014, 2013, doi: 10.1117/1.jbo.18.4.046014.
5. J. Jagtap et al., "Quantitative Mueller matrix fluorescence spectroscopy for precancer detection," *Opt. Lett.*, vol. 39, no. 2, pp. 243–246, 2014, doi: 10.1364/OL.39.000243.
6. K. Kettunen, "Food safety enforcement at the local level in Finland: Risk-basis, efficacy and consistency," University of Helsinki, Helsinki, Finland, 2018.
7. WHO/FAO, "Diet, nutrition and the prevention of chronic diseases," 2003. Accessed: Apr.09, 2020. [Online]. Available: http://www.who.int/dietphysicalactivity/publications/trs916/download/en/.
8. M. Mladenov, S. Penchev, and M. Deyanov, "Optical methods for food quality and safety assessment – a review," *Inf. Commun. Control Syst. Technol.*, vol. 1, no. 2014, pp. 44–56, 2014.
9. M. Kamruzzaman, Y. Makino, and S. Oshita, "Non-invasive analytical technology for the detection of contamination, adulteration, and authenticity of meat, poultry, and fish: A review," *Anal. Chim. Acta*, vol. 853, no. 1, pp. 19–29, 2015, doi: 10.1016/j.aca.2014.08.043.
10. D. Dave and A. E. Ghaly, "Meat spoilage mechanisms and preservation techniques: A critical review," *Am. J. Agric. Biol. Sci.*, vol. 6, no. 4, pp. 486–510, 2011, doi: 10.3844/ajabssp.2011.486.510.
11. X. Zhao, H. Zhuang, S. C. Yoon, Y. Dong, W. Wang, and W. Zhao, "Electrical impedance spectroscopy for quality assessment of meat and fish: A review on basic principles measurement methods, and recent advances," *J. Food Qual.*, vol. 2017, 2017, doi: 10.1155/2017/6370739.
12. D. Yang, A. Lu, D. Ren, and J. Wang, "Detection of total viable count in spiced beef using hyperspectral imaging combined with wavelet transform and multiway partial least squares algorithm," *J. Food Saf.*, vol. 38, no. 1, pp. 1–13, 2018, doi: 10.1111/jfs.12390.
13. K. H. Eom, K. H. Hyun, S. Lin, and J. W. Kim, "The meat freshness monitoring system using the smart RFID tag," *Int. J. Distrib. Sens. Networks*, vol. 2014, 2014, doi: 10.1155/2014/591812.
14. G. ElMasry and S. Nakauchi, "Prediction of meat spectral patterns based on optical properties and concentrations of the major constituents," *Food Sci. Nutr.*, vol. 4, no. 2, pp. 269–283, 2016, doi: 10.1002/fsn3.286.
15. A. de la Cadena, S. Stolik, and J. M. de la Rosa, "A diffuse reflectance spectroscopy system to study biological tissues," *Proc. SPIE*, vol. 8785, pp. 1514–1521, Nov. 2013, [Online]. Available: https://doi.org/10.1117/12.2026477.
16. I. S. Saidi, S. L. Jacques, and F. K. Tittel, "Mie and Rayleigh modeling of visible- light scattering in neonatal skin," *Appl. Opt.*, vol. 34, no. 31, p. 7410, 1995, doi: 10.1364/ao.34.007410.
17. T. Avsievich, R. Zhu, A. Popov, A. Bykov, and I. Meglinski, "The advancement of blood cell research by optical tweezers," *Rev. Phys.*, p. 100043, 2020, doi: 10.1016/j.revip.2020.100043.

18. A. A. Blokhina, V. A. Ryzhova, V. V. Korotaev, and M. A. Kleshchenok, "The meat product quality control by a polarimetric method," *Proc. SPIE*, vol. 11053, p. 110534D, 2019, doi: 10.1117/12.2265844.

19. G. Zaccanti and D. Contini, "Photon migration and imaging of biological tissues," in *Trends in Optics (Research, Developments and Applications)*, A. Consortini, Ed. San Diego: Academic Press, 1996, pp. 51–61.

20. S. D. Gupta, N. Ghosh, and A. Banerjee, *Wave Optics: Basic Concepts and Contemporary Trends*. Boca Raton, FL: CRC Press, 2015.

21. P. Tománek, J. Mikláš, H. M. Abubaker, and L. Grmela, "Optical sensing of polarization states changes in meat due to the ageing," *AIP Conf. Proc.*, vol. 1288, no. November 2010, pp. 127–131, 2010, doi: 10.1063/1.3521343.

22. H. M. Abubaker, P. Tománek, and L. Grmela, "Measurement of dynamic variations of polarized light in processed meat due to aging," *Proc. SPIE*, vol. 8073, p. 80730U, 2011 doi: 10.1117/12.886836.

23. M. Sarkar, N. Gupta, and M. Assaad, "Monitoring of fruit freshness using phase information in polarization reflectance spectroscopy," *Appl. Opt.*, vol. 58, no. 23, p. 6396, 2019, doi: 10.1364/ao.58.006396.

24. H. M. Abubaker, "Study of Scattering and Polarization of Light in Biological Tissue," BRNO University of Technology, 2013.

25. H. J. Swatland, "Basic Science for Carcass Grading," Ontario, Canada: University of Guelph, Guelph, 2012. [Online]. Available: http://www3.sympatico.ca/howard.swatland/Brazil.htm.

26. E. Tornberg, "Effects of heat on meat proteins - Implications on structure and quality of meat products," *Meat Sci.*, vol. 70, no. 3, pp. 493–508, 2005, doi: 10.1016/j.meatsci.2004.11.021.

27. J. T. Alander, V. Bochko, B. Martinkauppi, S. Saranwong, and T. Mantere, "A review of optical nondestructive visual and near-infrared methods for food quality and safety," *Int. J. Spectrosc.*, vol. 2013, pp. 1–36, 2013, doi:10.1155/2013/341402.

28. G. Offer et al., "The Structural Basis of the Water-Holding, Appearance and Toughness of Meat and Meat Products," 1989. Accessed: Apr. 10, 2020. [Online]. Available: http://digitalcommons.usu.edu/foodmicrostructurehttp://digitalcommons.usu.edu/f oodmicrostructure/vol8/iss1/17.

29. E. J. G. Furtado et al., "Prediction of pH and color in pork meat using VIS-NIR near-infrared spectroscopy (NIRS)," *Food Sci. Technol.*, vol. 39, no. 1, pp. 88–92, 2019, doi: 10.1590/fst.27417.

30. A. H. Hoving-Bolink et al., "Perspective of NIRS measurements early post mortem for prediction of pork quality," *Meat Sci.*, vol. 69, no. 3, pp. 417–423, 2005, doi: 10.1016/j.meatsci.2004.08.012.

31. S. Andrés, A. Silva, A. L. Soares-Pereira, C. Martins, A. M. Bruno-Soares, and I. Murray, "The use of visible and near infrared reflectance spectroscopy to predict beef *M. longissimus thoracis et lumborum* quality attributes," *Meat Sci.*, vol. 78, no. 3, pp. 217–224, 2008, doi: 10.1016/j.meatsci.2007.06.019.

32. G. H. Geesink et al., "Prediction of pork quality attributes from near infrared reflectance spectra," *Meat Sci.*, vol. 65, no. 1, pp. 661–668, 2003, doi: 10.1016/S0309-1740(02)00269-3.

33. H. Z. Chen, M. Zhang, B. Bhandari, and C. hui Yang, "Development of a novel colorimetric food package label for monitoring lean pork freshness," *LWT*, vol. 99, pp. 43–49, 2019, doi: 10.1016/j.lwt.2018.09.048.

34. J. R. Andersen, C. Borggaard, A. J. Rasmussen, and L. P. Houmøller, "Optical measurements of pH in meat," *Meat Sci.*, vol. 53, no. 2, pp. 135–141, 1999, doi: 10.1016/S0309-1740(99)00045-5.

35. D. O. Andrăşescu, "Study and determination of meat products quality," *J. Agroaliment. Process. Technol.*, vol. 20, no. 4, pp. 363–368, 2014, [Online]. Available: http://journal-of-agroalimentary.ro/admin/articole/25009L53_Vol_20(4)_2014_363_368.pdf.

36. J. L. Damez and S. Clerjon, "Meat quality assessment using biophysical methods related to meat structure," *Meat Sci.*, vol. 80, no. 1, pp. 132–149, 2008, doi: 10.1016/j.meatsci.2008.05.039.

37. D. Alomar, C. Gallo, M. Castañeda, and R. Fuchslocher, "Chemical and discriminant analysis of bovine meat by near infrared reflectance spectroscopy (NIRS)," *Meat Sci.*, vol. 63, no. 4, pp. 441–450, 2003, doi: 10.1016/S0309-1740(02)00101-8.

38. J. P. Wold, F. Lundby, and B. Egelandsdal, "Quantification of connective tissue (hydroxyproline) in ground beef by autofluorescence spectroscopy," *J. Food Sci.*, vol. 64, no. 3, pp. 377–383, 1999, doi: 10.1111/j.1365-2621.1999.tb15045.x.

39. A. Suleimenova, "Biochemical and Sensory Profile of Meat," University of Eastern Finland, 2016.

40. M. C. Hunt, "Meat color measurements guidelines," *Amsa*, vol. 33, no. 8, 2012, doi: 10.1007/s11786-018-0341-9.

41. Y. Liu and Y. R. Chen, "Analysis of visible reflectance spectra of stored, cooked and diseased chicken meats," *Meat Sci.*, vol. 58, no. 4, pp. 395–401, 2001, doi: 10.1016/S0309-1740(01)00041-9.

42. R. A. Mancini and M. C. Hunt, "Current research in meat color," *Meat Sci.*, vol. 71, no. 1, pp. 100–121, 2005, doi: 10.1016/j.meatsci.2005.03.003.

43. G. G. Giddings, "Reduction of ferrimyoglobin in meat," *C R C Crit. Rev. Food Technol.*, vol. 5, no. 2, pp. 143–173, 1974, doi: 10.1080/10408397409527173.

44. K. Chao, Y. Liu, Y. R. Chen, D. W. Thayer, and W. R. Hruschka, "Characterization of spectral variations of irradiated chicken breasts with 2D-correlation spectroscopy," *Appl. Eng. Agric.*, vol. 18, no. 6, pp. 745–750, 2002.

45. S. P. Suman and P. Joseph, "Myoglobin chemistry and meat color," *Annu. Rev. Food Sci. Technol.*, vol. 4, no. 1, pp. 79–99, 2013, doi: 10.1146/annurev-food-030212-182623.

46. R. Alfano and S. Lingyan, "Evolution of the supercontinuum light source," *Photonics Spectra*, pp. 1–14, 2018. [Online]. Available: https://www.photonics.com/Articles/Evolution_of_the_Supercontinuum_Light_So urce/a62821.

47. S. K. V. Sekar et al., "Diffuse optical characterization of collagen absorption from 500 to 1700 nm.," *J. Biomed. Opt.*, vol. 22, no. 1, p. 15006, Jan. 2017, doi: 10.1117/1.JBO.22.1.015006.

48. J. Tang, C. Faustman, and T. A. Hoagland, "Krzywicki revisited: Equations for spectrophotometric determination of myoglobin redox forms in aqueous meat extracts," *J. Food Sci.*, vol. 69, no. 9, pp. C717–C720, 2004, doi: 10.1111/j.1365-2621.2004.tb09922.x.

49. B. Savenije, G. H. Geesink, J. G. P. Van Der Palen, G. Hemke, D. Hopkins, and A. Ouali, "Prediction of pork quality using visible/near-infrared reflectance spectroscopy," *Meat Sci.*, vol. 73, no. 1, pp. 181–184, 2006, doi: 10.1016/j.meatsci.2005.11.006.

50. Y. Hu, K. Guo, T. Suzuki, G. Noguchi, and T. Satake, "Quality evaluation of fresh pork using visible and near-infrared spectroscopy with fiber optics in interactance mode," *Am. Soc. Agric. Biol. Eng. ISSN*, vol. 51, no. 3, pp. 1029–1033, 2008.

51. H. J. Swatland, "Physical measurements of meat quality: Optical measurements, pros and cons," *Meat Sci.*, vol. 36, no. 1–2, pp. 251–259, 1994, doi: 10.1016/0309-1740(94)90044-2.

52. G. Lindahl, "Colour characteristics of fresh pork," Swedish University of Agricultural Sciences, 2005.

53. C. L. Tsai, J. C. Chen, and W. J. Wang, "Near-infrared absorption property of biological soft tissue constituents," *J. Med. Biol. Eng.*, vol. 21, no. 1, pp. 7–14, 2001.

54. Y. H. Hui et al., *Handbook of Meat and Meat Processing*, 2nd ed. Boca Raton, FL: CRS Press, 2012.

55. L. M. Kandpal, J. Lee, J. Bae, S. Lohumi, and B. K. Cho, "Development of a low- cost multi-waveband LED illumination imaging technique for rapid evaluation of fresh meat quality," *Appl. Sci.*, vol. 9, no. 5, 2019, doi: 10.3390/app9050912.

56. Y. Xu et al., "A novel hyperspectral microscopic imaging system for evaluating fresh degree of pork," *Korean J. Food Sci. Anim. Resour.*, vol. 38, pp. 362–375, 2018, doi: 10.5851/kosfa.2018.38.2.362.

57. R. R. Anderson and J. A. Parrish, "The optics of human skin," *J. Invest. Dermatol.*, vol. 77, no. 1, pp. 13–19, 1981, doi: 10.1111/1523-1747.ep12479191.

58. G. Downey and D. Beauchêne, "Discrimination between fresh and frozen-then- thawed beef m. longissimus dorsi by combined visible-near infrared reflectance spectroscopy: A feasibility study," *Meat Sci.*, vol. 45, no. 3, pp. 353–363, 1997, doi: 10.1016/S0309-1740(96)00127-1.

59. Y. Liu, B. G. Lyon, W. R. Windham, C. E. Realini, T. D. D. Pringle, and S. Duckett, "Prediction of color, texture, and sensory characteristics of beef steaks by visible and near infrared reflectance spectroscopy. A feasibility study," *Meat Sci.*, vol. 65, no. 3, pp. 1107–1115, 2003, doi: 10.1016/S0309-1740(02)00328-5.

60. N. Prieto et al., "On-line application of visible and near infrared reflectance spectroscopy to predict chemical-physical and sensory characteristics of beef quality," *Meat Sci.*, vol. 83, no. 1, pp. 96–103, 2009, doi: 10.1016/j.meatsci.2009.04.005.

61. D. Cozzolino, I. Murray, J. R. Scaife, and R. Paterson, "Study of dissected lamb muscles by visible and near infrared reflectance spectroscopy for composition assessment," *Anim. Sci.*, vol. 70, no. 3, pp. 417–423, 2000, doi: 10.1017/S1357729800051766.

62. D. Pérez-Marín, E. De Pedro Sanz, J. E. Guerrero-Ginel, and A. Garrido-Varo, "A feasibility study on the use of near-infrared spectroscopy for prediction of the fatty acid profile in live Iberian pigs and carcasses," *Meat Sci.*, vol. 83, no. 4, pp. 627–633, 2009, doi: 10.1016/j.meatsci.2009.07.012.

63. R. M. García-Rey, J. García-Olmo, E. De Pedro, R. Quiles-Zafra, and M. D. Luque De Castro, "Prediction of texture and colour of dry-cured ham by visible and near infrared spectroscopy using a fiber optic probe," *Meat Sci.*, vol. 70, no. 2, pp. 357–363, 2005, doi: 10.1016/j.meatsci.2005.02.001.

64. M. Lin, M. Al-Holy, M. Mousavi-Hesary, H. Al-Qadiri, A. G. Cavinato, and B. A. Rasco, "Rapid and quantitative detection of the microbial spoilage in chicken meat by diffuse reflectance spectroscopy (600–1100 nm)," *Lett. Appl. Microbiol.*, vol. 39, no. 2, pp. 148–155, 2004, doi: 10.1111/j.1472-765X.2004.01546.x.

65. G. Ripoll, P. Albertí, B. Panea, J. L. Olleta, and C. Sañudo, "Near-infrared reflectance spectroscopy for predicting chemical, instrumental and sensory quality of beef," *Meat Sci.*, vol. 80, no. 3, pp. 697–702, 2008, doi: 10.1016/j.meatsci.2008.03.009.

66. J. Girón, E. Ivorra, A. J. Sánchez, I. Fernández-Segovia, J. M. Barat, and R. Grau, "Preliminary study using visible and SW-NIR analysis for evaluating the loss of freshness in commercially packaged cooked ham and Turkey ham," *Czech J. Food Sci.*, vol. 32, no. 4, pp. 376–383, 2014.

67. C. Alamprese, M. Casale, N. Sinelli, S. Lanteri, and E. Casiraghi, "Detection of minced beef adulteration with turkey meat by UV-vis, NIR and MIR spectroscopy," *LWT - Food Sci. Technol.*, vol. 53, no. 1, pp. 225–232, 2013, doi: 10.1016/j.lwt.2013.01.027.

68. R. Grau, A. J. Sánchez, J. Girón, E. Iborra, A. Fuentes, and J. M. Barat, "Non-destructive assessment of freshness in packaged sliced chicken breasts using SW-NIR spectroscopy," *Food Res. Int.*, vol. 44, no. 1, pp. 331–337, 2011, doi: 10.1016/j.foodres.2010.10.011.

69. A. Rady and A. Adedeji, "Assessing different processed meats for adulterants using visible-near-infrared spectroscopy," *Meat Sci.*, vol. 136, no. October 2017, pp. 59–67, 2018, doi: 10.1016/j.meatsci.2017.10.014.

70. D. K. Pedersen, S. Morel, H. J. Andersen, and S. B. Engelsen, "Early prediction of water-holding capacity in meat by multivariate vibrational spectroscopy," *Meat Sci.*, vol. 65, no. 1, pp. 581–592, 2003, doi: 10.1016/S0309-1740(02)00251-6.

71. D. I. Ellis, D. Broadhurst, D. B. Kell, J. J. Rowland, and R. Goodacre, "Rapid and quantitative detection of the microbial spoilage of meat by fourier transform infrared spectroscopy and machine learning," *Appl. Environ. Microbiol.*, vol. 68, no. 6, pp. 2822–2828, 2002, doi: 10.1128/AEM.68.6.2822-2828.2002.

72. A. A. Argyri, E. Z. Panagou, P. A. Tarantilis, M. Polysiou, and G. J. E. Nychas, "Rapid qualitative and quantitative detection of beef fillets spoilage based on Fourier transform infrared spectroscopy data and artificial neural networks," *Sensors Actuators, B Chem.*, vol. 145, no. 1, pp. 146–154, 2010, doi: 10.1016/j.snb.2009.11.052.

73. A. Hassoun, A. Sahar, L. Lakhal, and A. Aït-Kaddour, "Fluorescence spectroscopy as a rapid and non-destructive method for monitoring quality and authenticity of fish and meat products: Impact of different preservation conditions," *LWT*, vol. 103, pp. 279–292, 2019, doi: 10.1016/j.lwt.2019.01.021.

74. S. P. Aubourg, "Recent advances in assessment of marine lipid oxidation by using fluorescence," *J. Am. Oil Chem. Soc.*, vol. 76, no. 4, pp. 409–419, 1999, doi: 10.1007/s11746-999-0018-2.

75. J. P. Wold, M. Mielnik, M. K. Pettersen, K. Aaby, and P. Baardseth, "Rapid assessment of rancidity in complex meat products by front face fluorescence spectroscopy," *J. Food Sci.*, vol. 67, no. 6, pp. 2397–2404, 2002, doi: 10.1111/j.1365-2621.2002.tb09560.x.

76. É. Dufour, J. P. Frencia, and E. Kane, "Development of a rapid method based on front-face fluorescence spectroscopy for the monitoring of fish freshness," *Food Res. Int.*, vol. 36, no. 5, pp. 415–423, 2003, doi: 10.1016/S0963-9969(02)00174-6.

77. I. Latka et al., "In-vivo Raman spectroscopy: From basics to applications," *J. Biomed. Opt.*, vol. 23, no. 7, 2020, doi: 10.1117/1.JBO.23.7.

78. A. M. Herrero, "Raman spectroscopy a promising technique for quality assessment of meat and fish: A review," *Food Chem.*, vol. 107, no. 4, pp. 1642–1651, 2008, doi: 10.1016/j.foodchem.2007.10.014.

79. R. Scheier, J. Köhler, and H. Schmidt, "Identification of the early post-mortem metabolic state of porcine *M. semimembranosus* using Raman spectroscopy," *Vib. Spectrosc.*, vol. 70, pp. 12–17, 2014, doi: 10.1016/j.vibspec.2013.10.001.

80. D. I. Ellis, D. Broadhurst, S. J. Clarke, and R. Goodacre, "Rapid identification of closely related muscle foods by vibrational spectroscopy and machine learning," *Analyst*, vol. 130, no. 12, pp. 1648–1654, 2005, doi: 10.1039/b511484e.

81. M. Nache, R. Scheier, H. Schmidt, and B. Hitzmann, "Non-invasive lactate- and pH-monitoring in porcine meat using Raman spectroscopy and chemometrics," *Chemom. Intell. Lab. Syst.*, vol. 142, pp. 197–205, 2015, doi: 10.1016/j.chemolab.2015.02.002.

82. H. Al Ebrahim, K. Sowoidnich, and H. D. Kronfeldt, "Raman spectroscopic differentiation of beef and horse meat using a 671 nm microsystem diode laser," *Appl. Phys. B Lasers Opt.*, vol. 113, no. 2, pp. 159–163, 2013, doi: 10.1007/s00340-013-5677-x.

83. I. M. Mileusnić, J. Z. Š. Rosic, J. S. Munćan, S. B. Dogramadzi, and L. R. Matija, "Computer assisted rapid nondestructive method for evaluation of meat freshness," *FME Trans.*, vol. 45, no. 4, pp. 597–602, 2017, doi: 10.5937/fmet1704597M.

84. J. L. Damez, S. Clerjon, S. Abouelkaram, and J. Lepetit, "Beef meat electrical impedance spectroscopy and anisotropy sensing for non-invasive early assessment of meat ageing," *J. Food Eng.*, vol. 85, no. 1, pp. 116–122, 2008, doi: 10.1016/j.jfoodeng.2007.07.026.

85. J. L. Damez and S. Clerjon, "Quantifying and predicting meat and meat products quality attributes using electromagnetic waves: An overview," *Meat Sci.*, vol. 95, no. 4, pp. 879–896, 2013, doi: 10.1016/j.meatsci.2013.04.037.

86. E. Zherebtsov et al., "Hyperspectral imaging of human skin aided by artificial neural networks," *Biomed. Opt. Express*, vol. 10, no. 7, p. 3545, 2019, doi: 10.1364/boe.10.003545.

87. Z. Xiong, D. W. Sun, H. Pu, W. Gao, and Q. Dai, "Applications of emerging imaging techniques for meat quality and safety detection and evaluation: A review," *Crit. Rev. Food Sci. Nutr.*, vol. 57, no. 4, pp. 755–768, 2017, doi: 10.1080/10408398.2014.954282.

88. G. Elmasry, D. F. Barbin, D. W. Sun, and P. Allen, "Meat quality evaluation by hyperspectral imaging technique: An overview," *Crit. Rev. Food Sci. Nutr.*, vol. 52, no. 8, pp. 689–711, 2012, doi: 10.1080/10408398.2010.507908.

89. D. Wu et al., "Application of Time series hyperspectral imaging (TS-HSI) for determining water distribution within beef and spectral kinetic analysis during dehydration," *Food Bioprocess Technol.*, vol. 6, no. 11, pp. 2943–2958, 2013, doi: 10.1007/s11947-012-0928-0.

90. J. Š. Rosić, M. Conte, J. Munćan, L. Matija, and D. Koruga, "Characterization of fullerenes thin film Oon glasses by UV/VIS/NIR and opto-magnetic imaging spectroscopy," *FME Trans.*, vol. 42, no. 2, pp. 172–176, 2014, doi: 10.5937/fmet1402172S.

91. T. Yaseen, D. W. Sun, and J. H. Cheng, "Raman imaging for food quality and safety evaluation: Fundamentals and applications," *Trends Food Sci. Technol.*, vol. 62, pp. 177–189, 2017, doi: 10.1016/j.tifs.2017.01.012.

92. M. S. Kim, A. M. Lefcourt, and Y.-R. Chen, "Multispectral laser-induced fluorescence imaging system for large biological samples," *Appl. Opt.*, vol. 42, no. 19, pp. 3927–3934, Jul. 2003, doi: 10.1364/ao.42.003927.

93. D. Burfoot, D. Tinker, R. Thorn, and M. Howell, "Use of fluorescence imaging as a hygiene indicator for beef and lamb carcasses in UK slaughterhouses," *Biosyst. Eng.*, vol. 109, no. 3, pp. 175–185, 2011, doi: 10.1016/j.biosystemseng.2011.03.002.

94. B. Cho, M. S. Kim, K. Chao, K. Lawrence, B. Park, and K. Kim, "Detection of fecal residue on poultry carcasses by laser-induced fluorescence imaging," *J. Food Sci.*, vol. 74, no. 3, pp. E154–E159, Apr. 2009, doi: 10.1111/j.1750-3841.2009.01103.x.

95. A. Veberg et al., "Measurement of lipid oxidation and porphyrins in high oxygen modified atmosphere and vacuum-packed minced turkey and pork meat by fluorescence spectra and images," *Meat Sci.*, vol. 73, no. 3, pp. 511–520, 2006, doi: 10.1016/j.meatsci.2006.02.001.

96. J. P. Wold and K. Kvaal, "Mapping lipid oxidation in chicken meat by multispectral imaging of autofluorescence," *Appl. Spectrosc.*, vol. 54, no. 6, pp. 900–909, 2000, doi: 10.1366/0003702001950300.

97. L. Nanni Costa, C. Stelletta, C. Cannizzo, M. Gianesella, D. Pietro Lo Fiego, and M. Morgante, "The use of thermography on the slaughter-line for the assessment of pork and raw ham quality," *Ital. J. Anim. Sci.*, vol. 6, no. Suppl. 1, pp. 704–706, 2007, doi: 10.4081/ijas.2007.1s.704.

98. B. K. Cho and J. M. K. Irudayaraj, "Foreign object and internal disorder detection in food materials using noncontact ultrasound imaging," *J. Food Sci.*, vol. 68, no. 3, pp. 967–974, 2003, doi: 10.1111/j.1365-2621.2003. tb08272.x.

99. P. Pallav, D. A. Hutchins, and T. H. Gan, "Air-coupled ultrasonic evaluation of food materials," *Ultrasonics*, vol. 49, no. 2, pp. 244–253, 2009, doi: 10.1016/j.ultras.2008.09.002.

100. C. L. Hansen, F. van der Berg, S. Ringgaard, H. Stødkilde-Jørgensen, and A. H. Karlsson, "Diffusion of NaCl in meat studied by 1H and 23Na magnetic resonance imaging," *Meat Sci.*, vol. 80, no. 3, pp. 851–856, 2008, doi: 10.1016/j.meatsci.2008.04.003.

101. J.-L. Damez, S. Clerjon, R. Labas, J. Danon, F. Peyrin, and J. Bonny, "Microstructure characterization of meat by quantitative MRI," in *58th International Congress of Meat Science and Technology*, Aug. 2012, p. p17.

102. S. Yoon et al., "Deep optical imaging within complex scattering media," *Nat. Rev. Phys.*, vol. 2, no. 3, pp. 141–158, 2020, doi: 10.1038/s42254-019-0143-2.

103. K. C. Hadley and I. A. Vitkin, "Optical rotation and linear and circular depolarization rates in diffusively scattered light from chiral, racemic, and achiral turbid media," *J. Biomed. Opt.*, vol. 7, no. 3, p. 291, 2002, doi: 10.1117/1.1483880.

104. M. Kupinski et al., "Polarimetric information for pre-cancer detection from uterine cervix specimens," in *Biophotonics Congress: Optics in the Life Sciences Congress 2019 (BODA, BRAIN, NTM, OMA, OMP)*, OSA Technical Digest, Optica Publishing Group, paper JT4A.47, 2019, doi: 10.1364/ BODA.2019.JT4A.47.

105. A. Pierangelo et al., "Use of Mueller polarimetric imaging for the staging of human colon cancer," *Opt. Biopsy IX*, vol. 7895, no. July 2016, p. 78950E, 2011, doi: 10.1117/12.878248.

106. N. G. Khlebtsov, I. L. Maksimova, I. Meglinski, L. V. Wang, and V. V. Tuchin, "Introduction to light scattering by biological objects," in *Handbook of Optical Biomedical Diagnostics, Second Edition, Volume 1: Light-Tissue Interaction*, V.V. Tuchin, Ed. Bellingham: SPIE PRESS, 2016, pp. 1–160.

107. J. Qi and D. S. Elson, "Mueller polarimetric imaging for surgical and diagnostic applications: A review," *J. Biophotonics*, vol. 10, no. 8, pp. 950–982, 2017, doi: 10.1002/jbio.201600152.

108. K. U. Spandana, K. K. Mahato, and N. Mazumder, "Polarization-resolved Stokes- Mueller imaging: A review of technology and applications," *Lasers Med. Sci.*, vol. 34, no. 7, pp. 1283–1293, 2019, doi: 10.1007/s10103-019-02752-1.

109. O. Angelsky, A. Ushenko, Y. Ushenko, V. Pishak, and A. Peresunko, "Statistical, correlation, and topological approaches in diagnostics of the structure and physiological state of birefringent biological tissues," in

Handbook of Photonics for Biomedical Science. Series: Series in Medical Physics and Biomedical Engineering, V. Tuchin, Ed. Boca Raton, FL: CRC Press, 2010, pp. 283–322.

110. B. Kunnen, C. Macdonald, A. Doronin, S. Jacques, M. Eccles, and I. Meglinski, "Application of circularly polarized light for non-invasive diagnosis of cancerous tissues and turbid tissue-like scattering media," *J. Biophotonics*, vol. 8, no. 4, pp. 317–323, 2015, doi: 10.1002/jbio.201400104.

111. M. Borovkova, A. Bykov, A. Popov, and I. Meglinski, "Role of scattering and birefringence in phase retardation revealed by locus of Stokes vector on Poincaré sphere," *J. Biomed. Opt.*, vol. 25, no. 5, p. 057001, 2020, doi: 10.1117/1.JBO.25.5.057001.

112. R. Uberna, "New polarization generator/analyzer for imaging Stokes and Mueller polarimetry," *SPIE Newsroom*, pp. 5–7, 2006, doi: 10.1117/2.1200608.0366.

113. L. Qiu et al., "Multispectral scanning during endoscopy guides biopsy of dysplasia in Barrett's esophagus," *Nat. Med.*, vol. 16, no. 5, pp. 603–606, 2010, doi: 10.1038/nm.2138.

114. S. L. Jacques, J. C. Ramella-Roman, and K. Lee, "Imaging skin pathology with polarized light," *J. Biomed. Opt.*, vol. 7, no. 3, p. 329, 2002, doi: 10.1117/1.1484498.

115. E. Du et al., "Characteristic features of mueller matrix patterns for polarization scattering model of biological tissues," *J. Innov. Opt. Health Sci.*, vol. 7, no. 1, pp. 1–9, 2013, doi: 10.1142/S1793545813500284.

116. A. De Martino, E. Garcia-Caurel, B. Laude, and B. Drévillon, "General methods for optimized design and calibration of Mueller polarimeters," *Thin Solid Films*, vol. 455–456, pp. 112–119, 2004, doi: 10.1016/j.tsf.2003.12.052.

117. V. V. Tuchin, *Handbook of Coherent-Domain Optical Methods: Biomedical Diagnostics, Environmental Monitoring, and Materials Science*, 2nd ed. New York: Springer-Verlag New York, 2013.

118. S. Alali and A. Vitkin, "Polarized light imaging in biomedicine: Emerging Mueller matrix methodologies for bulk tissue assessment," *J. Biomed. Opt.*, vol. 20, no. 6, p. 061104, 2015, doi: 10.1117/1.jbo.20.6.061104.

119. C. He et al., "Quantitatively differentiating microstructures of tissues by frequency distributions of Mueller matrix images," *J. Biomed. Opt.*, vol. 20, no. 10, p. 105009, 2015, doi: 10.1117/1.jbo.20.10.105009.

120. M. Peyvasteh et al., "3D Mueller-matrix-based azimuthal invariant tomography of polycrystalline structure within benign and malignant soft-tissue tumours," *Laser Phys. Lett.*, vol. 17, no. 11, p. 9, 2020, doi: 10.1088/1612-202X/abbee0.

121. H. He et al., "Monitoring microstructural variations of fresh skeletal muscle tissues by Mueller matrix imaging," *J. Biophotonics*, vol. 10, no. 5, pp. 664–673, 2017, doi: 10.1002/jbio.201600008.

122. A. Pierangelo et al., "Polarimetric imaging of uterine cervix: A case study," *Opt. Express*, vol. 21, no. 12, p. 14120, 2013, doi: 10.1364/oe.21.014120.

123. W. Sheng et al., "Quantitative analysis of 4×4 mueller matrix transformation parameters for biomedical imaging," *Photonics*, vol. 6, no. 1, pp. 1–14, 2019, doi: 10.3390/PHOTONICS6010034.
124. T. Liu et al., "Comparative study of the imaging contrasts of Mueller matrix derived parameters between transmission and backscattering polarimetry," *Biomed. Opt. Express*, vol. 9, no. 9, p. 4413, 2018, doi: 10.1364/boe.9.004413.
125. M. Borovkova et al., "Complementary analysis of Mueller-matrix images of optically anisotropic highly scattering biological tissues," *J. Eur. Opt. Soc.*, vol. 14, no. 1, pp. 4–11, 2018, doi: 10.1186/s41476-018-0085-9.
126. J. Zhou, H. He, Y. Wang, and H. Ma, "Identification and quantitative evaluation of the fiber structure in the pathological tissue using Mueller matrix microscope," *Opt. Tomogr. Spectrosc. Tissue XII*, vol. 10059, no. February 2017, p. 1005926, 2017, doi: 10.1117/12.2251325.
127. S. Forward, A. Gribble, S. Alali, A. A. Lindenmaier, and I. A. Vitkin, "Flexible polarimetric probe for 3×3 Mueller matrix measurements of biological tissue," *Sci. Rep.*, vol. 7, no. 1, pp. 1–12, 2017, doi: 10.1038/s41598-017-12099-8.
128. K. Rajkumar, P. Sunethri, P. V. K. Rao, and V. Padmaja, "Mueller matrix imaging polarimetry - For tissue imaging," in *2015 International Conference on Industrial Instrumentation and Control (ICIC)*, pp. 1540–1543, 2015, doi: 10.1109/IIC.2015.7150994.
129. P. H. Lissberger, "Ellipsometry and polarised light," *Nature*, vol. 269, no. 5625, p. 270, 1977, doi: 10.1038/269270a0.
130. A. Vitkin, N. Ghosh, and A. de Martino, "Tissue polarimetry," in *Photonics: Scientific Foundations, Technology and Applications*, vol. 4, D. L. Andrews, Ed. Hoboken, NJ: John Wiley & Sons, Inc., 2015, pp. 239–321.
131. A. Mendoza-Galván, E. Muñoz-Pineda, S. J. L. Ribeiro, M. V. Santos, K. Järrendahl, and H. Arwin, "Mueller matrix spectroscopic ellipsometry study of chiral nanocrystalline cellulose films," *J. Opt.*, vol. 20, no. 2, p. 024001, 2018, doi: 10.1088/2040-8986/aa9e7d.
132. R. A. Chipman, W. S. T. Lam, and G. Young, *Polarized Light and Optical Systems*. Boca Raton, FL: CRC Press, 2018.
133. S. J. Matcher, "Signal quantification and localization in tissue near-infrared spectroscopy," in *Handbook of Optical Biomedical Diagnostics*, 2nd ed., V. V. Tuchin, Ed. Bellingham, Washington: SPIE PRESS, 2016, p. 1410.
134. D. Dashdorj, V. K. Tripathi, S. Cho, Y. Kim, and I. Hwang, "Dry aging of beef; review," *J. Anim. Sci. Technol.*, vol. 58, no. 1, pp. 1–11, 2016, doi: 10.1186/s40781-016-0101-9.
135. V. Sierra, N. Aldai, P. Castro, K. Osoro, A. Coto-Montes, and M. Oliván, "Prediction of the fatty acid composition of beef by near infrared transmittance spectroscopy," *Meat Sci.*, vol. 78, no. 3, pp. 248–255, 2008, doi: 10.1016/j.meatsci.2007.06.006.
136. B. M. Nicolaï et al., "Nondestructive measurement of fruit and vegetable quality by means of NIR spectroscopy: A review," *Postharvest Biol. Technol.*, vol. 46, no. 2, pp. 99–118, 2007, doi: 10.1016/j.postharvbio.2007.06.024.

137. M. Peyvasteh, A. Popov, A. Bykov, and I. Meglinski, "Meat freshness revealed by visible to near-infrared spectroscopy and principal component analysis," *J. Phys. Commun.*, vol. 4, no. 9, p. 95011, 2020, doi: 10.1088/2399-6528/abb322.
138. D. Wangpraseurt, S. L. Jacques, T. Petrie, and M. Kühl, "Monte Carlo modeling of photon propagation reveals highly scattering coral tissue," *Front. Plant Sci.*, vol. 7, no. September, pp. 1–10, 2016, doi: 10.3389/fpls.2016.01404.
139. I. Meglinski and S. J. Matcher, "The application of the Monte Carlo technique for estimation of the detector depth sensitivity for the skin oxygenation measurements," *Monte Carlo Methods Appl.*, vol. 6, no. 1, pp. 15–26, 2000, [Online]. Available: https://econpapers.repec.org/RePEc:bpj:mcmeap:v:6:y:2000:i:1:p:15-26:n:2.
140. V. Dremin, E. Zherebtsov, A. Bykov, A. Popov, A. Doronin, and I. Meglinski, "Influence of blood pulsation on diagnostic volume in pulse oximetry and photoplethysmography measurements," *Appl. Opt.*, vol. 58, no. 34, pp. 9398–9405, 2019, doi: 10.1364/AO.58.009398.
141. A. Doronin and I. Meglinski, "Peer-to-peer Monte Carlo simulation of photon migration in topical applications of biomedical optics," *J. Biomed. Opt.*, vol. 17, no. 9, p. 0905041, 2012, doi: 10.1117/1.jbo.17.9.090504.
142. I. V Meglinsky and S. J. Matcher, "Modelling the sampling volume for skin blood oxygenation measurements.," *Med. Biol. Eng. Comput.*, vol. 39, no. 1, pp. 44–50, Jan. 2001, doi: 10.1007/BF02345265.
143. I. Meglinski, A. N. Bashkatov, E. A. Genina, D. Y. Churmakov, and V. V Tuchin, "Study of the possibility of increasing the probing depth by the method of reflection confocal microscopy upon immersion clearing of near-surface human skin layers," *Quantum Electron.*, vol. 32, no. 10, pp. 875–882, 2002, doi: 10.1070/qe2002v032n10abeh002309.
144. A. N. Bashkatov, E. A. Genina, and V. V. Tuchin, "Optical properties of skin, subcutaneous, and muscle tissues: A review," *J. Innov. Opt. Health Sci.*, vol. 4, no. 1, pp. 9–38, 2011, doi: 10.1142/S1793545811001319.
145. G. Destefanis, M. T. Barge, A. Brugiapaglia, and S. Tassone, "The use of principal component analysis (PCA) to characterize beef," *Meat Sci.*, vol. 56, no. 3, pp. 255–259, 2000, doi: 10.1016/S0309-1740(00)00050-4.
146. C. Syms, "Principal components analysis," in *Encyclopedia of Ecology*, Sven Erik Jørgensen and Brian D. Fath, Eds. Oxford: Elsevier, 2008, pp. 2940–2949.
147. I. Tazi, N. L. Isnaini, M. Mutmainnah, and A. Ainur, "Principal component analysis (PCA) method for classification of beef and pork aroma based on electronic nose," *Indones. J. Halal Res.*, vol. 1, no. 1, pp. 5–8, 2019, doi: 10.15575/ijhar.v1i1.4155.
148. X. Y. Tian, Q. Cai, and Y. M. Zhang, "Rapid classification of hairtail fish and pork freshness using an electronic nose based on the PCA method," *Sensors*, vol. 12, no. 1, pp. 260–277, 2012, doi: 10.3390/s120100260.
149. D. Yang, D. He, A. Lu, D. Ren, and J. Wang, "Detection of the freshness state of cooked beef during storage using hyperspectral imaging," *Appl. Spectrosc.*, vol. 71, no. 10, pp. 2286–2301, 2017, doi: 10.1177/0003702817718807.

150. M. Michalczuk et al., "Application of the support sensory system and principal component analysis to compare meat of chickens of two genotypes," *CyTA - J. Food*, vol. 16, no. 1, pp. 667–671, Jan. 2018, doi: 10.1080/19476337.2018.1448457.

151. R. A. Chipman, E. A. Sornsin, and J. L. Pezzaniti, "Mueller matrix imaging polarimetry: An overview," in *International Symposium on Polarization Analysis and Applications to Device Technology*, 1996, vol. 2873, no. August 1996, pp. 5–12, doi: 10.1117/12.246186.

152. S.-Y. Lu and R. A. Chipman, "Interpretation of Mueller matrices based on polar decomposition," *J. Opt. Soc. Am. A*, vol. 13, no. 5, p. 1106, 1996, doi: 10.1364/josaa.13.001106.

153. C. He et al., "Characterizing microstructures of cancerous tissues using multispectral transformed Mueller matrix polarization parameters," *Biomed. Opt. Express*, vol. 6, no. 8, p. 2934, 2015, doi: 10.1364/boe.6.002934.

154. J. Gil and R. Ossikovski, *Polarized Light and the Mueller Matrix Approach*. Boca Raton: CRC Press, 2016.

155. M. Peyvasteh, A. Popov, A. Bykov, A. Pierangelo, and T. Novikova, "Evolution of raw meat polarization-based properties by means of Mueller matrix imaging," *J. Biophotonics*, vol. 14, no. 5, p. e202000376, 2021.

156. T. Novikova et al., "Multi-spectral Mueller Matrix Imaging Polarimetry for Studies of Human Tissues," in *Biomedical Optics 2016*, 2016, p. TTh3B.2, doi: 10.1364/translational.2016.tth3b.2.

157. M. Borovkova et al., "Evaluating β-amyloidosis progression in Alzheimer's disease with Mueller polarimetry," *Biomed. Opt. Express*, vol. 11, no. 8, p. 4509, 2020, doi: 10.1364/boe.396294.

158. T. Novikova et al., "The origins of polarimetric image contrast between healthy and cancerous human colon tissue," *Appl. Phys. Lett.*, vol. 102, no. 24, p. 241103, 2013, doi: 10.1063/1.4811414.

159. Y. A. Ushenko, "Laser autofluorescence polarimetry of optically anisotropic structures of biological tissues in cancer diagnostics," *Opt. Spectrosc.*, vol. 118, no. 6, pp. 1007–1016, 2015, doi: 10.1134/S0030400X15060235.

160. P. H. Westfall, "Kurtosis as peakedness," *Am. Stat.*, vol. 68, no. 3, pp. 191–195, 2014, doi: 10.1080/00031305.2014.917055.Kurtosis.

161. J. Broky and A. Dogariu, "Complex degree of mutual polarization in randomly scattered fields," *Opt. Express*, vol. 18, no. 19, pp. 20105–20113, 2010, doi: 10.1364/OE.18.020105.

162. A. G. Ushenko and V. P. Pishak, "Laser polarimetry of biological tissues: Principles and applications" in *Handbook of Coherent-Domain Optical Methods: Biomedical Diagnostics, Environmental Monitoring, and Materials Science*, V. V. Tuchin, Ed. New York: Springer, 2004, pp. 93–138. doi: 10.1007/0-387-29989-0_3.

163. T. Novikova, I. Meglinski, J. C. Ramella-roman, and V. V Tuchin, "Polarized light for biomedical applications," *J. Biomed. Opt.*, vol. 21, no. 7, p. 071001, 2016, doi: 10.1117/1.JBO.21.7.071001.

164. M. Peyvasteh, A. Dubolazov, A. Popov, A. Ushenko, Y. A. Ushenko, and I. Meglinski, "Two-point Stokes vector diagnostic approach for characterization of optically anisotropic biological tissues," *J. Phys. D. Appl. Phys.*, vol. 53, no. 2020, p. 395401, 2020, doi: 10.1088/1361-6463/ab9571.

165. T. T. Tower and R. T. Tranquillo, "Alignment maps of tissues: I. Microscopic elliptical polarimetry," *Biophys. J.*, vol. 81, no. 5, pp. 2954–2963, Nov. 2001, doi: 10.1016/S0006-3495(01)75935-8.

166. N. Ghosh, "Tissue polarimetry: Concepts, challenges, applications, and outlook," *J. Biomed. Opt.*, vol. 16, no. 11, p. 110801, 2011, doi: 10.1117/1.3652896.

167. V. O. Ushenko, "Spatial-frequency polarization phasometry of biological polycrystalline networks," *Opt. Mem. Neural Networks*, vol. 22, no. 1, pp. 56–64, 2013, doi: 10.3103/S1060992X13010050.

168. N. K. Das, R. Dey, S. Chakraborty, P. K. Panigrahi, I. Meglinski, and N. Ghosh, "Quantitative assessment of submicron scale anisotropy in tissue multifractality by scattering Mueller matrix in the framework of Born approximation," *Opt. Commun.*, vol. 413, pp. 172–178, Apr. 2018, doi: 10.1016/j.optcom.2017.11.082.

169. Y. A. Ushenko, T. M. Boychuk, V. T. Bachynsky, and O. P. Mincer, "Diagnostics of structure and physiological state of birefringent biological tissues: Statistical, correlation and topological approaches," in *Handbook of Coherent-Domain Optical Methods: Biomedical Diagnostics, Environmental Monitoring, and Materials Science*, 2nd ed., V. V. Tuchin, Ed. New York: Springer, 2013, pp. 107–148.

170. V. A. Ushenko and M. S. Gavrylyak, "Azimuthally invariant Mueller-matrix mapping of biological tissue in differential diagnosis of mechanisms protein molecules networks an sotropy," *Proc. SPIE*, vol. 8812, p. 88120Y, 2013, doi: 10.1117/12.2023686.

171. V. O. Ushenko, "Two-dimensional Mueller matrix phase tomography of self- similarity birefringence structure of biological tissues," *Proc. SPIE*, vol. 8487, p. 84870W, 2012, doi: 10.1117/12.928481.

172. V. A. Ushenko, N. D. Pavlyukovich, and L. Trifonyuk, "Spatial-frequency azimuthally stable cartography of biological polycrystalline networks," *Int. J. Opt.*, vol. 2013, p. 683174, 2013, doi: 10.1155/2013/683174.

173. Y. A. Ushenko, M. P. Gorskii, A. V Dubolazov, A. V Motrich, V. A. Ushenko, and M. I. Sidor, "Spatial-frequency Fourier polarimetry of the complex degree of mutual anisotropy of linear and circular birefringence in the diagnostics of oncological changes in morphological structure of biological tissues," *Quantum Electron.*, vol. 42, no. 8, pp. 727–732, 2012, doi: 10.1070/qe2012v042n08abeh014825.

174. Y. A. Ushenko, "Investigation of formation and interrelations of polarization singular structure and Mueller-matrix images of biological tissues and diagnostics of their cancer changes," *J. Biomed. Opt.*, vol. 16, no. 6, pp. 1–9, 2011, doi: 10.1117/1.3585689.

175. S. Andrés, I. Murray, E. A. Navajas, A. V. Fisher, N. R. Lambe, and L. Bünger, "Prediction of sensory characteristics of lamb meat samples by near infrared reflectance spectroscopy," *Meat Sci.*, vol. 76, no. 3, pp. 509–516, 2007, doi: 10.1016/j.meatsci.2007.01.011.

176. D. F. Barbin et al., "Prediction of chicken quality attributes by near infrared spectroscopy," *Food Chem.*, vol. 168, pp. 554–560, 2015, doi: 10.1016/j.foodchem.2014.07.101.

177. J. M. Hughes, F. M. Clarke, P. P. Purslow, and R. D. Warner, "Meat color is determined not only by chromatic heme pigments but also by the physical structure and achromatic light scattering properties of the muscle," *Compr. Rev. Food Sci. Food Saf.*, vol. 19, no. 1, pp. 44–63, 2020, doi: 10.1111/1541-4337.12509.

178. S. L. Jacques, "Polarized light imaging of biological tissues," in *Handbook of Biomedical Optics*, N. R. David, A. Boas, C. Pitris, Eds. Boca Raton: CRC Press, 2011, pp. 649–69.

Index

www.ingramcontent.com/pod-product-compliance
Lightning Source LLC
Chambersburg PA
CBHW060552220326
41598CB00024B/3082